P9-EED-437

The American Diabetes Association
Guide to
HEALTHY
RESTAURANT
EATING

HOPE S.
WARSHAW,
MMSc, RD, CDE

Book Acquisitions	Robert J. Anthony
Editor	Aime M. Ballard
Production Director	Carolyn R. Segree
Production Coordinator	Peggy M. Rote
Desktop Publishing & Text Design	Harlowe Typography, Inc.
Cover Design	Wickham & Associates, Inc.

Printed in Canada
1 3 5 7 9 10 8 6 4 2

The suggestions and information contained in this publication are generally consistent with the *Clinical Practice Recommendations* and other policies of the American Diabetes Association, but they do not represent the policy or position of the Association or any of its boards or committees. Reasonable steps have been taken to ensure the accuracy of the information presented. However, the American Diabetes Association cannot ensure the safety or efficacy of any product or service described in this publication. Individuals are advised to consult a physician or other appropriate health care professional before undertaking any diet or exercise program or taking any medication referred to in this publication. Professionals must use and apply their own professional judgment, experience, and training and should not rely solely on the information contained in this publication before prescribing any diet, exercise, or medication. The American Diabetes Association—its officers, directors, employees, volunteers, and members—assumes no responsibility or liability for personal or other injury, loss, or damage that may result from the suggestions or information in this publication.

ADA titles may be purchased for business or promotional use or for special sales. For information, please write to: Lee M. Romano, Special Sales & Promotions, at the address below.

Published by American Diabetes Association, Inc., 1660 Duke Street, Alexandria, Virginia 22314.

Library of Congress Cataloging-in-Publication Data

Warshaw, Hope S., 1954–
    The American Diabetes Association guide to healthy restaurant eating / Hope S. Warshaw.
        p.   cm.
    ISBN 1-58040-004-3 (pbk.)
    1. Diabetes—Diet therapy.   2. Food exchange lists.
3. Restaurants.   I. Title.
RC662.W3155   1998
616.4′620654—dc21

98-35395
CIP

*To people with diabetes who, on a daily basis,
strive to control blood glucose to stay healthy
and prevent diabetes complications.
May the knowledge and information
you gain from this book help you
stay healthy and complication-free.*

— HSW

Contents

Alphabetical Index of Restaurants

Acknowledgments

This book would have been impossible to create without the cooperation and assistance from many people at the corporate headquarters of nearly 60 restaurant chains. On behalf of people with diabetes who will use and benefit from the information in the pages ahead, I am indebted to these restaurant chains for making all or some of their nutrition information available. These restaurants set an example of public responsibility to the rest of the chain restaurant industry.

No book is completed by just the author alone. In this case, many manuscript pages and a large nutrient database became a book with many people's ideas and countless hours. Thanks first goes to Aime Ballard, my editor at the American Diabetes Association. She worked tirelessly to make this book a winner, while she kept a smile on her face. Thanks also goes to Patti Geil, MS, RD, FADA, CDE, David Kelly, MD, and Virginia Peragallo-Ditko, RN, MA, CDE, who reviewed this manuscript for ADA and provided valuable input. Thanks to others at ADA who supported this effort: Robert J. Anthony, Acquisitions Manager; Susan Lau, Publisher; and Len Boswell, Director of Book Marketing.

Thanks also to people who assisted with the development of the nutrient database—Debbie Rowland, RD, and Alicia Parks.

A last thanks goes to my professional colleagues who lent their ears and ideas to make this book the best it could be. They continue to be a source of inspiration and encouragement.

Today's Diabetes Eating Goals

During the 1990s the diabetes eating goals underwent a minor revolution. In fact, the phrase "a diabetic diet" is now a misnomer. No such diet exists. No longer must you ax sugary foods and sweets from your list of desirables. Now you can savor the taste of a few slices of pizza at your local pizza parlor or cruise to the drive-thru for a hamburger and french fries when time is not on your side. The bottom line is, the current diabetes eating goals encourage you to eat healthfully and to do what it takes to keep your blood glucose in the normal range as much as possible. The end goal, of course, is to prevent or slow down long-term diabetes complications, such as eye, heart, and kidney problems. These occur, to a great degree, because of high blood glucose levels day after day.

Diabetes Eating Goals in a Nutshell

In 1994 the American Diabetes Association (ADA) put forth these six nutrition goals:

1. Hold blood glucose (blood sugar) as near to normal as possible. Balance what you eat with insulin or diabetes pills (if you need diabetes medicine to control your blood glucose) and physical activity.
2. Keep or get your blood lipid (blood fat) levels as close to normal as possible. Blood lipids include cho-

lesterol, low-density lipoproteins (LDL) ("bad" cholesterol), high-density lipoproteins (HDL) ("good" cholesterol), and triglycerides (the form in which your body stores fat in fat cells for ready energy).

3. Eat enough calories to stay at or get to a healthy weight for you. If you are a child or teenager or if you are pregnant or breastfeeding, eat enough calories to grow and develop.

4. Prevent or treat problems caused by high or low blood glucose. For instance, eat on time to prevent low blood glucose (hypoglycemia).

5. Prevent, slow down, or treat long-term diabetes problems. For example, eat less saturated fat to prevent heart problems, or eat a moderate amount of protein to slow kidney problems.

6. Improve your overall health by choosing foods and eating the way all Americans are encouraged to eat. This means eating what you know is healthy for your whole family.

Those are the nutrition goals. But what foods should you eat to reach these goals? Here are general pointers to focus on:

- Eat more (6 or more servings) grains, beans, and starchy vegetables each day.
- Eat more fruits and vegetables. Strive for at least 5 servings a day from a combination of fruits and vegetables. More is better!
- Include at least 2 servings of fat-free or low-fat dairy foods—milk, yogurt, and cheese—within your calorie allotment. That's for calcium.
- Eat a moderate amount of meat and other protein foods. Two 3-oz servings each day is enough for

most people. Not only does eating less meat help you eat less protein, it also makes it easier for you to eat less total fat, saturated fat, and cholesterol.

- Go light on fats and oils (especially those high in saturated fat, such as coconut and palm oils).
- Limit foods high in cholesterol (such as whole milk dairy foods, egg yolks, and organ meats).
- Eat small amounts of sugary foods and sweets only once in a while. If you have some pounds to shed or your blood sugar or blood fats are not in a good range, you'll need to eat sweets even more sparingly. If you're on the slim side, calories are on your side to splurge on sweets a bit more often if you want to.
- Drink no more than one alcoholic drink a day if you are a woman and two drinks a day if you are a man. One drink is defined as 1½ oz of hard liquor (a shot), 12 oz of beer, or 6 oz of wine.

Everybody Sings the Same Song

Take note: ADA recommendations for healthy eating echo the way all Americans are encouraged to eat—even Americans at risk for heart disease or some cancers. Whether it's the American Heart Association, the American Cancer Society, or the U.S. Government, every organization sings the same nutrition song.

This means that as a person with diabetes, you don't need to stick out like a sore thumb because you strive to eat healthfully. That's not to make healthy eating sound simple or not to acknowledge that at times you feel like a fish swimming upstream because so many Americans chow down on downright unhealthy foods. Remember, it's not easy to eat healthfully. And that may be particularly true with restaurant foods.

How Much Should You Eat?

Base what you eat each day on what you like to eat, as long as you eat these foods in reasonable amounts. The quantities of food you eat and times you eat must match your lifestyle and schedule. Another critical element is what foods and times for meals and snacks work best to help you keep your blood glucose, blood lipids, and blood pressure in control. Lastly, what's best for your diabetes is what allows you to feel good day to day and what helps prevent or slow down the development of diabetes problems.

No set number of calories is right for everyone with diabetes. The number of calories you need depends on many factors. A few of them are your height, your age, your current weight and whether you want to lose weight or are at a healthy weight, your daily activity level, the type of exercise you do, and more. Always have a meal plan and method of meal planning that fits you and your lifestyle. To develop a meal plan you are comfortable with and one that factors in your individual needs, work with a registered dietitian (RD) with diabetes expertise (preferably a certified diabetes educator, CDE). A dietitian can help you learn how to work almost any food into your meal plan or to solve meal planning dilemmas (for instance, maybe you travel several days a week and eat all your meals in restaurants). A book called *Diabetes Meal Planning Made Easy*, published by the ADA, gives more in-depth information about how much and what you should eat.

Myriad Approaches to Meal Planning

Once you know what and how much you should eat, you and your dietitian can zero in on a meal planning approach that fits your needs. If you want a simple approach, for example, then the diabetes food pyramid may be best for you. Or if you will test your blood glucose several times a day and do some math, then you might opt for carbohydrate counting.

You may be familiar with the diabetes exchange system as the way people with diabetes learn to plan meals. The ADA and The American Dietetic Association's *Exchange Lists for Meal Planning* date back to 1950. The exchange system has been revised a number of times. The last revision was in 1995. Today, the exchange system is no longer the only way to do diabetes meal planning. You can use the diabetes food pyramid, carbohydrate gram counting, fat gram counting, or the point system, to name a few options. The right meal planning approach for you is the one that you can learn and put to work. One approach might be right for you when you first develop diabetes, then down the road another approach may work best.

Any Meal Planning Approach Works in Restaurants

No matter which meal planning approach you use, you can take advantage of the information in this book. If you opt for the exchange system or the diabetes food pyramid, use the food servings or exchanges noted in the charts. If you do carbohydrate counting, then the grams of carbohydrate and grams of dietary fiber are where you want to focus. Zero in on the calories and fat if fat gram counting is part of your meal planning method.

Help Is Nearby

Whether you have just found out you have diabetes or you have been doing the diabetes balancing act for years, you can always learn more. Get to know a diabetes educator. Your diabetes educator will help you tailor your diabetes management plan and offer tips for dealing with diabetes. The following resources are a good start to link you up with quality diabetes care:

- To find diabetes educators (who may be dietitians, nurses, pharmacists, counselors, or other health professionals) near you, call the American Association of Diabetes Educators toll-free at 1-800-TEAMUP4 (1-800-832-6874).
- To find a Recognized Diabetes Education Program (a teaching program approved by the American Diabetes Association) near you, call 1-800-DIABETES (1-800-342-2383), look at ADA's Internet homepage *<http://www.diabetes.org>*, or go straight to *<http://www.diabetes.org/education/eduprogram.asp>*.
- To find a registered dietitian with expertise in diabetes (RD, CDE) near you, call The American Dietetic Association's National Center for Nutrition and Dietetics at 1-800-366-1655 or look at its Internet homepage *<http://www.eatright.org/>* and click on "Find a Dietitian."

Here's more good news: It may now be easier for you to take advantage of the services of a diabetes educator or diabetes education program. Medicare now covers diabetes education in many new settings for those with Medicare part B or managed care. In most cases, this may include nutrition education by a registered dietitian with diabetes expertise. Also, in more than half the states across the country, those private insurers and managed care organizations that are regulated by the state must pay for diabetes education. If you have questions about whether or not your diabetes education will be covered, contact your health care company, your state insurance commissioner's office, the local Medicare office, or the American Diabetes Association.

Restaurant Pitfalls and Strategies for Self-Defense

To eat out healthfully is no small task. You need power and perseverance. It's tough enough to eat healthfully in your own house. But even more challenges confront you when you pick and choose from a menu and are not able to sneak a peek in the kitchen. You can't march into the kitchen and hold the cook's hand when he or she ladles more butter or shakes more salt onto your once healthy vegetables. Healthy restaurant eating is, no doubt, a challenge. That's because there are lots of pitfalls—from plate-piled portions to fat, fat everywhere. The good news is that you can eat healthfully in 99% of restaurants. All you have to do is learn the pitfalls of restaurant eating and tuck the strategies to eat more healthfully in restaurants under your belt.

Pitfalls of Restaurant Eating

- **You think of restaurant ventures as special occasions.** Yes, once upon a time, people only ate in restaurants to celebrate a birthday, Mother's Day, or an anniversary. Not today. The average American eats four meals away from home each week. And you may top that number. When you eat that many meals away from home each week, your waistline quickly spreads if you eat as if each meal is a special occasion. Today, restaurant meals for most people are just part of our fast-paced life. They're hardly special occasions.

- **You're not the cook.** The cook is in the kitchen and you can't peek. Your methods of control are to ask questions about the food on the menu, to make special requests to get an item delivered the way you want it, and to practice portion control when you order and eat.

- **Fats are here, there, and everywhere.** Remember, fat makes food taste good and stay moist. Restaurants, therefore, love it. Extra fat is in high-fat ingredients, such as butter, sour cream, or cream; in high-fat foods, such as cheese, bacon, or potato chips; and in high-fat cooking methods, such as deep-fat frying, breading and frying, and sautéing. And it's at the table in fried Chinese noodles, tortilla chips, or butter. You need to master the craft of a fat sleuth.

- **Sodium can skyrocket.** Along with fat, salt makes food taste good. So many restaurants pour it aplenty. If you're watching your sodium intake, you'll need to shy away from certain items and make some special requests.

- **Portions are oversized.** Restaurants, especially table-service restaurants, simply serve too much food. Restaurants, and many Americans, believe more is better.

- **Meat (protein) is front and center.** A primary focus of the American diner is summed up in the catch-phrase "Where's the beef?" Whether it is fish, chicken, or beef, the protein often takes center stage in restaurant meals. And most plates contain too much of it. A steak is often 8 oz or more cooked. A chicken breast is often a whole chicken breast. Your goal is to put the meat on the side of your plate.

Americans Eat Out: How Much and When?

An average American today spends almost half of every food dollar on food eaten away from home. In 1950, according to the National Restaurant Association, the average American spent only a quarter of his or her food dollar eating away from home. The average American today eats four meals out of the house each week. Lunch is the meal eaten out most often, with dinner a close second. Breakfast is eaten out least often. And men eat out more than women. Fast-food restaurants—from hamburger joints to pizza and sub shops—represent about a quarter of all restaurants. As for ethnic food, Americans' favorites are Mexican, Chinese, and Italian.

Let's face it, restaurant meals—eaten in or out—are just part of dealing with our fast-paced world. You might ask, "Is that a problem if I have diabetes?" The answer is no, as long as you learn to eat healthy restaurant meals most of the time. And remember, whether you eat in the restaurant or take food out to the soccer field, your office, or the kitchen table, you need to contemplate the same decisions when you make menu choices. In fact, you have to make similar choices in today's supermarkets, because they have begun to look a bit like restaurants with ready-to-eat meal components, complete meals, sandwiches, and salad bars. Of course, one advantage in the supermarket is that the nutrition facts stare you in the face. Not so in restaurants.

Ten Strategies for Eating Out Healthfully

1. **Develop a can-do attitude.** Too many of us think in negative equations: Eating out equals pigging out; a restaurant meal must be a special occasion; eating out means blowing your diet. These attitudes defeat your efforts to eat healthfully. It's time to develop a can-do attitude about restaurant meals. Build confidence to believe that you can enjoy a healthy meal when you eat out. Slowly begin to change how you order and the types of restaurants in which you choose to eat.

2. **Decide when to eat out—or not.** Take a look at how often you eat out. If the count verges on the excessive, then ask yourself why you eat out so frequently and how you can reduce your restaurant meals. If you eat out more frequently, then you need to keep splurges to a minimum. If you eat out only once a month, you might take a few more liberties—perhaps with an alcoholic drink or a dessert.

3. **Zero in on the site.** Seek out restaurants that offer at least a smattering of healthier options. Remember, there is an advantage to eating in chain restaurants. You can master the menu and plan ahead, no matter which one of the chain's locations you pop into.

4. **Set your game plan.** On your way to the restaurant—whether it's a quick fast-food lunch or a leisurely weekend dinner—envision a healthy and enjoyable outcome. Plan your order, or at least what you might have if you aren't familiar with the restaurant, before you cross the threshold. Don't become a victim of hasty choices.

5. **Become a fat sleuth.** Learn to focus on fats. Fat is the densest form of calories, and it often gets lost in the sauce, so to speak—or on the salad, on the bread, or in the chips. Watch out for high-fat ingredients—butter, cream, sour cream. Be alert for high-fat foods—cheese, avocado, sausage. Steer clear of high-fat preparation methods—frying of any kind. Look out for high-fat dishes—Mexican chimichangas, broccoli with cheese sauce, or stuffed potato skins, for starters.

6. **Let your food plan be your guide.** Keep a miniaturized version of your food plan with you. Choose foods with your meal plan in mind. Try to fulfill each food group with menu items or substitute foods to make your meal complete. For instance, replace a serving of milk or a fruit serving, which are often hard to get in restaurants, with another starch serving so that you will keep your carbohydrate intake consistent—an important goal.

7. **Practice portion control from the get go.** The best way not to eat too much is to order less. Order with your stomach in mind, not your eyes. You need to outsmart the menu to get the right amount of food for you.

8. **Be creative with the menu.** You outsmart the menu by being creative. Remember, no sign at the entrance says, "All who enter must order an entree." Your options are to take advantage of appetizers, soups, and salads; to split menu items, including the entree, with your dining partner; to order one or two fewer dishes than the number of people at the table and eat family style; or to mix and match two entrees to achieve nutritional balance. For example, in a steak house, one person

orders the steak, baked potato, and salad bar and the other orders just the potato and salad bar, then they split the steak. In an Italian restaurant, one person orders pasta with a tomato-based sauce and the other orders a chicken or veal dish with a vegetable.

9. **Get foods made to order.** Don't be afraid to ask for what you want, even in a fast-food restaurant. Restaurants today need your business and want you back. Make sure your requests are practical—leave an item such as potato chips off the plate; substitute mustard for mayonnaise on a sandwich; make a sandwich on whole-wheat bread rather than on a croissant; or serve the salad dressing on the side. Restaurants can abide by these requests. However, don't expect to have your special requests greeted with a smile at noon in a fast-food restaurant or when you try to remake a menu item. Be reasonable and pleasant.

10. **Know when enough is enough.** Many of us grew up being members of the clean-plate club. Now you need to reserve a membership in the "leave-a-few-bites-on-your-plate club." To keep from overeating, don't order too much, order creatively, and push your plate away when you meet your calorie needs. Remember, take-home containers are at-the-ready in most restaurants.

Diabetes Dining Dilemmas

Lots of people who eat restaurant meals have concerns about their health and need to ask questions about this entree or that salad. As a person with diabetes, your questions and special requests are nothing out of the ordinary. However, as someone with diabetes, you deal with additional dining dilemmas, particularly if you take a diabetes medication that can cause low blood glucose (sulfonylureas, repaglinide [Prandin], or insulin). Other diabetes pills, such as metformin (Glucophage), acarbose (Precose), and troglitazone (Rezulin), do not cause low blood glucose if you take them alone, so you can be more flexible. Following are some diabetes dining dilemmas and some solutions.

Delayed Meals

You might schedule a restaurant meal later than your regular mealtime. Perhaps it's a weekend-morning gathering for pancakes, an evening dinner meeting, or a rendezvous with your spouse or a friend. Eating later than usual is fine as long as you manage the situation and don't let your blood glucose get too low. Generally, if you take repaglinide as your only diabetes medication, you should just take the pill when you eat your delayed meal. If you take another diabetes medication or medications, here's what you should do.

If you delay your meal about 1 hour, you need to:

1. Take your diabetes medicine at your usual meal-time.
2. Eat 15 grams of carbohydrate (1 carbohydrate serving or exchange) at your usual mealtime.
3. Keep quick and easy carbohydrate foods at the ready in places such as your desk, briefcase, purse, locker, or glove compartment.

Note: If you usually take a sulfonylurea diabetes pill, repaglinide, or insulin before the meal you delay (such as dinner), you may choose to delay taking the medicine until just before the meal. Check with your doctor or diabetes educator to learn what is best for you.

If you delay your meal over 1½ hours, you have several options. The option you choose depends on how often you take insulin and/or sulfonylurea diabetes pills.

If you take sulfonylureas or insulin only in the morning:

1. Eat your next snack at the usual time of the meal that has been delayed.
2. Eat the delayed meal at your usual snack time.
3. Do not eat another snack after the delayed meal.

Example: Your usual lunch is at 12:00 noon, but today you will eat at 1:30 p.m.

(1) Eat your afternoon snack at 12:00 noon.
(2) Eat your regular lunch at 1:30 p.m. and then continue on your routine as usual.

If you take insulin before breakfast and before dinner and use a mixture of short-acting (regular) insulin (do not use this option if you take lispro [Humalog]) and intermediate-acting insulin (NPH or lente), premixed insulin (70/30), or a sulfonylurea, you have two options.

OPTION 1

1. Take your insulin or pills as usual before the regular time you eat your evening meal.
2. Eat your evening snack at your usual mealtime.
3. Eat your dinner at the delayed time.

Example: Your usual dinnertime is 6:00 p.m., but tonight you will eat at 7:45 p.m.

   (1) Take your insulin or sulfonylurea at 5:30 p.m.
   (2) Eat your evening snack at 6:00 p.m.
   (3) Eat your dinner at 7:45 p.m.

OPTION 2

Wait to take insulin until 30 minutes before the delayed meal. (Note: If you take the very quick-acting insulin lispro [Humalog], always take this insulin only when you know you are about to eat.)

1. Eat your regular meal at the delayed dinnertime.
2. Have your regular snack before bed.

   Example: Your usual dinnertime is 6:00 p.m., but tonight you will eat at 7:30 p.m.

   (1) Take insulin at 7:00 p.m.
   (2) Eat dinner at 7:30 p.m.
   (3) Eat your regular evening snack before bed.

OPTION 3

If you take insulin twice a day and use a mixture of short-acting insulin (regular) and intermediate-acting insulin (NPH or lente) before your evening meal, you have one more option, which involves splitting your dose into two shots.

1. Take your intermediate-acting insulin at your usual dinnertime because it won't start acting for 1–2 hours.
2. Eat 15 grams of carbohydrate or half of your evening snack at your regular mealtime.
3. Take short-acting (regular) insulin 30 minutes before the delayed meal. If you take lispro (Humalog), you should take this insulin only once you know you will eat.
4. Eat your regular meal plus the rest of your snack at the delayed time.
5. Eat another night snack only if your blood glucose test suggests you need it.

   Example: Your usual dinnertime is 6:30 p.m., but tonight you will eat at 8:00 p.m.

   (1) Take intermediate-acting (NPH or lente) insulin at 6:00 p.m.
   (2) Eat a small box of raisins or half your evening snack at 6:30 p.m.
   (3) Take short-acting (regular) insulin at 8:00 p.m.
   (4) Eat dinner at 8:00 p.m.
   (5) Test your blood glucose before bed. If it is less than 100 mg/dl, eat your regular night snack, even if you have eaten some food from this snack earlier in the evening.

If you take short-acting (regular) or very quick-acting (lispro) insulin before all your meals, here's what you can do.

1. Take your short-acting (regular) insulin 30 minutes before you eat the delayed meal. If you take lispro (Humalog), then take it when you know you're about to eat.
2. Take your intermediate-acting insulin at the usual time you take it.
3. If your blood glucose gets too low before the delayed meal, eat 15 grams of carbohydrate to increase your blood glucose.

   Example: Your lunch is usually at 12:30 p.m., but today you will eat at 2:00 p.m.

   (1) Take regular insulin at 1:30 p.m.
   (2) Eat lunch at 2:00 p.m.
   (3) If your blood glucose gets low before the delayed mealtime, eat a small piece of fruit or four to six crackers.

These options offer you general rules of thumb. Check with your doctor or diabetes educator to learn what is best for you. Regardless of changes that you make to account for mealtime delays, always carry some easy-to-eat carbohydrate with you. Glucose tablets or gel, crackers, juice, pretzels, milk, yogurt, diabetes nutrition bars, or dried fruit are just a few suggestions. Life is unpredictable. You never know what will happen in restaurants. The restaurant might not have your reservation, they might not be able to seat you quickly, your meal-mate might be late, the kitchen might be slow, or there may be a mix up with your order. And the list goes on. As the saying goes, "It's better to be safe than sorry."

Alcohol Use

No one needs to drink alcohol. Clearly there are numerous downsides. Alcohol is high in calories (unhealthy calories). It can raise blood lipid levels. It can cause low blood glucose if you take sulfonylureas, repaglinide, or insulin. And it can cause problems if you take metformin (Glucophage). It can lead to health problems with overuse, can slow your responses, and can be dangerous if you drink and drive. However, if your blood glucose and blood lipids are in good control and you drink sensibly, there is no reason you cannot enjoy some alcohol. And a common time to drink alcohol is when you eat in a restaurant. Here's how to drink smartly with diabetes. If you drink alcohol and take a sulfonylurea, repaglinide, or insulin, all of which can cause blood glucose to get too low, pay particular attention to these rules of thumb.

Tips to Sip By

- Don't drink when your blood glucose is too low.
- Remember that alcohol can cause low blood glucose soon after you drink it (if your medicine is working hardest and/or you need to eat). It can continue to cause low blood glucose 8–12 hours after you drink it, especially if you drink in excess and take too much medicine or don't eat enough.
- Don't drink on an empty stomach. Either munch on a carbohydrate source (popcorn or pretzels) as you drink or wait to drink until you get your meal.
- Alcohol can also make blood glucose too high. This is true for anyone with diabetes, no matter how they control it. High blood glucose can be caused by the

calories from carbohydrate in the alcoholic beverage, such as wine or beer, or in a mixer, such as orange juice.

- Avoid mixers that add lots of carbohydrates and calories—tonic water, regular soda, syrups, juices, and liqueurs.
- Check your blood glucose to help you decide whether you should drink and when you need to eat something.
- Wear or carry identification that states you have diabetes.
- Sip a drink to make it last.
- Have a noncaloric, nonalcoholic beverage by your side to quench your thirst.
- If you do not take a diabetes medicine that can cause low blood glucose and you have some pounds to shed, substitute an alcoholic drink for fats in your meal plan.
- If you do not have pounds to shed, then just have an occasional drink and don't worry about the extra calories.
- Do not drive for several hours after you drink alcohol. Never drink and drive.

Sugars and Sweets

It is common to want a sweet dessert to end a restaurant meal. As with alcohol, it's probably part of the special occasion psychology. As you know by now, you can fit sweets into your diabetes food plan as long as you substitute them for other foods or compensate for their extra carbohydrates, fat, and calories with your diabetes medicines to keep your blood glucose close to normal. To set healthy goals with sweets, you also need to consider your weight and blood fats. Work with a dietitian to figure out how to fit sweets into your meal plan. In the meantime, here are a few pointers.

Hints for Sweet Tooths

- Prioritize your personal diabetes goals. Which is most important for you: blood glucose control, weight loss, or lower blood fats? Your priorities dictate how you strike a balance with sugars and sweets.
- Choose a few favorite desserts. Decide how often to eat them and how to fit them into your meal plan.
- Perhaps it is best for you to limit desserts just to when you eat in restaurants. That way you keep sweets out of your home.
- Split a dessert in a restaurant.
- Take advantage of smaller portions available in restaurants or ice cream spots—kiddie, small, or regular are the words to look for.
- Use the nutrition information you find in this book and information you find in restaurants to learn about the calorie, carbohydrate, fat, saturated fat, and cholesterol content of desserts.
- When you eat a sweet, check your blood glucose 1–2 hours later to see how it has been affected by the treat. You might find, for instance, that because of the fat content, the same quantity of ice cream raises your blood glucose more slowly than does frozen yogurt, which contains less fat and more carbohydrate.
- Keep an eye on your glycated hemoglobin (your longer-range blood glucose measure, also known as hemoglobin A1c or glycosylated hemoglobin) and your blood fat (lipid) levels to see whether eating more sweets leads to an unwanted rise in these numbers.

These are basic guidelines and suggestions to deal with diabetes dining dilemmas. Each person with diabetes is different, and more diabetes medicines and medicine combinations are in use today than ever before. So talk with your doctor or diabetes educator to get specific information pertinent to the way you manage your diabetes.

Restaurants Help or Hinder Your Healthy Eating Efforts

The pendulum swings back and forth. During the 1980s and early 1990s, when the voices of people concerned about what they ate and about their health were loud, restaurants gave in. Lower-calorie and lower-fat menu items were introduced. Restaurateurs willingly made lower-fat milk and lighter-caloric salad dressings available. Some chain and independent restaurants even marked their menus with little hearts or other notations to indicate which menu items met specific health criteria.

Now the pendulum in restaurants has swung back toward a lax attitude about healthy eating. Witness, McDonald's no longer carries the McLean hamburger or meal-sized salads. Taco Bell's Border Lights line bombed because it was introduced toward the end of the health craze. We've entered the era of new giant burgers, super-sized meals, and more all-you-can-eat buffets. But don't blame it on the restaurants. They cannot stock menu items that customers don't order. Unfortunately, a majority of Americans cast all health and nutrition cares to the wind when they set foot in a restaurant.

No doubt the "no cares nutrition attitude" makes it harder for people who remain health conscious. But don't feel pessimistic. What does remain from the

1980s and early 1990s is the availability of lower-fat milk, lighter-calorie salad dressings, lower-fat frozen desserts, and greater ease in making special requests. With skills and a bit of fortitude, you can eat healthfully at most restaurants. Granted, you still have to pick and choose among the menu offerings.

Your voice still matters and can make a difference. If you and thousands of other people with concerns about their health continue to make special requests, eventually your voices will be heard loud and clear. Maybe then the pendulum will once again swing toward an abundant supply of healthy menu items.

Chains That Give the Nutrition Lowdown

For this book, menu and nutrition information was sought from about 80 large family and chain restaurants—from large hamburger chains to smaller Italian table-service chains. (See "How This Book Can Work for You" to find more information about the restaurant selection process we used.) A notation is made by each restaurant that provides a nutrition information pamphlet to consumers.

Generally, the fast-food hamburger chains—from the large McDonald's and Burger King to the smaller Whataburger and Rally's Hamburgers—provide nutrition information. Other categories of restaurants that give nutrition information are pizza chains, chicken chains, large Mexican restaurant chains, dessert and ice cream chains, sub and sandwich shops, large quick-service seafood chains, and donut and bagel shops.

The types of restaurants that, for the most part, either do not have or do not give out nutrition information are steak houses, family restaurants (such as Applebee's or Shoney's), and dinner houses (such as Chili's Grill and Bar and T.G.I. Friday's). Several of these restaurants are willing to provide nutrition information for only healthier menu items. This shows that they can provide information if they so desire. Many of these restaurants were contacted and chose not to provide information for this guide.

Why don't some restaurants provide nutrition information? There are a few reasons. First, it's expensive to obtain nutritional analyses on all menu items. Second, restaurants that do not provide information tend to change their menus frequently. As soon as they would print nutrition information, it would need to be revised. Third, they want you to stay blindfolded to the nutrition lowdown on their foods. An important point here is that you—a person with diabetes concerned about your health—need to keep asking for nutrition information at restaurants that don't give it.

How to Get the Latest Nutrition Lowdown

If you do not find a particular restaurant chain in this book or there is a new menu item introduced for a restaurant that is included, here are a few hints on how to get the nutrition information.

- Ask for nutrition information at the location you frequent. You might get lucky and have a nutrition pamphlet put right into your hands. Sometimes they have run out or just don't keep them in stock. Make sure you check the date on the nutrition pamphlet to be sure it is current.

- If the restaurant does not have the information, ask where you can call or write for it. You might need to call or write the corporate headquarters and have them send you a pamphlet.
- Several of the large chains, such as McDonald's, Burger King, and Wendy's, have Internet homepages. They publish nutrition information on their websites.

A Bit of Help from Your Government

The nutrition facts panel on most canned and packaged foods in the supermarket hardly seems new. But you only started to see it in 1994. How come the same type of nutrition labeling is not required for restaurants? There are a number of reasons. The most important reason is that the content of menu items varies too much and that menu items change often. However, as part of the Nutrition Labeling and Education Act (NLEA), which is the federal legislation that changed the nutrition label and increased the number of foods with information, restaurants must comply with several aspects of this law.

In January 1993, NLEA regulations required restaurants to provide nutrition information to customers when nutrition and health claims were made on signs and placards. Menu claims were exempt at that point. Since May 1997, if any restaurant makes a health claim about a food, that it is "low-fat" for instance, the nutrition information has to comply with the meaning of the term according to the NLEA. This helps you know that when you see the word "healthy" to describe a can of beans or a fast-food sandwich, it has the same meaning. Restaurants from small one-unit sandwich shops to McDonald's will have to abide. Table 1 gives terms

TABLE 1 Meaning of Nutrition Claims on Restaurant Menus, Signs, and Placards*

Nutrition Claim	Meaning
Cholesterol-Free	Less than 2 mg of cholesterol per serving and 2 g or less of saturated fat per serving
Low-Cholesterol	20 mg or less of cholesterol per serving and 2 g or less of saturated fat per serving
Fat-Free	Less than 0.5 g of fat per serving
Low-Fat	3 g or less of fat per serving
Light or Lite	Cannot be used by restaurants as a nutrient content claim, but can be used to describe a menu item, such as "lighter fare" or "light size"
Sodium-Free	Less than 5 mg of sodium per serving
Low-Sodium	140 mg or less of sodium per serving
Sugar-Free	Less than 0.5 g of sugar per serving
Low-Sugar	May not be used as a nutrient claim
Healthy	The food item is low in fat, low in saturated fat, has limited amounts of cholesterol and sodium, and provides significant amounts of one or more key nutrients—vitamins A and C, iron, calcium, protein, or fiber.
Heart Healthy (These claims will indicate that a diet low in saturated fat and cholesterol may reduce the risk of heart disease.)	The item is low in fat, saturated fat, cholesterol, and provides without fortification (added nutrients) significant amounts of one or more key nutrients—vitamins A and C, iron, calcium, protein, or fiber. OR The item is low in fat, saturated fat, cholesterol, and provides without fortification (added nutrients) significant amounts of one or more key nutrients—vitamins A and C, iron, calcium, protein—and is a significant source of soluble fiber.

*The definitions of these claims are the same as for food labels in the supermarket.

you might see on restaurant menu items and their definitions.

The new law permits restaurants to

- Make specific claims about a menu item's nutritional content.
- Make one of the allowed health claims about the relationship between a nutrient or food and a disease or health condition. The criteria to make the health claim must be met.

If the restaurant makes a nutrition or health claim, it must provide you with the nutrition information to back it up. The claim can be substantiated by a nutrition database, nutrition information in the cookbook from which the recipe was made, or another source that provides nutrition information. Further, restaurants do not have to give you the information in the nutrition label format you are familiar with from the supermarket. They can provide it in any format they choose.

How This Book Can Work for You

You might open this book and be thrilled to see many restaurants you frequent. Then again, you might wonder why a certain restaurant that you've never laid eyes on is included, or why your favorite hamburger or pizza stop is nowhere to be found. Each July, a restaurant trade association magazine, *Restaurants and Institutions*, publishes a list of the top 400 restaurant chains. The 80 largest chains were culled from a recent list. The restaurants were selected based on the number of locations they operate and whether the business was growing or in the red.

These 80 restaurant chains were sent a letter requesting menu and/or nutrition information for this book. In the end, nearly 60 restaurant chains responded with sufficient menu and/or nutrition information to warrant their inclusion. Just before we put the finishing touches on this book, each restaurant received a copy of the information to be included. Each restaurant was given an opportunity to change or update their information, and most did. Therefore, what you see here is the most up-to-date menu and nutrition information for these chain restaurants.

If one of your favorite restaurants is not included, it is for one of the following reasons:

- The restaurant might not have been willing or able to provide sufficient menu and/or nutrition information to warrant their inclusion.

- The restaurant chain may not be large enough around the country, although it appears to you that in your area there's an outlet on every corner.
- The restaurant might not have wanted to be included.

If you don't find a particular restaurant in the book, there are still ways for you to use the information to your advantage. First, find similar types of restaurants. Next, compare similar foods. For example, if you're going to a local pizza parlor and you want to make an educated guess about the nutrients in a medium slice of cheese pizza, then look at cheese pizza from two to three restaurants in the pizza chapter and take an average. That will give you a reasonable guess of the nutrition lowdown for your pizza.

Where to Look

Clearly, you know to look in Burgers and More to find McDonald's or Wendy's, or Pizza, Pasta, and All Else Italian to find Domino's or Pizza Hut. But because Boston Market's menu today includes more than just chicken, you might not guess that it is in the section with chicken chains. Let's just say we used the "best-fit" approach. Nine times out of 10 you'll guess correctly. But if you don't find a restaurant in the chapter where you think it should be, then check the alphabetical listing of restaurants right after the table of contents.

Close but Not Exact

You should be aware that the nutrition information from restaurants is close but not exact. Many restaurants sent letters or have notes on their nutrition information that state their nutrition information is based on the specified ingredients and preparation. However, the same restaurant has locations all over the country, and different regions purchase their ingredients and foods from various food wholesalers. For example, a Wendy's in California might purchase lettuce, tomatoes, and hamburger buns from one food supplier, whereas a Wendy's in Connecticut will buy foods from another company. The nutrition analysis of these items is close, but not identical. Most importantly for you, the nutrition information from restaurants is close enough to help you to make food decisions and manage your blood glucose.

Restaurant foods are also prepared by different people. Even in the same restaurant, on different days you might get more or less cheese on your pizza, more pickles or ketchup on your hamburger, or a slightly smaller or larger steak even though you order the 6-oz filet. Wherever humans are involved, portions can't be exact. Consider these differences if one day you notice that your blood glucose goes up more or less than you expect from a restaurant meal you've eaten again and again.

Restaurants are concerned that you know their nutrition information is close but not exact. That's because they have been called on the carpet by some public interest groups who evaluate their food for its nutrients and find that the foods they choose to sample do not exactly match the nutrition information published by the restaurant.

What's In, What's Out

Nutrition information that was made available by the restaurants is included in the pages ahead. Some restaurants provided nutrition information for only their "core menu items," the items that every one of their outlets must serve. An outlet you visit might serve a few foods that are not part of the core menu. So you might find foods that are not included in this book.

Also, there are two categories of items that are not listed separately in the information provided for each restaurant. The first is beverages. The only beverages included for individual restaurants are milk and fruit juice (most often orange juice). Regularly sweetened drinks, such as carbonated beverages (soda, or pop), lemonade, noncarbonated fruit drinks, and the like, are out because from a nutrition standpoint, they are loaded with sugar and provide next to no nutritional value. Most restaurants also serve a similar variety of noncaloric beverages. To avoid repeating information on the same products, we've put the nutrition information for the most commonly served regular and diet beverages in Table 2.

The second category of items not listed for individual restaurants is common condiments, such as ketchup, mustard, mayonnaise, honey, etc. Don't despair, we've put the nutrition information for these condiments in Table 3.

The Nutrition Numbers Ahead

All the nutrition information you need to know to fit foods into your meal plan is in the pages ahead, unless certain information was not available from the restaurant. Whether you use the diabetes exchange system or the diabetes food pyramid, do carbohydrate counting or fat gram counting for meal planning, the numbers are here. This is the nutrition information you'll find, in this order:

TABLE 2 Nutrition Information for Beverages

Beverage	Amount	Cal.	Fat (g)	Sat. Fat (g)	Chol. (mg)	Sod. (mg)	Carb. (g)	Pro. (g)	Servings/Exchanges
Beer (regular)	12 oz	140	0	0	0	11	13	1	1 carb., 2 fat*
Beer (light)	12 oz	99	0	0	0	18	5	1	2 fat*
Coffee, black (regular and decaffeinated)	8 oz	5	0	0	0	4	1	0	free
Coke (regular)	12 oz	144	0	0	0	6	43	0	3 carb.
Coke (diet)	12 oz	1	0	0	0	6	0	0	free
Iced Tea	12 oz	4	0	0	0	6	1	0	free
Liquor (any type)	1 1/2 oz	96	0	0	0	0	0	0	2 fat*
Lemonade (regular)	12 oz	160	0	0	0	0	42	0	3 carb.
Milk (whole)	8 oz	150	8	5	33	120	12	8	1 whole milk
Milk (reduced-fat/2%)	8 oz	120	5	3	18	122	12	8	1 low-fat milk

(Continued)

TABLE 2 Nutrition Information for Beverages (*Continued*)

Beverage	Amount	Cal.	Fat (g)	Sat. Fat (g)	Chol. (mg)	Sod. (mg)	Carb. (g)	Pro (g)	Servings/Exchanges
Milk (fat-free/skim)	8 oz	86	0	0	4	126	12	8	1 fat-free milk
Orange Juice	8 oz	112	0	0	0	2	27	2	2 fruit
Pepsi (regular)	12 oz	144	0	0	0	6	43	0	3 carb.
Pepsi (diet)	12 oz	1	0	0	0	6	0	0	free
Sprite (regular)	12 oz	148	0	0	0	3	37	0	2 1/2 carb.
Sprite (diet)	12 oz	1	0	0	0	6	0	0	free
Tea (hot, nothing added)	8 oz	2	0	0	0	7	1	0	free
Wine, white	4 oz	80	0	0	0	6	1	0	2 fat*
Wine, red	4 oz	80	0	0	0	114	3	1	2 fat*

*Talk to your diabetes educator or physician about whether you can work alcoholic beverages into your meal plan and how to do so.

TABLE 3 Nutrition Information for Condiments

Condiment	Amount	Cal.	Fat (g)	Sat. Fat (g)	Chol. (mg)	Sod. (mg)	Carb. (g)	Pro. (g)	Servings/Exchanges
Bacon, thinly sliced	1 slice	36	3	1	5	101	0	2	1 fat
Butter	1 tsp	30	4	2	10	39	0	0	1 fat
Cheese, American	1-oz slice	106	9	6	27	405	1	6	1 high-fat meat
Cheese, Swiss	1-oz slice	107	8	5	26	74	1	8	1 high-fat meat
Cheese, mozzarella, whole-milk	1 oz/4 cups shredded	80	6	4	22	106	1	6	1 medium-fat meat
Cream Cheese (regular)	1 Tbsp	50	5	3	15	45	1	1	1 fat
Cream Cheese (light)	1 Tbsp	30	3	2	5	80	1	2	1/2 fat
Half & Half	1/2 oz/1 Tbsp	20	2	1	6	6	1	0	free
Honey	1 tsp	22	0	0	0	0	6	0	1/2 carb.
Honey Mustard	1 tsp	15	1	n/a	n/a	75	2	0	free

(Continued)

TABLE 3 **Nutrition Information for Condiments** (*Continued*)

Condiment	Amount	Cal.	Fat (g)	Sat. Fat (g)	Chol. (mg)	Sod. (mg)	Carb. (g)	Pro. (g)	Servings/Exchanges
Ketchup	1 Tbsp	16	0	0	0	137	4	0	free
Margarine (regular stick)	1 tsp	34	4	1	0	44	0	0	1 fat
Margarine (regular tub)	1 tsp	34	4	1	0	51	0	0	1 fat
Margarine (light)	1 tsp	17	2	0	0	17	0	0	free
Mayonnaise (regular)	1 Tbsp	100	11	2	8	78	0	0	2 fat
Mayonnaise (light)	1 Tbsp	40	4	0	5	15	1	0	1 fat
Mustard	1 tsp	5	0	0	0	65	0	0	free
Non-Dairy Creamer	1/2 oz/1 Tbsp	16	1	0	0	5	2	0	free
Olive Oil	1 tsp	40	5	2	0	0	0	0	1 fat
Pancake Syrup (regular)	1 Tbsp	50	0	0	0	13	13	0	1 carb.
Pancake Syrup (light)	1 Tbsp	25	0	0	0	56	7	0	1/2 carb.

Pancake Syrup (low-calorie)	1 Tbsp	23	0	0	0	57	6	0	1/2 carb.
Relish, pickle-type	1 Tbsp	19	0	0	0	164	5	0	free
Salsa, tomato-based	1 Tbsp	3	0	0	0	112	1	0	free
Sour Cream (regular)	1 Tbsp	31	3	2	6	8	1	0	1/2 fat
Sour Cream (light)	1 Tbsp	18	1	0	5	10	1	1	free
Soy Sauce	1 tsp	3	0	0	0	343	1	0	free
Vinegar (all types)	1 tsp	2	0	0	0	0	1	0	free

n/a, not available

- Calories
- Fat (in grams) and
  - Percentage of calories from fat. Look at this in relation to grams of fat. Keep in mind that the percentage of calories from fat might be high, but the grams of fat might be low, or vice versa.
  - Saturated fat (in grams). Saturated fat is the type of fat that raises blood cholesterol levels. You should keep your saturated fat intake to 10% or less of your total calories.

- Cholesterol (in milligrams)
- Sodium (in milligrams)
- Carbohydrate (in grams)
  - Dietary fiber (in grams). Dietary fiber is a component of carbohydrate. Generally, Americans don't eat enough dietary fiber. Try to eat 20–35 grams of dietary fiber each day. If you count carbohydrates, you might have been taught to subtract grams of dietary fiber from your carbohydrate count if a serving of the food has more than 5 grams of dietary fiber.

- Protein (in grams)
- Food servings/exchanges. Servings and exchanges are virtually the same. They have been calculated using the *1995 Exchange Lists for Meal Planning*, published by the ADA and The American Dietetic Association, and the book *Diabetes Meal Planning Made Easy*, published by ADA in 1996.

A "best-fit" approach was used to calculate servings or exchanges. There is no one right way to fit restaurant foods into your meal plan. Figuring out what food group the grams of carbohydrate come from is the biggest challenge to figuring servings or exchanges. This is how we approached it: When it appears that the grams of carbohydrate come from a starch—be it potato, bread, or starchy vegetable— we've called the servings or exchanges starches. If the carbohydrate comes from vegetable, fruit, or milk, we've designated the servings or exchanges as such.

A new food group in the *1995 Exchange Lists for Meal Planning* is the "other carbohydrate" group. This group contains foods such as sweets, frozen desserts, spaghetti sauce, jam, and maple syrup, to name a few. The calories and carbohydrates in many of these foods come from simple sugars. Therefore, in calculating the servings or exchanges for this book, we've called foods that fit into the "other carbohydrate" group "carb." Exchanges for fast-food shakes and frozen and regular desserts, for example, are calculated as carbs.

When it comes to meat dishes, we've tried to calculate the servings or exchanges based on the group that the meat itself fits into regardless of how it's prepared. For example, fish fillet sandwiches and chicken fingers are considered to fall into the lean meat group even though they have a lot of fat by the time they are served. On the other hand, sausage in any form is classified as a high-fat meat because that's the food group sausage fits into.

Putting It All Together

Perhaps one of the hardest parts of meal planning is figuring out how to put together healthy, well-balanced meals. This is a particular challenge in restaurants. To show you that it is easy to design healthier meals in all of these restaurants, we've come up with two sample meals for each restaurant. We applied the following criteria to put together the meals. (Please note that the criteria might be less strict than what you would consider for a healthy meal at home. That's because restaurant meals tend to be higher in calories, fat, etc.

The Light 'n Lean Choice

- 400–700 calories (based on about 1,200–1,600 calories per day)
- 30–40% of calories from fat
- 100–200 milligrams of cholesterol (total per day should be 300 milligrams or less)
- 1,000–2,000 milligrams of sodium (total per day should be 2,400–3,000 milligrams)

The Healthy 'n Hearty Choice

- 600–1,000 calories (based on about 1,800–2,400 calories per day)
- 30–40% of calories from fat
- 100–200 milligrams of cholesterol (total per day should be 300 milligrams or less)
- 1,000–2,000 milligrams of sodium (total per day should be 2,400–3,000 milligrams)

Healthiest Bets

With nutrition information in hand, we've also made it easy for you to zero in on healthier restaurant offerings. We've marked these "Healthiest Bets" with a ✔. The only restaurants that do not have any Healthiest Bets marked are those that did not provide sufficient nutrition information to determine the healthier dishes. Remember, foods that are not marked as Healthiest Bets are not necessarily foods you should never eat. Healthiest Bets just steer you toward healthier choices.

When you're putting together healthy meals, don't look at only the Healthiest Bets. You can feel free to mix and match healthier and less healthy foods to make up overall healthy meals. That's why you'll see some Healthiest Bets and some less healthy items mixed and matched in the sample meals for each restaurant. Also, what's most important is that you eat a healthy balance over the course of the day and from week to week. So if you want a juicy hamburger and french fries for lunch one day a month, go ahead and enjoy.

The Healthiest Bets were chosen on the basis of the following criteria:

- Breakfast entrees: Less than 400 calories per serving, with less than 15 grams of fat (3 fat exchanges [about 30% fat]) and 1,000 milligrams of sodium.
- Lunch or dinner entrees: Less than 600–750 calories, with less than 20 grams of fat (4 fat exchanges [about 30% fat]) and 1,000 milligrams of sodium.
- Pizza, sandwiches, hamburgers, etc.: Less than 500 calories per reasonable serving (for example, 2 slices of pizza), 20 grams of fat (4 fat exchanges [about 30% fat]), and 1,000 milligrams of sodium.
- Side items: For items such as fruit, vegetables (raw and cooked), grains, legumes, starches, and meats, no more than 5 grams of fat (1 fat exchange). For fried items, such as french fries, hash browns, and onion rings, less than 10 grams of fat (2 fat exchanges); less than 500 milligrams of sodium per serving.
- Soups: Less than 10 grams of fat (2 fat exchanges) and 1,000 milligrams of sodium per serving.

- Salad dressings and condiments: Less than 50 calories, 5 grams of fat (1 fat exchange), and 250 milligrams of sodium per tablespoon.
- Breads (such as rolls, biscuits, bagels, donuts, muffins, and pretzels): Less than 400 calories, 10 grams of fat (2 fat exchanges), and 800 milligrams of sodium per serving.
- Desserts: Less than 300 calories, 10 grams of fat (2 fat exchanges), and 30 grams of carbohydrate per serving.
- Beverages (such as milk, juice, milk shakes, and special coffees): Less than 300 calories, 30 grams of carbohydrate, and 5 grams of fat (1 fat exchange). Less than 400 milligrams of sodium. (Coffee, though minimal in calories, was not checked as one of the Healthiest Bets.)

Healthier Picks

As mentioned above, some restaurants—mainly those in the sections Sit-Down American Fare and Steak Houses—provide little nutrition information or only provide information for their healthier menu items. If one of these restaurants was willing to be included in this book and provided us with a menu, we made a list of Healthier Picks—menu items that appear to be healthier than others. We've also added suggestions for special requests or substitutions to make these items even healthier.

Bon Appétit!

Bagels, Coffees, Snacks, and More

RESTAURANTS

Auntie Anne's Hand-Rolled Soft Pretzels

Bruegger's Bagels

Dunkin' Donuts

Manhattan Bagel Company

Starbucks

Note: Restaurants in this chapter devote their menu to bagels, donuts, coffee, and pretzels. Look in Burgers, Fries, and More for fast-food breakfasts. Look in Sit-Down American Fare for restaurants that serve breakfast and brunch as well as lunch and dinner. Look in Subs and Sandwiches for Au Bon Pain, which also serves breakfast items.

The healthy meal choices for the restaurants in this section will have slightly fewer calories and other nutrients than the criteria noted on page 42. That's because meals you eat in these restaurants are most likely breakfasts, light meals, or snacks.

NUTRITION PROS

- Bagels are the rage. That's great because they are low in fat—as long as you apply spreads thinly and wisely.
- Light cream cheese spreads are available in most bagel shops.
- Soft-baked pretzels unadulterated with lots of fat or sugar are a healthy snack or side item.
- Pretzels and bagels are a source of dietary fiber.

Healthy Tips

* Stick with coffee without a lot of added cream, whole milk, or sugar. They add fat and empty calories.
* Try a soft-baked pretzel as an accompaniment to a sandwich or salad.
* Opt for one of the light bagel spreads, but keep in mind that they are hardly calorie or fat free. Spread them thinly.
* Cake donuts have slightly less fat than yeast donuts.
* Do eat breakfast. Skipping breakfast just keeps your engine in low gear and helps you rationalize overeating at meals during the rest of the day. Plus, if you take diabetes medications to lower your blood sugar, skipping breakfast is not a smart move.
* Steer clear of tuna, chicken, or seafood salads. They're chock full of fat. Stick with unadulterated meats and cheese.
* Read the fine print when you see the words "low-fat," "fat-free," or "sugar-free." They don't mean "no calories" or "no carbohydrate." In fact, some of these foods can contain more carbohydrate and/or more calories than the regular food.
* If jam or jelly is an option, take it. Jams and jellies have no fat. Spread them thinly all the same.

- No longer is it donuts-only at Dunkin' Donuts and other donut shops. They serve bagels, low-fat muffins, and various coffees too.
- Muffin mania has died down, but you'll find them at some breakfast spots. Often low-fat muffins are up for grabs. Even regular muffins are a better choice than some donuts or loaded bagels.
- English muffins and yeast rolls are healthy choices as long as you spread a light amount of butter or margarine.

NUTRITION CONS

- Bagels can quickly become high fat and high calorie if they are topped with a quarter inch of high-fat cream cheese or spread.
- Bagels in most bagels shops average 3–4 oz and 250–340 calories. They're often equal to about three or four slices of bread, not two.
- Pretzels sound healthy, but their calories and fat rise when they are rolled in lots of glaze or butter, or dipped in cheese sauce, cream cheese, or caramel.
- Croissants are high fat by nature—that's how they become flaky. You add insult to injury when you stuff a croissant with items such as bacon, sausage, cheese, tuna salad, or chicken salad.
- Donuts are high in fat (but surprisingly, not as bad as you might think). Save them for a once in a while splurge.
- Biscuits are loaded with fat. When sausage, bacon, egg, and/or cheese is sandwiched between them, they give you your fat for one day in one fell swoop.

■ The newfangled coffees—latte, mocha, or Starbucks' Frappuccino—are not just coffee. The sugar is blended through and through.

■ One of the quickest and most healthy breakfast foods—dry or cooked cereal with fat-free (skim) milk—is rarely served.

Get It Your Way

★ Order bagel spreads on the side so that you can control how much is spread.

★ Order butter or margarine on the side.

★ Opt for fat-free (skim) milk in specialty coffees.

★ Order a sandwich on a bagel or roll, not on a high-fat croissant.

Auntie Anne's Hand-Rolled Soft Pretzels

❖Auntie Anne's Hand-Rolled Soft Pretzels provides nutrition information for all of its menu items in a brochure.

Light 'n Lean Choice

Jalapeno Pretzel, without butter

Calories	270	Sodium (mg)	780
Fat (g)	1	Carbohydrate (g)	58
% calories from fat	3	Fiber (g)	2
Saturated fat (g)	0	Protein (g)	8
Cholesterol (mg)	0		

Exchanges: 4 starch

Healthy 'n Hearty Choice

Sour Cream & Onion Pretzel, without butter

Calories	310	Sodium (mg)	920
Fat (g)	1	Carbohydrate (g)	66
% calories from fat	3	Fiber (g)	2
Saturated fat (g)	0	Protein (g)	9
Cholesterol (mg)	0		

Exchanges: 4 1/2 starch

(*Continued*)

Auntie Anne's Hand-Rolled Soft Pretzels

	Amount	Cal.	Fat (g)	% Cal. Fat	Sat. Fat (g)	Chol. (mg)	Sod. (mg)	Carb. (g)	Fiber (g)	Pro. (g)	Servings/Exchanges
DIPS											
Caramel Dip	1.5 oz	135	3	20	1.5	5	110	27	0	1	2 carb.
✓Cheese Sauce	1 oz	70	5	64	4	15	400	2	0	3	1 fat
Chocolate Flavored Dip	1.25 oz	130	4	28	1.5	2	65	24	1	1	1 1/2 carb., 1 fat
✓Marinara Sauce	1 oz	10	0	0	0	0	130	3	0	0	free
✓Philadelphia Brand Light Cream Cheese	0.75 oz	45	4	70	2.5	15	105	1	0	2	1 fat
✓Philly Flavors Pineapple Cream Cheese	0.75 oz	70	6	77	4	20	70	3	0	1	1 fat
✓Philly Flavors Strawberry Cream Cheese	0.75 oz	70	6	77	4	20	70	3	0	1	1 fat

✔Sweet Mustard	1 oz	60	2	23	1	40	120	8	0	1	1/2 carb.
DUTCH ICE											
Kiwi-Banana Dutch Ice (large)	18 oz	250	0	0	0	0	40	57	0	0	4 carb
✔Kiwi-Banana Dutch Ice (regular)	12 oz	160	0	0	0	0	25	38	0	0	2 1/2 carb.
Lemonade Dutch Ice (large)	18 oz	405	0	0	0	0	0	99	1	0	6 1/2 carb.
Lemonade Dutch Ice (regular)	12 oz	270	0	0	0	0	0	66	0	0	4 1/2 carb.
Mocha Dutch Ice (large)	18 oz	500	14	24	11.5	0	135	95	0	0	6 carb 3 fat
Mocha Dutch Ice (regular)	12 oz	340	9	24	7.5	0	90	63	0	0	4 carb 2 fat
Orange Creme Dutch Ice (large)	18 oz	360	0	0	0	0	45	83	0	0	5 1/2 carb.
Orange Creme Dutch Ice (regular)	12 oz	240	0	0	0	0	30	55	0	0	3 1/2 carb.
Raspberry Dutch Ice (large)	18 oz	220	0	0	0	0	40	51	1	0	3 1/2 carb.
✔Raspberry Dutch Ice (regular)	12 oz	150	0	0	0	0	25	34	1	0	2 carb.
Strawberry Dutch Ice (large)	18 oz	280	0	0	0	0	50	65	1	0	4 carb.

(Continued)

✔ = Healthiest Bets; n/a = not available

DUTCH ICE (*Continued*)	Amount	Cal.	Fat (g)	% Cal. Fat	Sat. Fat (g)	Chol. (mg)	Sod. (mg)	Carb. (g)	Fiber (g)	Pro. (g)	Servings/Exchanges
✔Strawberry Dutch Ice (regular)	12 oz	190	0	0	0	0	35	43	0	0	3 carb.
PRETZELS WITH BUTTER											
✔Almond	1	400	8	18	5	20	400	72	2	9	5 starch, 1 fat
Cinnamon Sugar	1	450	9	18	5	25	430	83	3	8	4 1/2 starch, 1 carb., 2 fat
✔Garlic	1	350	5	11	2.5	10	850	68	2	9	4 1/2 starch, 1 fat
✔Glazin' Raisin	1	510	4	7	2	10	480	107	4	11	5 starch, 2 carb., 1 fat
Jalapeno	1	310	5	13	2.5	10	940	59	2	8	4 starch, 1 fat
✔Original	1	370	4	10	2	10	930	72	3	10	5 starch, 1 fat
Sesame	1	410	12	26	4	15	860	64	7	12	4 starch, 2 fat
Sour Cream & Onion	1	340	5	13	3	10	930	66	2	9	4 1/2 starch, 1 fat
Whole Wheat	1	370	5	11	1.5	10	1120	72	7	11	5 starch, 1 fat

PRETZELS WITHOUT BUTTER

✔Almond	1	350	2	4	0.5	0	390	72	2	9	4 starch, 1 carb.
✔Cinnamon Sugar	1	350	2	5	0	0	410	74	2	9	4 starch, 1 carb.
✔Garlic	1	320	1	3	0	0	830	66	2	9	4 1/2 starch
Glazin' Raisin	1	470	1	1	0	0	460	104	3	11	5 starch, 2 carb.
✔Jalapeno	1	270	1	3	0	0	780	58	2	8	4 starch
✔Original	1	340	1	3	0	0	900	72	3	10	5 starch
Sesame	1	350	6	15	1	0	840	63	3	11	4 starch, 1 fat
Sour Cream & Onion	1	310	1	3	0	0	920	66	2	9	4 1/2 starch
Whole Wheat	1	350	2	3	0	0	1100	72	7	11	5 starch

✔ = Healthiest Bets; n/a = not available

Notes

Bruegger's Bagels

❖Bruegger's Bagels provided nutrition information for all of its menu items.

Light 'n Lean Choice

Sundried Tomato Bagel
Light Herb Garlic Cream Cheese
(order on side; use 2 Tbsp)

Calories......................340	Sodium (mg) 565	
Fat (g) 6	Carbohydrate (g).........58	
% calories from fat..16	Fiber (g) 2	
Saturated fat (g)........2	Protein (g) 13	
Cholesterol (mg) 25		

Exchanges: 4 starch, 1 fat

Healthy 'n Hearty Choice

Chicken Fajita Bagel Sandwich

Calories......................460	Sodium (mg) 830
Fat (g) 10	Carbohydrate (g).........66
% calories from fat..20	Fiber (g) 3
Saturated fat (g).....4.5	Protein (g) 28
Cholesterol (mg) 80	

Exchanges: 4 1/2 starch, 2 lean meat, 1 fat

Bruegger's Bagels

	Amount	Cal.	Fat (g)	% Cal. Fat	Sat. Fat (g)	Chol. (mg)	Sod. (mg)	Carb. (g)	Fiber (g)	Pro. (g)	Serving/Exchanges
BAGELS											
✓Blueberry	1	300	2	6	0	0	480	60	2	10	4 starch
✓Cinnamon Raisin	1	290	2	3	0	0	400	60	3	10	4 starch
✓Cranberry Orange	1	290	1	3	0	0	470	61	2	10	4 starch
✓Egg	1	280	1	3	0.5	25	510	57	3	10	4 starch
✓Everything	1	290	2	6	0	0	700	58	2	11	4 starch
✓Garlic	1	280	2	4	0	0	440	57	2	10	4 starch
✓Honey Grain	1	300	3	8	0.5	0	390	58	3	11	4 starch
✓Onion	1	280	2	4	0	0	430	57	2	10	4 starch
✓Pesto	1	280	2	6	0	0	480	55	2	10	3 1/2 starch

✓ = Healthiest Bets; n/a = not available

(Continued)

BAGELS (*Continued*)	Amount	Cal.	Fat (g)	% Cal. Fat	Sat. Fat (g)	Chol. (mg)	Sod. (mg)	Carb. (g)	Fiber (g)	Pro. (g)	Servings/Exchanges
✓Plain	1	280	2	5	0	0	430	56	2	10	4 starch
✓Poppy Seed	1	280	2	5	0	0	440	57	2	11	4 starch
✓Pumpernickel	1	280	2	5	0	0	390	56	4	11	4 starch
Salt	1	270	2	6	0	0	1670	55	2	10	3 1/2 starch
✓Sesame	1	290	3	7	0	0	440	57	2	11	4 starch
✓Spinach Herb	1	280	1	3	0	0	490	56	3	11	4 starch
✓Sun Dried Tomato	1	280	2	5	0	0	490	56	3	10	4 starch
✓Wheat Bran	1	280	2	6	0	0	410	55	5	10	3 1/2 starch
CREAM CHEESES											
✓Bacon Scallion	1 scoop	100	8	72	4.5	25	95	3	0	2	1 1/2 fat
✓Chive	1 scoop	100	9	81	4.5	25	85	2	0	2	2 fat
✓Garden Veggie	1 scoop	100	8	72	4.5	25	100	4	0	2	1 1/2 fat

✔ Honey Walnut	1 scoop	100	8	72	4.5	25	95	3	0	2	1 1/2 fat
✔ Jalapeno	1 scoop	100	9	81	5	30	100	3	0	2	2 fat
✔ Light Garden Veggie	1 scoop	50	4	60	2.5	15	60	2	0	3	1 fat
✔ Light Herb Garlic	1 scoop	60	4	60	2	25	75	2	0	3	1 fat
✔ Light Plain	1 scoop	70	5	57	3	15	95	3	0	4	1 fat
✔ Light Strawberry	1 scoop	60	4	50	2	10	70	3	0	3	1 fat
✔ Plain	1 scoop	100	9	81	6	35	65	2	0	2	2 fat
✔ Salmon	1 scoop	100	9	81	4	25	100	2	0	2	2 fat
✔ Wildberry	1 scoop	100	9	81	5	25	85	4	0	2	2 fat

SANDWICHES

✔ Chicken Fajita	1	460	10	20	4.5	80	830	66	3	28	4 1/2 starch, 2 lean meat, 1 fat

(Continued)

✔ = Healthiest Bets; n/a = not available

SANDWICHES *(Continued)*	Amount	Cal.	Fat (g)	% Cal. Fat	Sat. Fat (g)	Chol. (mg)	Sod. (mg)	Carb. (g)	Fiber (g)	Pro. (g)	Servings/Exchanges
Herby Turkey	1	510	13	23	5	45	1100	67	3	30	4 1/2 starch, 2 lean meat, 1 fat
Hot Shot Turkey	1	450	8	16	3.5	45	1090	68	3	26	4 1/2 starch, 2 lean meat
✔Leonardo da Veggie	1	420	11	24	6	30	690	62	3	19	4 starch, 1 medium-fat meat, 1 fat
Santa Fe Turkey	1	450	9	18	4	45	1040	63	3	27	4 starch, 2 lean meat, 1/2 fat

✔ = Healthiest Bets; n/a = not available

Notes

Dunkin' Donuts

❖Dunkin' Donuts provides nutrition information for all of its menu items in a brochure.

Light 'n Lean Choice

Lowfat Bran Muffin

Calories......................260	Sodium (mg) 440
Fat (g) 2	Carbohydrate (g).........59
% calories from fat ...7	Fiber (g) 4
Saturated fat (g)........0	Protein (g) 4
Cholesterol (mg) 0	

Exchanges: 4 starch

Healthy 'n Hearty Choice

2 Glazed Yeast Donuts

Calories......................320	Sodium (mg) 400
Fat (g) 14	Carbohydrate (g).........46
% calories from fat..39	Fiber (g) 2
Saturated fat (g)........4	Protein (g) 6
Cholesterol (mg) 0	

Exchanges: 3 carb., 3 fat

(*Continued*)

Dunkin' Donuts

BAGELS	Amount	Cal.	Fat (g)	% Cal. Fat	Sat. Fat (g)	Chol. (mg)	Sod. (mg)	Carb. (g)	Fiber (g)	Pro. (g)	Servings/Exchanges
✔Blueberry	1	330	1	3	0	0	640	70	3	11	4 1/2 starch
✔Cinnamon Raisin	1	340	1	8	0	0	470	72	4	11	5 starch
✔Egg	1	340	2	5	0	40	670	69	3	12	4 1/2 starch
✔Everything	1	340	2	5	0	0	680	68	3	12	4 1/2 starch
✔Garlic	1	330	1	3	0	0	670	69	3	12	4 1/2 starch
✔Onion	1	320	1	0	0	0	650	66	3	12	4 1/2 starch
✔Plain	1	330	1	0	0	0	690	68	3	12	4 1/2 starch
✔Poppy	1	340	3	8	0	0	680	68	3	12	4 1/2 starch
✔Pumpernickel	1	340	2	5	0	0	660	70	3	11	4 1/2 starch
Salt	1	320	1	3	0	0	3170	65	3	11	4 starch

✔ Sesame	1	350	0	10	0	0	660	66	3	13	4 1/2 starch
✔ Whole Wheat	1	320	2	6	0	0	630	63	5	12	4 starch

BEVERAGES

Coffee Coolatta (18% Fat Cream)	16 oz	370	22	54	14	75	70	44	0	3	3 carb, 4 fat
✔ Coffee Coolatta (2% Milk)	16 oz	210	2	9	1.5	10	85	45	0	4	3 carb
✔ Coffee Coolatta (Skim Milk)	16 oz	190	0	0	0	2	85	45	0	4	3 carb
✔ Coffee Coolatta (Whole Milk)	16 oz	230	4	16	2.5	15	80	45	0	4	3 carb 1 fat
Hazelnut Coolatta (18% Fat Cream)	16 oz	370	22	54	13	75	70	42	0	3	3 carb, 4 fat
✔ Hazelnut Coolatta (2% Milk)	16 oz	210	2	9	1.5	10	85	43	0	4	3 carb.
✔ Hazelnut Coolatta (Skim Milk)	16 oz	200	0	0	0	2	85	43	0	4	3 carb.
✔ Hazelnut Coolatta (Whole Milk)	16 oz	230	4	16	2.5	15	80	43	0	4	3 carb., 1 fat
Mocha Coolatta (18% Fat Cream)	16 oz	380	22	52	13	75	70	42	0	3	3 carb., 1 fat
✔ Mocha Coolatta (2% Milk)	16 oz	220	2	8	1.5	10	80	43	0	4	3 carb.

✔ = Healthiest Bets; n/a = not available

(Continued)

BEVERAGES (Continued)	Amount	Cal.	Fat (g)	% Cal. Fat	Sat. Fat (g)	Chol. (mg)	Sod. (mg)	Carb. (g)	Fiber (g)	Pro. (g)	Servings/Exchanges
✔Mocha Coolatta (Skim Milk)	16 oz	200	0	0	0	2	85	43	0	4	3 carb.
✔Mocha Coolatta (Whole Milk)	16 oz	230	4	16	2.5	15	80	43	0	4	3 carb., 1 fat
Vanilla Coolatta (18% Fat Cream)	16 oz	380	22	52	13	75	70	42	0	3	3 carb., 4 fat
✔Vanilla Coolatta (2% Milk)	16 oz	220	2	8	1.5	10	85	43	0	4	3 carb
✔Vanilla Coolatta (Skim Milk)	16 oz	200	0	0	0	2	85	43	0	4	3 carb.
✔Vanilla Coolatta (Whole Milk)	16 oz	230	4	16	2.5	15	80	43	0	4	3 carb, 1 fat
BREAKFAST CROISSANT SANDWICHES											
Egg & Cheese	1	430	27	57	9	280	640	30	0	16	2 starch, 1 medium-fat meat, 4 fat
Egg, Bacon & Cheese	1	500	34	61	12	290	930	30	0	20	2 starch, 2 medium-fat meat, 5 fat
Egg, Ham & Cheese	1	530	29	49	9	295	1080	30	0	23	2 starch, 2 medium-fat meat, 4 fat

	Amount	Cal.	Fat (g)	% Fat Cal.	Sat. Fat (g)	Chol. (mg)	Sod. (mg)	Carb. (g)	Fiber (g)		Exchanges
Egg, Sausage & Cheese	1	630	49	70	15	320	1180	30	0	24	2 starch, 3 medium-fat meat, 7 fat

BROWNIES

	Amount	Cal.	Fat (g)	% Fat Cal.	Sat. Fat (g)	Chol. (mg)	Sod. (mg)	Carb. (g)	Fiber (g)		Exchanges
Blondie w/ Chocolate Chips	1	300	13	39	3	25	150	41	1	4	3 carb., 2 1/2 fat
Fudge	1	290	13	40	3	35	85	37	0	5	2 1/2 carb., 2 1/2 fat
Peanut Butter Blondie	1	330	18	49	4	25	300	36	1	6	2 1/2 carb., 3 1/2 fat

CAKE DONUTS

	Amount	Cal.	Fat (g)	% Fat Cal.	Sat. Fat (g)	Chol. (mg)	Sod. (mg)	Carb. (g)	Fiber (g)		Exchanges
✔Blueberry	1	230	10	39	2.5	0	240	30	1	4	2 carb., 2 fat
Blueberry Crumb	1	260	11	38	3	0	260	36	1	4	2 1/2 carb., 2 fat
Butternut	1	340	20	53	5	0	360	35	2	4	2 carb., 4 fat
Chocolate	1	210	14	60	3	0	270	19	1	3	1 carb., 3 fat
Chocolate Coconut	1	250	15	54	5	0	270	25	2	3	1 1/2 carb., 3 fat
Chocolate Glazed	1	250	14	50	3	0	280	29	1	3	2 carb., 3 fat

(Continued)

✔ = Healthiest Bets; n/a = not available

CAKE DONUTS (Continued)	Amount	Cal.	Fat (g)	% Cal. Fat	Sat. Fat (g)	Chol. (mg)	Sod. (mg)	Carb. (g)	Fiber (g)	Pro. (g)	Servings/Exchanges
Cinnamon	1	300	19	57	4	0	350	29	1	3	2 carb., 4 fat
Coconut	1	320	20	56	5	0	360	32	1	3	2 carb., 4 fat
Double Chocolate	1	260	14	48	3	0	280	30	1	3	2 carb., 3 fat
Old Fashioned	1	280	19	61	4	0	350	24	1	3	1 1/2 carb., 4 fat
Peanut	1	340	22	58	4	0	360	32	2	5	2 carb., 4 fat
Powdered	1	310	19	55	4	0	350	30	1	3	2 carb., 4 fat
Sugared	1	310	20	58	4	0	380	28	1	4	2 carb., 4 fat
Toasted Coconut	1	320	19	53	5	0	360	33	1	3	2 carb., 4 fat
Whole Wheat Glazed	1	230	11	43	2.5	0	340	31	2	3	2 carb., 2 fat
CAKE MUNCHKINS											
Butternut	3	230	11	43	4	0	210	30	2	2	2 carb., 2 fat
✔Chocolate Glazed	3	180	10	50	2	0	240	22	1	2	1 1/2 carb., 2 fat

Cinnamon	4	240	13	49	2.5	0	290	29	1	3	2 carb, 2 1/2 fat
Coconut	3	200	11	50	4	0	220	22	1	2	1 1/2 carb., 2 fat
✔Glazed	3	220	9	37	2	0	220	32	1	2	2 carb, 2 fat
✔Plain	4	200	12	54	2.5	0	290	21	1	3	1 1/2 carb, 2 fat
Powdered Sugar	4	240	13	49	2.5	0	290	28	1	3	2 carb 2 1/2 fat
✔Toasted Coconut	3	210	11	47	3	0	220	26	1	2	1 1/2 carb, 2 fat

COFFEES

Dark Roast	10 oz	5	0	0	0	0	5	1	0	0	free
French Vanilla	10 oz	5	0	0	0	0	5	1	0	0	free
Hazelnut	10 oz	5	0	0	0	0	10	1	0	0	free
Regular Blend	10 oz	5	0	0	0	0	5	1	0	0	free

COOKIES

Chocolate Chocolate Chunk	1	200	11	50	6	30	160	26	1	2	2 carb,, 2 fat

✔ = Healthiest Bets; n/a = not available

(Continued)

COOKIES *(Continued)*	Amount	Cal.	Fat (g)	% Cal. Fat	Sat. Fat (g)	Chol. (mg)	Sod. (mg)	Carb. (g)	Fiber (g)	Pro. (g)	Servings/Exchanges
Chocolate Chunk	1	200	10	45	6	30	150	26	1	2	1 1/2 carb., 2 fat
Chocolate Chunk w/ Nuts	1	200	11	50	6	30	150	25	1	2	1 1/2 carb., 2 fat
Chocolate White Chocolate Chunk	1	200	11	50	6	30	160	25	1	2	1 1/2 carb., 2 fat
✓Oatmeal Raisin Pecan	1	190	9	43	5	25	150	27	0	2	2 carb., 2 fat
Peanut Butter Chocolate Chunk w/ Nuts	1	210	13	56	6	25	110	23	1	4	1 1/2 carb., 2 fat
Peanut Butter Chocolate Chunk w/ Peanuts	1	210	12	51	5	30	140	22	0	4	1 1/2 carb., 2 fat
CREAM CHEESES											
✓Classic Lite	1 oz/2 Tbsp	60	5	75	3	15	115	3	0	3	1 fat
✓Classic Plain	1 oz/2 Tbsp	100	10	90	6	30	110	1	0	2	2 fat
✓Garden Veggie	1 oz/2 Tbsp	90	9	90	5	25	200	2	0	2	2 fat

✔ Savory Chive	1 oz/2 Tbsp	100	10	90	6	30	125	2	0	2	2 fat
✔ Smoked Salmon	1 oz/2 Tbsp	100	9	81	5	30	95	1	0	2	2 fat
✔ Strawberry	1 oz/2 Tbsp	100	9	81	5	25	100	5	0	1	2 fat
CROISSANTS											
Almond	1	360	21	53	5	10	300	38	2	6	2 1/2 starch, 4 fat
Cheese	1	240	15	56	3	5	260	28	0	6	2 starch, 3 fat
Chocolate	1	370	23	56	8	10	260	40	1	5	2 starch, 1/2 carb, 4 1/2 fat
Plain	1	270	17	57	4	5	260	27	0	4	2 starch, 3 fat
CRULLERS/STICKS											
Dunkin' Donut Cruller	1	240	14	53	3	0	370	26	2	4	1 1/2 carb., 3 fat
Glazed Chocolate Cruller	1	410	24	53	6	0	350	46	3	4	3 carb., 5 fat
Glazed Cruller	1	340	14	37	3	0	320	49	2	3	3 carb., 3 fat
Jelly Stick	1	330	14	38	3	0	350	48	3	3	3 carb., 3 fat

(Continued)

✔ = Healthiest Bets; n/a = not available

CRULLERS/STICKS (*Continued*)	Amount	Cal.	Fat (g)	% Cal. Fat	Sat. Fat (g)	Chol. (mg)	Sod. (mg)	Carb. (g)	Fiber (g)	Pro. (g)	Servings/Exchanges
Plain Cruller	1	260	14	49	3	0	300	29	2	3	2 carb., 3 fat
Powdered Cruller	1	290	15	47	4	0	300	35	2	3	2 carb., 3 fat
Sugar Cruller	1	270	14	47	3	0	300	31	2	3	2 carb., 3 fat
FANCIES											
Apple Fritter	1	300	13	39	3	0	320	41	2	5	3 carb., 2 1/2 fat
Apple Tart	1	290	10	31	3	0	330	45	1	5	3 carb., 2 fat
Apple Turnover	1	350	15	39	4	0	340	49	2	5	3 carb., 3 fat
Bismark	1	310	14	41	4	0	260	42	1	4	3 carb., 3 fat
Blueberry Tart	1	300	10	30	3	0	320	48	2	5	3 carb., 2 fat
Blueberry Turnover	1	370	15	36	4	0	330	54	2	5	3 1/2 carb., 3 fat
Bow Tie	1	250	10	36	3	0	300	35	1	5	2 carb., 2 fat
Chocolate Frosted Coffee Roll	1	290	14	43	3	0	300	38	2	5	2 1/2 carb., 3 fat

Item											
Cinnamon Raisin Coffee Roll	1	330	13	35	3	0	300	48	3	5	3 carb, 2 1/2 fat
Coffee Roll	1	280	13	42	3	0	300	35	2	5	2 carb, 2 1/2 fat
Eclair	1	290	12	37	3	0	280	42	1	4	3 carb, 2 fat
Glazed Fritter	1	290	13	40	3	0	300	39	2	5	2 1/2 carb, 2 1/2 fat
Lemon Tart	1	280	11	35	3	0	340	43	1	5	3 carb, 2 fat
Lemon Turnover	1	350	15	39	4	0	360	48	2	5	3 carb, 3 fat
Maple Frosted Coffee Roll	1	300	13	39	3	0	300	40	2	5	2 1/2 carb, 2 1/2 fat
Raspberry Tart	1	310	10	29	3	0	350	51	2	5	3 1/2 carb, 2 fat
Raspberry Turnover	1	380	15	36	4	0	370	57	2	5	4 carb, 3 fat
Strawberry Tart	1	310	10	29	3	0	340	51	1	5	3 1/2 carb, 2 fat
Strawberry Turnover	1	380	15	36	4	0	360	57	2	5	4 carb, 3 fat
Vanilla Frosted Coffee Roll	1	300	13	39	3	0	300	40	2	5	2 1/2 carb, 2 fat

(Continued)

	Amount	Cal.	Fat (g)	% Cal. Fat	Sat. Fat (g)	Chol. (mg)	Sod. (mg)	Carb. (g)	Fiber (g)	Pro. (g)	Servings/Exchanges
LOWFAT MUFFINS											
✔Apple n' Spice	1	220	2	8	0	0	480	50	1	3	3 1/2 starch
✔Banana	1	240	2	8	0	0	380	54	1	3	3 1/2 starch
✔Blueberry	1	230	2	8	0	0	370	51	1	3	3 starch
✔Bran	1	260	2	7	0	0	440	59	4	4	4 starch
✔Cherry	1	230	2	8	0	0	380	53	0	3	3 1/2 starch
✔Corn	1	250	2	7	0	0	460	55	1	4	3 1/2 starch
✔Cranberry Orange	1	230	2	8	0	0	380	53	1	3	3 starch
LUNCH CROISSANT SANDWICHES											
Broccoli & Cheese	1	370	21	51	6	20	680	36	2	10	2 starch, 1 veg., 1 high-fat meat, 2 fat

	Amount	Calories	Fat (g)	% Calories from Fat	Saturated Fat (g)	Cholesterol (mg)	Sodium (mg)	Carbohydrate (g)	Fiber (g)	Protein (g)	Servings/Exchanges
Chicken Salad	1	540	31	52	7	75	710	37	-	27	2 1/2 starch, 3 lean meat, 4 fat
Ham & Cheese	1	710	32	41	13	85	1840	29	C	33	2 starch, 4 medium-fat meat, 2 fat
Roast Beef & Cheese	1	490	27	50	8	30	680	28	0	31	2 starch, 4 medium-fat meat, 1 fat
Seafood Salad	1	480	26	49	6	50	1020	45	1	16	3 starch, 2 lean meat, 3 fat
Tuna Salad	1	540	30	50	6	50	1140	39	1	30	2 1/2 starch, 3 lean meat, 4 fat

MISCELLANEOUS

	Amount	Calories	Fat (g)	% Calories from Fat	Saturated Fat (g)	Cholesterol (mg)	Sodium (mg)	Carbohydrate (g)	Fiber (g)	Protein (g)	Servings/Exchanges
✔ English Muffin	1	130	1	7	0.5	0	520	26	1	4	2 starch
✔ French Roll (Baked)	1	140	1	4	0	0	220	27	1	5	2 starch

(Continued)

✔ = Healthiest Bets; n/a = not available

MUFFINS

	Amount	Cal.	Fat (g)	% Cal. Fat	Sat. Fat (g)	Chol. (mg)	Sod. (mg)	Carb. (g)	Fiber (g)	Pro. (g)	Servings/Exchanges
✔Apple n' Spice	1	330	10	27	2.5	35	330	54	2	5	3 1/2 starch, 2 fat
Banana Nut	1	340	12	32	3	35	210	53	2	6	3 1/2 starch, 2 fat
✔Blueberry	1	310	10	29	2.5	35	190	51	2	5	3 1/2 starch, 2 fat
Cherry	1	330	11	30	2.5	35	210	53	1	5	3 1/2 starch, 2 fat
Chocolate Chip	1	400	16	36	6	35	190	63	2	5	4 starch, 3 fat
Corn	1	350	14	36	0.5	50	310	51	2	6	3 1/2 carb., 3 fat
Cranberry Orange Nut	1	310	11	32	2.5	30	180	51	2	5	3 1/2 starch, 2 fat
✔Honey Raisin Bran	1	330	10	27	0	15	360	57	4	5	4 starch, 2 fat
Lemon Poppy Seed	1	360	13	33	3	40	440	57	1	6	4 starch, 2 1/2 fat
✔Oat Bran	1	290	11	34	1	0	330	44	1	4	3 starch, 2 fat

SOUPS

✓Beef Barley	227 g	90	1	10	0	10	970	15	0	7	1 carb.
✓Beef Noodle	227 g	90	1	10	0	20	980	12	0	8	1 carb., 1 very lean meat
✓Chicken Noodle	227 g	80	2	23	0	15	890	12	0	6	1 carb.
✓Chile	227 g	170	6	32	2.5	20	860	20	0	8	1 carb., 1 lean meat, 1/2 fat
Chile con Carne w/ Beans	227 g	300	15	45	0	45	690	25	0	17	1 1/2 carb., 2 lean meat, 2 fat
Cream of Broccoli	227 g	200	11	50	6	25	1050	17	0	8	1 carb., 2 fat
✓Cream of Potato	227 g	190	10	47	5	25	770	19	1	6	1 carb., 2 fat
Harvest Vegetable	227 g	80	2	23	0	0	1120	12	0	4	1 carb.
✓Manhattan Clam Chowder	227 g	70	1	13	0	5	890	11	1	5	1/2 carb., 1 very lean meat
✓Minestrone	227 g	100	1	9	0	0	900	16	2	5	1 carb.
New England Clam Chowder	227 g	200	10	45	3	30	1050	16	0	10	1 carb., 1 lean meat, 1 fat

✓ = Healthiest Bets; n/a = not available

(Continued)

SOUPS (Continued)	Amount	Cal.	Fat (g)	% Cal. Fat	Sat. Fat (g)	Chol. (mg)	Sod. (mg)	Carb. (g)	Fiber (g)	Pro. (g)	Servings/Exchanges
✔Split Pea w/ Ham	227 g	190	9	43	3	15	830	20	0	8	1 carb., 1 medium-fat meat, 1 fat

YEAST DONUTS

	Amount	Cal.	Fat (g)	% Cal. Fat	Sat. Fat (g)	Chol. (mg)	Sod. (mg)	Carb. (g)	Fiber (g)	Pro. (g)	Servings/Exchanges
✔Apple Crumb	1	250	11	40	3	0	270	34	1	4	2 carb., 2 fat
Apple n' Spice	1	230	10	39	2.5	0	250	31	1	4	2 carb., 2 fat
✔Bavarian Kreme	1	250	11	40	2.5	0	250	33	1	4	2 carb., 2 fat
Black Raspberry	1	240	10	38	2.5	0	260	32	1	4	2 carb., 2 fat
✔Boston Kreme	1	270	11	37	3	0	260	38	1	4	2 1/2 carb., 2 fat
✔Chocolate Frosted	1	210	8	34	2	0	230	31	1	4	2 carb., 1 1/2 fat
✔Chocolate Kreme Filled	1	320	16	45	4	0	250	39	1	4	2 1/2 carb., 3 fat
✔Glazed	1	160	7	39	2	0	200	23	1	3	1 1/2 carb., 1 fat
Jelly Filled	1	240	11	41	2.5	0	260	32	1	4	2 carb., 2 fat

Lemon	1	240	11	41	2.5	0	250	31	1	4	2 carb., 2 fat
✔ Maple Frosted	1	210	8	34	2	0	230	32	1	4	2 carb., 1 1/2 fat
✔ Marble Frosted	1	210	8	34	2	0	230	32	1	4	2 carb., 1 1/2 fat
Strawberry	1	240	10	38	2.5	0	250	32	1	4	2 carb., 2 fat
✔ Strawberry Frosted	1	220	8	33	2	0	230	32	1	4	2 carb., 1 1/2 fat
✔ Sugar Raised	1	170	7	37	2	0	220	23	1	4	1 1/2 carb., 1 fat
✔ Vanilla Frosted	1	220	8	33	2	0	230	32	1	4	2 carb., 1 1/2 fat
YEAST MUNCHKINS											
✔ Glazed Raised	4	210	7	30	1.5	0	170	36	1	3	2 carb., 1 fat
✔ Jelly	3	170	5	26	1	0	170	28	1	2	2 carb., 1 fat
✔ Lemon	3	160	6	34	1	0	160	23	1	2	1 1/2 carb., 1 fat
✔ Sugar Raised	6	210	10	43	2.5	0	250	26	2	4	2 carb., 2 fat

✔ = Healthiest Bets; n/a = not available.

Manhattan Bagel Company

❖Manhattan Bagel Company provides nutrition
information for only its bagels in a brochure.

Light 'n Lean Choice

Jalapeno Cheddar Bagel

Calories	260	Sodium (mg)	310
Fat (g)	2	Carbohydrate (g)	52
% calories from fat	7	Fiber (g)	2
Saturated fat (g)	0	Protein (g)	10
Cholesterol (mg)	0		

Exchanges: 3 1/2 starch

Healthy 'n Hearty Choice

Oat Bran, Raisin & Walnut Bagel

Calories	270	Sodium (mg)	450
Fat (g)	3	Carbohydrate (g)	54
% calories from fat	10	Fiber (g)	3
Saturated fat (g)	0	Protein (g)	10
Cholesterol (mg)	0		

Exchanges: 3 1/2 starch, 1/2 fat

Manhattan Bagel Company

	Amount	Cal.	Fat (g)	% Cal. Fat	Sat. Fat (g)	Chol. (mg)	Sod. (mg)	Carb. (g)	Fiber (g)	Pro. (g)	Serving/Exchanges
BAGELS											
✔Blueberry	1	260	1	4	0	0	530	54	2	9	3 1/2 starch
✔Cheddar Cheese	1	270	4	13	2	10	560	48	2	11	3 starch, 1 fat
✔Chocolate Chip	1	290	3	9	1.5	0	530	56	2	9	3 1/2 starch, 1/2 fat
✔Cinnamon Raisin	1	280	1	4	0	0	560	57	3	10	3 1/2 starch
✔Egg	1	270	2	6	0	0	710	53	2	10	3 1/2 starch
Everything	1	290	3	9	0	0	2000	54	3	11	3 1/2 starch, 1/2 fat
✔Garlic	1	270	1	4	0	0	560	55	2	10	3 1/2 starch
✔Jalapeno Cheddar	1	260	2	6	0	0	310	52	2	10	3 1/2 starch
✔Marble	1	260	1	4	0	0	540	52	3	10	3 1/2 starch

(Continued)

✔ = Healthiest Bets; n/a = not available

BAGELS *(Continued)*	Amount	Cal.	Fat (g)	% Cal. Fat	Sat. Fat (g)	Chol. (mg)	Sod. (mg)	Carb. (g)	Fiber (g)	Pro. (g)	Servings/Exchanges
✔Oat Bran	1	260	1	3	0	0	470	53	3	10	3 1/2 starch
✔Oat Bran, Raisin & Walnut	1	270	3	9	0	0	450	54	3	10	3 1/2 starch, 1/2 fat
✔Onion	1	270	1	2	0	0	560	55	2	10	3 1/2 starch
✔Plain	1	260	1	2	0	0	560	52	2	10	3 1/2 starch
✔Poppy	1	300	4	12	0.5	0	560	54	5	11	3 1/2 starch, 1 fat
✔Pumpernickel	1	250	1	4	0	0	530	52	3	10	3 1/2 starch
✔Rye	1	260	1	3	0	0	560	52	3	10	3 1/2 starch
Salt	1	260	1	2	0	0	7100	53	2	10	3 1/2 starch
✔Sesame	1	310	5	15	1	0	560	55	3	11	3 1/2 starch, 1 fat
✔Spinach	1	270	1	4	0	0	580	54	3	10	3 1/2 starch
✔Sundried Tomato	1	260	1	3	0	0	340	53	3	10	3 1/2 starch
✔Whole Wheat	1	260	1	4	0	0	470	52	3	10	3 1/2 starch

✔ = Healthiest Bets; n/a = not available

Starbucks

❖Starbucks provided nutrition information for some of its coffees.

Light 'n Lean Choice

Cappuccino (nonfat milk)

Calories......................80
Fat (g) 0
   % calories from fat ...0
   Saturated fat (g) ....n/a
Cholesterol (mg) 5

Sodium (mg) 110
Carbohydrate (g).........11
   Fiber (g) ....n/a
Protein (g) 7

Exchanges: 1 fat-free milk

Healthy 'n Hearty Choice

Caffè Latte (nonfat milk)

Calories......................120
Fat (g) 1
   % calories from fat ...4
   Saturated fat (g) ....n/a
Cholesterol (mg) 5

Sodium (mg) 170
Carbohydrate (g).........17
   Fiber (g) ....n/a
Protein (g) 12

Exchanges: 1 fat-free milk

(*Continued*)

Starbucks

BEVERAGES

	Amount	Cal.	Fat (g)	% Cal. Fat	Sat. Fat (g)	Chol. (mg)	Sod. (mg)	Carb. (g)	Fiber (g)	Pro. (g)	Servings/Exchanges
✔Caffè Americano	12 oz	10	0	0	n/a	0	10	2	n/a	0	free
✔Caffè Latte (nonfat milk)	12 oz	120	1	4	n/a	5	170	17	n/a	12	1 fat-free milk
Caffè Latte (whole milk)	12 oz	210	11	47	n/a	45	160	17	n/a	11	1 whole milk, 1 fat
Caffè Mocha w/ whipping cream (nonfat milk)	12 oz	260	12	42	n/a	40	170	32	n/a	12	1 fat-free milk, 1 carb., 2 fat
Caffè Mocha w/ whipping cream (whole milk)	12 oz	340	21	56	n/a	70	160	31	n/a	12	1 whole milk, 1 carb., 2 1/2 fat
✔Cappuccino (nonfat milk)	12 oz	80	0	0	n/a	5	110	11	n/a	7	1 fat-free milk
Cappuccino (whole milk)	12 oz	140	7	45	n/a	30	105	11	n/a	7	1 whole milk

✔Coffee Frappuccino	12 oz	200	3	14	n/a	0	170	39	n/a	6	2 1/2 carb., 1/2 fat
Drip Coffee	12 oz	10	0	0	n/a	0	10	1	n/a	1	free
✔Mocha Frappuccino	12 oz	230	3	12	n/a	0	180	44	n/a	6	3 carb., 1/2 fat

✔ = Healthiest Bets; n/a = not available

Notes

Burgers, Fries, and More

RESTAURANTS

Burger King
Carl's Jr.
Dairy Queen/Brazier
Hardee's
Jack in the Box
McDonald's
Rally's Hamburgers
Wendy's
Whataburger

NUTRITION PROS

- Small portions are plentiful as long as you know and use the small-portion words, such as regular, small, junior, and single.
- There's no waiting for food. You order, then eat.
- No foods greet you at the table. What you order is what you eat. This puts you in the driver's seat.
- You can fill up on fiber from multigrain buns and baked potatoes.
- It's easy to add to your 5-a-day (fruits and vegetables) with an entree or a side salad.
- Salad dressing is served on the side. There's no need for a special request.
- Healthier cold drinks flow freely: low-fat (1%) or fat-free (skim) milk, fruit juice, water, unsweetened ice tea, diet soft drinks.
- Low-fat and low-calorie or fat-free salad dressings are now common. Keep in mind that these salad

dressings are not calorie free. They can also be high in sodium.

- Healthier dessert options include low-fat frozen yogurt in a cone or dish, low-fat milkshakes, or fat-free muffins.
- Honesty is their policy. Full disclosure of nutrition information is there for the asking.
- You know the menu well. You can have your order at the tip of your tongue when you walk in the door.

NUTRITION CONS

- Many menu items are high in fat. Cheese, cheese sauce, bacon, special sauce, and mayonnaise add fat.
- The large-portion words are all too frequent: large, jumbo, double, and triple are a few to watch out for.
- Sodium can skyrocket from salt on french fries, in special sauce, and in salad dressing.
- Chicken and fish start off healthy, but before you get to bite in, they are often buried in a crisp golden coating.
- Several fast-food restaurants have said so long to healthier options such as lean hamburgers, grilled chicken without special sauce, and salads.
- Biscuits are loaded with fat to begin with. Tuck sausage, bacon, egg, and/or cheese in the middle and you've just downed your fat grams for the day in one fell swoop.
- Fruit is nowhere to be found—other than in juice and between the pie crust.
- Vegetables are few and far between, just salad and a few bits of lettuce and tomato on some sandwiches.
- French fries or onion rings—deep fried of course—are still the traditional side.

- Super-sized and "value" meals push you to eat larger portions because you can buy more food for less.

Healthy Tips

★ Zero in on the words regular, junior, small, or single. These mean small portions.
▲ Try lower-calorie ketchup, mustard, or barbecue sauce as an option to higher-fat mayonnaise or special sauce.
★ Walk in rather than drive through. If you eat and drive, you hardly realize food has passed your lips.
★ Order less food to start. Remember, you can go back and get more in a flash.
★ Want fries, go ahead. But split a small order with your fast-food partner.

Get It Your Way

★ Work around busy times. This way you'll get your food your way with a smile on the order taker's face.
★ Be ready to wait. Fast-food restaurants are not set up for special requests.
★ Ask for simple changes: leave off the special sauce or mayonnaise; hold the pickles, bacon, or cheese; or hold the salt on the french fries.

Burger King

❖Burger King provides nutrition information for all of its menu items in a brochure.

Light 'n Lean Choice

Broiled Chicken Salad
Reduced Calorie Light Italian Dressing (*2 Tbsp*)
Croutons (*2 packages*)
Milk (2%)

Calories......................395	Sodium (mg)..........1,160
Fat (g) 16	Carbohydrate (g).........34
% calories from fat..25	Fiber (g) 3
Saturated fat (g)........7	Protein (g) 29
Cholesterol (mg).........95	

Exchanges: 1/2 starch, 1 veg., 1 low-fat milk, 3 lean meat

Healthy 'n Hearty Choice

Whopper Jr.
Garden Salad
Reduced Calorie Light Italian Dressing (*2 Tbsp*)
Orange Juice

Calories......................675	Sodium (mg) 1,000
Fat (g) 30	Carbohydrate (g).........72
% calories from fat..40	Fiber (g) 5
Saturated fat (g)......11	Protein (g) 30
Cholesterol (mg) 75	

Exchanges: 2 starch, 1 veg., 2 fruit, 3 medium-fat meat, 3 fat

Burger King

	Amount	Cal.	Fat (g)	% Cal. Fat	Sat. Fat (g)	Chol. (mg)	Sod. (mg)	Carb. (g)	Fiber (g)	Pro. (g)	Servings/Exchanges
BEVERAGES											
✔Milk, 2%	8 oz	130	5	35	3	20	120	12	0	8	1 low-fat milk
✔Tropicana Orange Juice	10 oz	140	0	0	0	0	0	33	0	2	2 fruit
BREAKFAST											
Biscuit	1	330	18	49	4	2	950	37	1	6	2 1/2 starch, 3 1/2 fat
Biscuit with Bacon, Egg, & Cheese	1	510	31	55	10	225	1530	39	1	19	2 1/2 starch, 2 medium-fat meat, 4 fat
Biscuit with Egg	1	420	24	51	6	205	1110	38	1	13	2 1/2 starch, 1 medium-fat meat, 4 fat

(*Continued*)

✔ = Healthiest Bets; n/a = not available

BREAKFAST (Continued)	Amount	Cal.	Fat (g)	% Cal. Fat	Sat. Fat (g)	Chol. (mg)	Sod. (mg)	Carb. (g)	Fiber (g)	Pro. (g)	Servings/Exchanges
Biscuit with Sausage	1	530	36	61	11	35	1350	38	1	13	2 1/2 carb., 2 high-fat meat, 5 fat
Croissan'wich w/ Sausage & Cheese	1	450	35	70	12	45	940	21	1	13	1 1/2 starch, 1 high-fat meat, 5 fat
Croissan'wich w/ Sausage, Egg & Cheese	1	550	42	69	14	250	1110	22	1	20	1 1/2 starch, 2 high-fat meat, 4 fat
French Toast Sticks	1 order	500	27	49	7	0	490	60	1	4	4 starch, 5 fat
Hash Browns (small)	1 order	240	15	56	6	0	440	25	2	2	2 starch, 3 fat
BURGERS											
Big King	1	660	43	59	18	135	920	29	1	40	2 starch, 5 medium-fat meat, 3 1/2 fat
✓Cheeseburger	1	380	19	45	9	65	770	28	1	23	2 starch, 2 medium-fat meat, 2 fat

Double Cheeseburger	1	600	36	54	17	135	1060	28	1	41	2 starch, 5 medium-fat meat, 2 fat
Double Cheeseburger with Bacon	1	640	39	55	18	145	1240	28	1	44	2 starch, 3 medium-fat meat, 5 fat
Double Whopper	1	870	56	58	19	170	940	45	3	46	3 starch, 5 medium-fat meat, 6 fat
Double Whopper with Cheese	1	960	63	59	24	195	1420	46	3	52	3 starch, 6 medium-fat meat, 6 1/2 fat
✔Hamburger	1	330	15	41	6	55	530	28	·	20	2 starch, 2 medium-fat meat, 1 fat
Whopper	1	640	39	55	11	90	870	45	3	27	3 starch, 3 medium-fat meat, 5 fat

(Continued)

✔ = Healthiest Bets; n/a = not available

BURGERS (Continued)	Amount	Cal.	Fat (g)	% Cal. Fat	Sat. Fat (g)	Chol. (mg)	Sod. (mg)	Carb. (g)	Fiber (g)	Pro. (g)	Servings/Exchanges
Whopper Jr.	1	420	24	51	8	60	530	29	2	21	2 starch, 2 medium-fat meat, 3 fat
Whopper Jr. with Cheese	1	460	28	55	10	75	770	29	2	23	2 starch, 2 medium-fat meat, 3 1/2 fat
Whopper with Cheese	1	730	46	57	16	115	1350	46	3	33	3 starch, 3 medium-fat meat, 6 fat
CONDIMENTS											
✔A.M. Express Dip	1 oz/2 Tbsp	80	0	0	0	0	20	21	0	0	1 1/2 carb.
✔A.M. Express Grape Jam	1/2 oz/1 Tbsp	30	0	0	0	0	0	7	0	0	1/2 carb.
✔A.M. Express Strawberry Jam	1/2 oz/1 Tbsp	30	0	0	0	0	5	8	0	0	1/2 carb.
✔Bacon Bits	3 g	15	1	60	0	3	70	0	0	1	free
✔Barbecue Dipping Sauce	1 oz/2 Tbsp	35	0	0	0	0	400	9	0	0	1/2 carb.

✔Bull's Eye Barbecue Sauce	1/2 oz/1 Tbsp	20	0	0	0	0	140	5	0	0	free
✔Croutons	1 pkg.	30	1	30	0	0	90	5	0	0	free
✔Honey Dipping Sauce	1 oz/2 Tbsp	90	0	0	0	0	10	23	0	0	1 1/2 carb.
King Sauce	1/2 oz/1 Tbsp	70	7	90	1	4	70	2	0	0	1 fat
Land O' Lakes Whipped Classic Blend	1 1/2 tsp	65	7	97	1	0	75	0	0	0	1 fat
Ranch Dipping Sauce	1 oz/2 Tbsp	170	17	90	3	0	200	2	0	0	3 fat
✔Sweet & Sour Dipping Sauce	1 oz/2 Tbsp	45	0	0	0	0	50	11	0	0	1 carb.
Tartar Sauce	1 oz/2 Tbsp	180	19	95	3	15	220	0	0	0	4 fat
DESSERTS											
Dutch Apple Pie	1	300	15	45	3	0	230	39	2	3	2 1/2 carb, 3 fat
OTHER ENTREES											
Chicken Tenders	8 pieces	350	22	57	7	65	940	17	1	22	1 starch 3 lean meat, 2 1/2 fat

(Continued)

✔ = Healthiest Bets; n/a = not available

	Amount	Cal.	Fat (g)	% Cal. Fat	Sat. Fat (g)	Chol. (mg)	Sod. (mg)	Carb. (g)	Fiber (g)	Pro. (g)	Servings/Exchanges
SALAD DRESSINGS											
Bleu Cheese	1 oz/2 Tbsp	160	16	90	4	30	260	1	0	2	3 fat
French	1 oz/2 Tbsp	140	10	64	2	0	190	11	0	0	1 carb., 2 fat
Ranch	1 oz/2 Tbsp	180	19	95	4	10	170	2	0	0	4 fat
✓Reduced Calorie Light Italian	1 oz/2 Tbsp	15	1	17	0	0	360	3	0	0	free
Thousand Island	1 oz/2 Tbsp	140	12	77	3	15	190	7	0	0	1/2 carb., 2 fat
SALADS											
✓Broiled Chicken Salad	1	190	8	38	4	75	500	9	3	20	2 veg., 2 lean meat, 1/2 fat
✓Garden Salad	1	100	5	45	3	15	110	7	3	6	1 veg., 1 medium-fat meat
✓Side Salad	1	60	3	45	2	5	55	4	2	3	1 veg., 1/2 fat
SANDWICHES											
BK Big Fish Sandwich	1	720	43	54	9	80	1180	59	3	23	4 sta·ch, 2 lean meat, 7 fat

BK Broiler Chicken Sandwich	1	530	26	44	5	105	1060	45	2	29	3 starch, 3 lean meat, 3 fat
Chicken Sandwich (fried)	1	710	43	55	9	60	1400	54	2	26	3 1/2 carb., 3 lean meat, 7 fat

S H A K E S

Chocolate Shake (medium)	10 oz	320	7	20	4	20	230	54	3	9	3 1/2 carb., 1 fat
Chocolate Shake (medium, syrup added)	10 oz	440	7	14	4	20	430	84	2	10	5 1/2 carb., 1 fat
Strawberry Shake (medium, syrup added)	12 oz	420	6	13	4	20	260	83	1	9	5 1/2 carb., 1 fat
✔ Vanilla Shake (medium)	10 oz	300	6	18	4	20	230	53	1	9	3 1/2 carb., 1 fat

S I D E S

French Fries (medium, salted)	1 order	370	20	49	5	0	240	43	3	5	3 starch, 4 fat
Onion Rings	1 order	310	14	41	2	0	810	41	6	4	2 1/2 starch, 3 fat

✔ = Healthiest Bets; n/a = not available

Carl's Jr.

❖Carl's Jr. provides nutrition information for all of its menu items in a brochure.

Light 'n Lean Choice

BBQ Chicken Sandwich
Garden Salad-To-Go
Fat Free French Salad Dressing (*2 Tbsp*)
Milk, 1% fat (*10 oz*)

Calories......................510	Sodium (mg)..........1,400
Fat (g) 9	Carbohydrate (g).........67
% calories from fat..16	Fiber (g) 5
Saturated fat (g)........5	Protein (g) 42
Cholesterol (mg) 80	

Exchanges: 2 starch, 1 veg., 1/2 carb., 1 low-fat milk, 4 very lean meat, 1/2 fat

Healthy 'n Hearty Choice

Jr. Hamburger
Baked Potato (*plain*)
Salsa (*2 packages for potato*)

Calories......................640	Sodium (mg) 820
Fat (g) 13	Carbohydrate (g).......106
% calories from fat..18	Fiber (g) 7
Saturated fat (g)........5	Protein (g) 24
Cholesterol (mg) 45	

Exchanges: 6 starch, 1 veg., 2 medium-fat meat, 1/2 fat

Carl's Jr.

	Amount	Cal.	Fat (g)	% Cal. Fat	Sat. Fat (g)	Chol. (mg)	Sod. (mg)	Carb. (g)	Fiber (g)	Pro. (g)	Servings/Exchanges
BEVERAGES											
✔Hot Chocolate	12 oz	110	2	16	2	0	80	22	1	2	1 1/2 carb.
✔Milk, 1% Fat	10 oz	150	3	18	2	15	180	18	0	14	1 1/2 low-fat milk
✔Orange Juice	10 oz	140	0	0	0	0	30	33	0	2	2 fruits
BREAKFAST											
Breakfast Burrito	1	480	30	56	13	465	750	26	2	27	2 starch, 3 medium-fat meat, 3 fat
✔Breakfast Quesadilla	1	310	16	46	6	230	670	27	2	14	2 starch, 1 medium-fat meat, 2 fat

(Continued)

✔ = Healthiest Bets; n/a = not available

BREAKFAST (*Continued*)	Amount	Cal.	Fat (g)	% Cal. Fat	Sat. Fat (g)	Chol. (mg)	Sod. (mg)	Carb. (g)	Fiber (g)	Pro. (g)	Servings/Exchanges
✔ English Muffin, w/ margarine	1	210	9	39	1	0	300	27	2	5	2 starch, 2 fat
French Toast Dips	1 order	370	20	49	2.5	0	430	42	1	6	3 starch, 4 fat
✔ Scrambled Eggs	1 order	160	11	62	3.5	425	125	1	0	13	2 medium-fat meat
Sunrise Sandwich (no bacon or sausage)	1	360	21	53	5	225	700	28	2	14	2 starch, 1 medium-fat meat, 3 fat
BURGERS											
Carl's Famous Star Hamburger	1	580	32	50	9	70	910	49	2	25	3 starch, 2 medium-fat meat, 4 fat
Double Western Bacon Cheeseburger	1	900	49	49	21	155	1770	64	2	51	4 starch, 6 medium-fat meat, 4 fat
✔ Jr. Hamburger	1	330	13	35	5	45	480	34	1	18	2 starch, 2 medium-fat meat, 1/2 fat

	Serving	Cal.	Fat Cal.	Fat (g)	Sat. Fat (g)	Chol. (mg)	Sod. (mg)	Carb. (g)	Fiber (g)	Sugar (g)	Exchanges
Super Star Hamburger	1	790	46	52	14	130	970	50	2	42	3 starch, 5 medium-fat meat, 4 fat
Western Bacon Cheeseburger	1	650	30	42	12	80	1430	63	2	32	4 starch, 3 medium-fat meat, 3 fat

CONDIMENTS

	Serving	Cal.	Fat Cal.	Fat (g)	Sat. Fat (g)	Chol. (mg)	Sod. (mg)	Carb. (g)	Fiber (g)	Sugar (g)	Exchanges
✔ BBQ Sauce	1 oz	50	0	0	0	0	270	11	0	1	1 carb.
✔ Grape Jelly	1/2 oz	35	0	0	0	0	0	9	0	0	1/2 carb.
✔ Honey Sauce	1 oz/2 Tbsp	90	0	0	0	0	0	22	0	0	1 1/2 carb.
✔ Mustard Sauce	1 oz	50	0	0	0	0	210	11	0	0	1 carb.
✔ Salsa	1 pkg.	10	0	0	0	0	160	2	0	0	free
✔ Strawberry Jam	1/2 oz	35	0	0	0	0	0	9	0	0	1/2 carb.
✔ Sweet N' Sour Sauce	1 oz	50	0	0	0	0	80	12	0	0	1 carb.
✔ Table Syrup	1 oz	90	0	0	0	0	0	21	0	0	1 1/2 carb.

✔ = Healthiest Bets; n/a = not available

(Continued)

	Amount	Cal.	Fat (g)	% Cal. Fat	Sat. Fat (g)	Chol. (mg)	Sod. (mg)	Carb. (g)	Fiber (g)	Pro. (g)	Servings/Exchanges
DESSERTS/MUFFINS											
Blueberry Muffin	1	340	14	37	2	40	340	49	1	5	3 starch, 3 fat
Bran Raisin Muffin	1	370	13	32	2	45	410	61	6	7	4 starch, 2 1/2 fat
Cheese Danish	1	400	22	50	5	15	390	49	1	5	3 carb., 4 fat
Cheesecake (Strawberry Swirl)	1	290	17	53	9	55	230	30	0	6	2 carb., 3 fat
✓Chocolate Cake	1	300	10	30	2.5	23	260	49	4	3	3 carb., 2 fat
Chocolate Chip Cookie	1	370	19	46	8	25	350	49	1	3	3 carb., 4 fat
POTATOES											
Bacon & Cheese Baked Potato	1	630	29	41	7	35	1700	76	6	20	5 starch, 1 high-fat meat, 4 fat
Broccoli & Cheese Baked Potato	1	530	21	36	4.5	15	950	74	7	11	5 starch, 4 fat
✓Plain Potato (no margarine)	1	290	0	0	0	0	20	68	6	6	4 1/2 starch

	Serving	Cal.	Fat (g)	% Fat Cal.	Sat. Fat (g)	Chol. (mg)	Sodium (mg)	Carb. (g)	Fiber (g)	Pro. (g)	Exchanges
✔Sour Cream & Chive Baked Potato	1	430	14	29	3	10	135	70	6	7	4 1/2 starch, 3 fat

SALAD DRESSINGS

	Serving	Cal.	Fat (g)	% Fat Cal.	Sat. Fat (g)	Chol. (mg)	Sodium (mg)	Carb. (g)	Fiber (g)	Pro. (g)	Exchanges
1000 Island	2 oz/4 Tbsp	230	23	90	3.5	20	420	5	0	1	4 1/2 fat
Blue Cheese	2 oz/4 Tbsp	320	35	98	6	25	370	1	0	2	7 fat
✔Fat Free French	2 oz/4 Tbsp	60	0	0	0	0	660	16	0	0	1 carb.
✔Fat Free Italian	2 oz/4 Tbsp	15	0	0	0	0	770	4	0	0	free
House	2 oz/4 Tbsp	220	22	90	3.5	20	440	3	0	1	4 fat

SALADS

	Serving	Cal.	Fat (g)	% Fat Cal.	Sat. Fat (g)	Chol. (mg)	Sodium (mg)	Carb. (g)	Fiber (g)	Pro. (g)	Exchanges
✔Chargrilled Chicken Salad-To-Go	1	200	7	32	3.5	75	440	12	3	25	2 veg., 3 lean meat
✔Garden Salad-To-Go	1	50	3	54	1.5	10	60	4	2	3	1 veg., 1/2 fat

SANDWICHES

	Serving	Cal.	Fat (g)	% Fat Cal.	Sat. Fat (g)	Chol. (mg)	Sodium (mg)	Carb. (g)	Fiber (g)	Pro. (g)	Exchanges
✔BBQ Chicken Sandwich	1	280	3	10	1	60	830	37	2	25	2 1/2 starch, 3 very lean meat

(Continued)

✔ = Healthiest Bets; n/a = not available

SANDWICHES (Continued)	Amount	Cal.	Fat (g)	% Cal. Fat	Sat. Fat (g)	Chol. (mg)	Sod. (mg)	Carb. (g)	Fiber (g)	Pro. (g)	Servings/Exchanges
Carl's Bacon Swiss Crispy Chicken Sandwich	1	720	36	45	10	75	1610	66	3	32	4 1/2 starch, 3 lean meat, 5 fat
Carl's Catch Fish Sandwich	1	510	27	48	7	80	1030	50	1	18	3 starch, 1 lean meat, 5 fat
Carl's Ranch Crispy Chicken Sandwich	1	620	29	42	6	50	1220	65	3	25	4 starch, 2 lean meat, 4 1/2 fat
Charbroiled Chicken Club Sandwich	1	460	22	43	7	90	1110	33	2	32	2 starch, 4 lean meat, 2 fat
Charbroiled Sante Fe Chicken Sandwich	1	510	31	55	7	95	1240	32	2	28	2 starch, 3 lean meat, 4 fat
Charbroiled Sirloin Steak Sandwich	1	580	26	40	5	85	1110	50	2	33	3 starch, 2 medium-fat meat, 3 fat
SHAKES											
Chocolate (small)	13.5 oz	390	7	16	5	30	280	74	0	9	5 carb., 1 fat

Strawberry (small)	13.5 oz	400	7	16	5	30	240	77	0	9	5 carb., 1 fat
Vanilla (small)	13.5 oz	330	8	22	5	35	250	54	0	11	3 1/2 carb., 1 1/2 fat

SIDES

✔Breadsticks	1 order	35	1	14	0	0	60	7	1	1	1/2 starch
✔Chicken Stars	6 pieces	280	19	61	4.5	40	330	15	0	12	1 starch, 1 lean meat, 3 fat
CrissCut Fries (large)	1 order	410	24	53	5	0	950	43	4	5	3 starch, 5 fat
✔Croutons	7 g	35	1	26	0	0	65	5	0	0	free
French Fries (regular)	1 order	290	14	43	3	0	170	37	3	5	2 1/2 starch, 3 fat
Hash Brown Nuggets	1 order	330	21	57	4.5	0	470	32	3	3	2 starch, 4 fat
Onion Rings	1 order	430	21	45	5	0	700	53	3	7	3 1/2 starch, 4 fat
Zucchini (fried)	1 order	340	19	54	4.5	0	860	37	2	5	2 1/2 starch, 4 fat

✔ = Healthiest Bets; n/a = not available

Notes

Dairy Queen/Brazier

❖Dairy Queen/Brazier provides nutrition
  information for all of its menu items in a brochure.

Light 'n Lean Choice

Chili Dog
Vanilla Cone (*small*)

Calories	510	Sodium (mg)	985
Fat (g)	23	Carbohydrate (g)	59
% calories from fat	20	Fiber (g)	2
Saturated fat (g)	11	Protein (g)	18
Cholesterol (mg)	55		

Exchanges: 1 1/2 starch, 2 1/2 carb., 1 high-fat meat,
2 fat

Healthy 'n Hearty Choice

Grilled Chicken Breast Fillet Sandwich
French Fries (*small*)
DQ Chocolate Soft Serve (*1/2 cup*)

Calories	670	Sodium (mg)	1,230
Fat (g)	25	Carbohydrate (g)	81
% calories from fat	34	Fiber (g)	6
Saturated fat (g)	8	Protein (g)	31
Cholesterol (mg)	65		

Exchanges: 4 starch, 1 1/2 carb., 3 lean meat, 3 fat

Dairy Queen/Brazier

	Amount	Cal.	Fat (g)	% Cal. Fat	Sat. Fat (g)	Chol. (mg)	Sod. (mg)	Carb. (g)	Fiber (g)	Pro. (g)	Servings/Exchanges
BLIZZARD											
Butterfinger (small)	12 oz	520	18	31	11	35	250	80	1	11	5 carb., 3 1/2 fat
Butterfinger (medium)	16 oz	750	26	31	16	50	360	115	1	16	7 1/2 carb., 5 fat
Chocolate Chip Cookie Dough (small)	12 oz	660	24	33	13	55	440	99	1	12	6 1/2 carb., 5 fat
Chocolate Chip Cookie Dough (medium)	16 oz	950	36	34	19	75	660	143	2	17	9 1/2 carb., 7 fat
Chocolate Sandwich Cookie (small)	12 oz	520	18	31	9	40	380	79	1	10	5 carb., 3 1/2 fat

(*Continued*)

✔ = Healthiest Bets; n/a = not available

BLIZZARD (*Continued*)	Amount	Cal.	Fat (g)	% Cal. Fat	Sat. Fat (g)	Chol. (mg)	Sod. (mg)	Carb. (g)	Fiber (g)	Pro. (g)	Servings/Exchanges
Chocolate Sandwich Cookie (medium)	16 oz	640	23	32	11	45	500	97	1	12	6 1/2 carb, 4 1/2 fat
Heath (small)	12 oz	560	21	34	14	45	380	82	1	10	5 carb, 4 fat
Heath (medium)	16 oz	820	33	36	20	60	580	119	1	14	8 carb, 6 1/2 fat
Reeses Peanut Butter Cup (small)	12 oz	590	24	37	13	45	320	81	1	14	5 carb, 5 fat
Reeses Peanut Butter Cup (medium)	16 oz	790	33	38	17	55	430	105	2	19	7 carb, 6 1/2 fat
Strawberry (small)	12 oz	400	11	25	7	35	190	66	1	9	4 1/2 carb, 2 fat
Strawberry (medium)	16 oz	570	16	25	11	50	260	95	1	12	6 carb, 3 fat
BURGERS											
DQ Homestyle Bacon Double Cheeseburger	1	610	36	53	18	130	1380	31	2	41	2 starch, 5 medium-fat meat, 2 fat

✓DQ Homestyle Cheeseburger	1	340	17	45	8	55	850	29	2	20	2 starch, 2 medium-fat meat, 1 fat
DQ Homestyle Deluxe Double Cheeseburger	1	540	31	52	16	115	1130	31	2	36	2 starch, 4 medium-fat meat, 2 fat
DQ Homestyle Deluxe Double Hamburger	1	440	22	45	10	90	680	29	2	30	2 starch, 3 medium-fat meat, 1 fat
DQ Homestyle Double Cheeseburger	1	540	31	52	16	115	1130	30	2	35	2 starch, 4 medium-fat meat, 2 fat
✓DQ Homestyle Hamburger	1	290	12	37	5	45	630	29	2	17	2 starch, 2 medium-fat meat
DQ Ultimate Burger	1	670	43	58	19	135	1210	29	2	40	2 starch, 5 medium-fat meat 3 1/2 fat

(Continued)

✔ = Healthiest Bets; n/a = not available

	Amount	Cal.	Fat (g)	% Cal. Fat	Sat. Fat (g)	Chol. (mg)	Sod. (mg)	Carb. (g)	Fiber (g)	Pro. (g)	Servings/Exchanges
FROZEN YOGURT											
Cup of Yogurt (medium)	1	230	1	4	0	5	150	48	0	8	3 carb.
✓DQ Nonfat Frozen Yogurt	1/2 cup	100	0	0	0	<5	70	21	0	3	1 1/2 carb.
Heath Breeze (medium)	16 oz	710	18	23	11	20	580	123	1	15	8 carb., 3 1/2 fat
Heath Breeze (small)	12 oz	470	10	19	6	10	380	85	1	11	5 1/2 carb., 1 fat
Strawberry Breeze (medium)	16 oz	460	1	2	1	10	270	99	1	13	6 1/2 carb.
Strawberry Breeze (small)	12 oz	320	1	3	0.5	5	190	68	1	10	4 1/2 carb.
Yogurt Cone (medium)	1	260	1	3	0.5	5	160	56	0	9	4 carb.
HOT DOGS											
✓Cheese Dog	1	290	18	56	8	40	950	20	1	12	1 starch, 1 high-fat meat, 1 1/2 fat

	Amount	Cal.	Fat (g)	Sat. Fat (g)	Chol. (mg)	Sod. (mg)	Carb. (g)	Fiber (g)	Exchanges/Choices
✔ Chili Dog	1	280	16	6	35	870	21	2	12	1 1/2 starch, 1 high-fat meat, 1 fat
Chili 'n' Cheese Dog	1	330	21	9	45	1090	22	2	14	1 1/2 starch, 1 high-fat meat, 2 fat
Hot Dog	1	240	14	5	25	730	19	1	9	1 starch, 1 high-fat meat, 1 fat
ICE CREAM										
Chocolate Cone (small)	1	240	8	5	20	115	37	0	6	2 1/2 carb., 1 1/2 fat
Chocolate Cone (medium)	1	340	11	7	30	160	53	0	8	3 1/2 carb., 2 fat
Dipped Cone (small)	1	340	17	9	20	130	42	1	6	3 carb., 3 fat
Dipped Cone (medium)	1	490	24	13	30	190	59	1	8	4 carb., 5 fat
✔ DQ Chocolate Soft Serve	1/2 cup	150	5	3.5	15	75	22	0	4	1 1/2 carb., 1 fat
✔ DQ Vanilla Soft Serve	1/2 cup	140	5	3	15	70	22	0	3	1 1/2 carb., 1 fat

✔ = Healthiest Bets; n/a = not available

(Continued)

ICE CREAM (*Continued*)	Amount	Cal.	Fat (g)	% Cal. Fat	Sat. Fat (g)	Chol. (mg)	Sod. (mg)	Carb. (g)	Fiber (g)	Pro. (g)	Servings/Exchanges
Vanilla Cone (small)	1	230	7	27	4.5	20	115	38	0	6	2 1/2 carb., 1 fat
Vanilla Cone (medium)	1	330	9	24	6	30	160	53	0	8	3 1/2 carb., 2 fat
Vanilla Cone (large)	1	410	12	26	8	40	200	65	0	10	4 carb., 2 fat
ICE CREAM BARS											
Buster Bar	1	450	28	56	12	15	280	41	2	10	3 carb., 5 1/2 fat
Chocolate Dilly Bar	1	210	13	56	7	10	75	21	0	3	1 1/2 carb., 2 1/2 fat
Chocolate Mint Dilly Bar	1	190	12	57	9	15	100	20	0	3	1 carb., 2 fat
DQ Caramel & Nut Bar	1	260	13	45	0	15	90	32	0	5	2 carb., 2 1/2 fat
✔DQ Fudge Bar, no sugar added	1	50	0	0	0	0	70	13	0	4	1 carb.
✔DQ Sandwich	1	150	5	30	2	5	115	24	1	3	1 1/2 carb., 1 fat
✔DQ Vanilla Orange Bar	1	60	0	0	0	0	40	17	0	2	1 carb.
Toffee Dilly Bar with Heath Pieces	1	210	12	51	9	15	100	24	0	3	1 1/2 carb., 2 fat

ICE CREAM CAKES

	Serving										Exchanges
DQ Frozen 10" Round Cake	1/12 cake	360	12	30	8	25	260	55	1	7	3 1/2 carb., 2 fat
DQ Frozen 8" Round Cake	1/8 cake	340	12	32	7	25	250	53	1	7	3 1/2 carb., 2 fat
DQ Frozen Heart Cake	1/10 cake	270	9	30	6	20	190	41	1	5	2 1/2 carb., 2 fat
DQ Frozen Log Cake	1/8 cake	280	9	29	6	15	220	43	1	5	3 carb., 1 fat
DQ Frozen Sheet Cake	1/20 cake	350	12	31	7	20	270	54	1	7	3 1/2 carb., 2 fat

ICE CREAM PIZZAS

	Serving										Exchanges
✔ Heath DQ Treatza Pizza	1/8 pizza	180	7	35	3.5	5	160	28	1	3	2 carb., 1 fat
✔ M&M DQ Treatza Pizza	1/8 pizza	190	7	33	4	5	160	29	1	3	2 carb., 1 fat
✔ Peanut Butter Fudge DQ Treatza Pizza	1/8 pizza	220	10	41	4.5	5	200	28	1	4	2 carb., 2 fat
✔ Strawberry-Banana DQ Treatza Pizza	1/8 pizza	180	6	30	3	5	140	29	1	3	2 carb., 1 fat

(Continued)

✔ = Healthiest Bets; n/a = not available

	Amount	Cal.	Fat (g)	% Cal. Fat	Sat. Fat (g)	Chol. (mg)	Sod. (mg)	Carb. (g)	Fiber (g)	Pro. (g)	Servings/Exchanges
MISCELLANEOUS											
✓DQ Lemon Freez'r	1/2 cup	80	0	0	0	0	10	20	0	0	1 carb.
✓Starkiss	1	80	0	0	0	0	10	21	0	0	1 1/2 carb.
OTHER ENTREES											
Chicken Strip Basket w/ Gravy*	1	1000	50	45	13	55	2260	102	5	35	7 starch, 2 lean meat, 9 fat
SANDWICHES											
✓Chicken Breast Fillet	1	430	20	42	4	55	760	37	2	24	2 1/2 starch, 2 medium-fat meat, 2 fat
Chicken Breast Fillet w/ Cheese	1	480	25	47	7	70	980	38	2	27	2 1/2 starch, 3 lean meat, 4 fat
✓Fish Fillet	1	370	16	39	3.5	45	630	39	2	16	2 1/2 starch, 1 lean meat, 3 1/2 fat

	Amount	Calories	Fat (g)	% Calories from Fat	Saturated Fat (g)	Cholesterol (mg)	Sodium (mg)	Carbohydrate (g)	Fiber (g)	Protein (g)	Choices/Exchanges
Fish Fillet w/ Cheese	1	420	21	45	6	60	850	40	2	19	2 1/2 starch, 2 lean meat, 3 fat
✔ Grilled Chicken Breast Fillet Sandwich	1	310	10	29	2.5	50	1040	30	3	24	2 starch, 3 lean meat
SHAKES AND MALTS											
Chocolate Malt (small)	1	650	16	22	10	55	370	111	0	15	7 carb., 3 fat
Chocolate Malt (medium)	1	880	22	23	14	70	500	153	0	19	10 carb., 4 fat
Chocolate Shake (small)	1	560	15	24	10	50	310	94	0	13	6 carb., 3 fat
Chocolate Shake (medium)	1	770	20	23	13	70	420	130	0	17	8 carb., 4 fat
Misty Slush (small)	1	220	0	0	0	0	20	56	0	0	4 carb.
Misty Slush (medium)	1	290	0	0	0	0	30	74	0	0	5 carb.
SIDES											
✔ French Fries (small)	1 order	210	10	43	2	0	115	29	3	3	2 starch, 2 fat
French Fries (medium)	1 order	350	18	46	3.5	0	630	42	3	4	3 starch, 3 1/2 fat

✔ = Healthiest Bets; n/a = not available

(Continued)

SIDES (Continued)	Amount	Cal.	Fat (g)	% Cal. Fat	Sat. Fat (g)	Chol. (mg)	Sod. (mg)	Carb. (g)	Fiber (g)	Pro. (g)	Servings/Exchanges
French Fries (large)	1 order	440	23	47	4.5	0	790	53	4	5	3 1/2 starch, 4 1/2 fat
Onion Rings	1 order	320	16	45	4	0	180	39	3	5	2 1/2 starch, 3 fat
SUNDAES											
Banana Split	1	510	12	21	8	30	180	96	3	8	6 carb., 2 fat
Chocolate Sundae (small)	1	280	7	23	4.5	20	140	49	0	5	3 carb., 1 fat
Chocolate Sundae (medium)	1	410	10	22	6	30	210	71	0	8	4 1/2 carb., 2 fat
Peanut Buster Parfait	1	730	31	38	17	35	400	99	2	16	6 1/2 carb., 6 fat
Strawberry Shortcake	1	430	14	29	9	60	360	70	1	7	4 1/2 carb., 3 fat
Yogurt Strawberry Sundae (medium)	1	280	1	3	0	5	160	61	1	8	4 carb.

✔ = Healthiest Bets; n/a = not available

The following are registered trademarks of American Dairy Queen Corporation: Dairy Queen, Dairy Queen/Brazier, Dilly, Blizzard, Breeze, Homestyle, Ultimate, Misty, Peanut Buster, Buster Bar, Starkiss, DQ Freez'r, DQ Treatzza Pizza, DQ Treatza Pizza. *Chicken Strip Basket with Gravy includes four breaded chicken strips, medium french fries, Texas toast, and gravy.

Hardee's

❖Hardee's provides nutrition information for all its menu items in a brochure.

Light 'n Lean Choice

Grilled Chicken Sandwich
Mashed Potatoes
Gravy
Chocolate Shake (*split*)

Calories......................625	Sodium (mg)..........1,675
Fat (g) 14	Carbohydrate (g).........89
% calories from fat..20	Fiber (g).................n/a
Saturated fat (g)........4	Protein (g) 34
Cholesterol (mg) 80	

Exchanges: 3 1/2 starch, 2 carb., 3 lean meat, 1/2 fat

Healthy 'n Hearty Choice

Regular Roast Beef Sandwich
French Fries (*split regular order*)
Cool Twist Cone

Calories......................670	Sodium (mg)..........1,135
Fat (g) 20	Carbohydrate (g).........83
% calories from fat..27	Fiber (g).................n/a
Saturated fat (g)........8	Protein (g) 24
Cholesterol (mg) 53	

Exchanges: 3 1/2 starch, 1 veg., 1 carb., 2 medium-fat meat, 2 1/2 fat

(*Continued*)

Hardee's

	Amount	Cal.	Fat (g)	% Cal. Fat	Sat. Fat (g)	Chol. (mg)	Sod. (mg)	Carb. (g)	Fiber (g)	Pro. (g)	Servings/Exchanges
BEVERAGES											
✔ Orange Juice	10 oz	140	0	0	0	0	5	34	n/a	2	2 fruit
BREAKFAST											
✔ Apple Cinnamon 'N' Raisin Biscuit	1	250	8	28	2	0	350	42	n/a	2	3 starch, 1 1/2 fat
Bacon, Egg and Cheese Biscuit	1	530	30	51	11	205	1420	45	n/a	17	3 starch, 1 medium-fat meat, 5 fat
Biscuit 'N' Gravy	1	530	30	51	9	15	1550	56	n/a	10	4 starch, 6 fat
Chicken Biscuit	1	590	27	41	7	45	1820	62	n/a	24	4 starch, 2 lean meat, 4 fat
Country Ham Biscuit	1	440	22	45	7	28	1710	44	n/a	14	3 starch, 1 medium-fat meat, 3 fat

	Amount										Exchanges/Choices
Frisco Breakfast Sandwich (ham)	1	450	22	44	8	226	1290	42	n/a	22	3 starch, 2 medium-fat meat, 2 fat
Ham Biscuit	1	410	20	44	8	25	1200	45	n/a	13	3 starch, 1 medium-fat meat, 3 fat
Jelly Biscuit	1	440	21	43	6	0	1000	57	n/a	6	3 starch, 1 carb., 3 fat
Regular Hash Rounds	16 pieces	230	14	55	3	0	560	24	n/a	3	1 1/2 starch, 3 fat
Rise 'N' Shine Biscuit	1	390	21	48	6	0	1000	44	n/a	6	3 starch, 4 fat
Sausage and Egg Biscuit	1	620	41	60	13	225	1370	45	n/a	19	3 starch, 1 high-fat meat, 6 fat
Sausage Biscuit	1	550	36	59	11	25	1300	44	n/a	12	3 starch, 1 high-fat meat, 5 fat
Steak Biscuit	1	580	32	50	10	30	1580	56	n/a	15	3 1/2 starch, 1 medium-fat meat, 5 fat

✔ = Healthiest Bets; n/a = not available

(Continued)

BREAKFAST (*Continued*)	Amount	Cal.	Fat (g)	% Cal. Fat	Sat. Fat (g)	Chol. (mg)	Sod. (mg)	Carb. (g)	Fiber (g)	Pro. (g)	Servings/Exchanges
Ultimate Omelet Biscuit	1	550	32	52	12	225	1350	45	n/a	20	3 starch, 2 medium-fat meat, 5 fat
BURGERS											
Big Deluxe	1	650	44	61	11	75	870	40	n/a	24	2 1/2 starch, 2 medium-fat meat, 7 fat
✓Cheeseburger	1	310	14	41	6	40	890	30	n/a	16	2 starch, 1 medium-fat meat, 2 fat
Classic Bacon Cheeseburger	1	760	50	59	17	105	1380	43	n/a	31	3 starch, 3 medium-fat meat, 7 fat
Classic Bacon Double Cheeseburger	1	1020	71	63	27	175	1780	45	n/a	48	3 starch, 6 medium-fat meat, 8 fat

	Amount	Calories	Fat (g)	% Fat Cal.	Sat. Fat (g)	Chol. (mg)	Sod. (mg)	Carb. (g)	Fiber (g)	Prot. (g)	Exchanges
Double Cheeseburger	1	470	26	50	11	80	1270	32	n/a	28	2 starch, 3 medium-fat meat, 3 fat
Frisco Burger	1	720	46	58	16	95	1340	43	n/a	33	3 starch, 3 medium-fat meat, 6 fat
✔ Hamburger	1	270	11	37	3	35	670	29	n/a	14	2 starch, 1 medium-fat meat, 1 fat
Monster Burger	1	1060	79	67	29	185	1860	37	n/a	49	2 1/2 starch, 6 medium-fat meat, 10 fat
Mushroom 'N' Swiss Burger	1	490	25	46	12	80	1100	39	n/a	28	2 1/2 starch, 3 medium-fat meat, 2 fat
CHICKEN											
Chicken Breast (fried)	1	370	15	36	4	75	1190	29	n/a	29	2 starch, 3 lean meat, 1 fat
✔ Chicken Leg (fried)	1	170	7	37	2	45	570	15	n/a	13	1 starch, 1 lean meat, 1 fat

(Continued)

✔ = Healthiest Bets; n/a = not available

CHICKEN (*Continued*)	Amount	Cal.	Fat (g)	% Cal. Fat	Sat. Fat (g)	Chol. (mg)	Sod. (mg)	Carb. (g)	Fiber (g)	Pro. (g)	Servings/Exchanges
✔Chicken Thigh (fried)	1	330	15	41	4	60	1000	30	n/a	19	2 starch, 2 lean meat, 2 fat
✔Chicken Wing (fried)	1	200	8	36	2	30	740	23	n/a	10	1 1/2 starch, 1 medium-fat meat, 1/2 fat
DESSERTS											
Cool Twist Cone (vanilla or chocolate)	1	180	2	10	1	10	120	34	n/a	4	2 carb.
✔Peach Cobbler (small)	1	310	7	20	1	0	360	60	n/a	2	4 carb., 1 fat
SANDWICHES											
Big Roast Beef Sandwich	1	460	24	47	9	70	1230	35	n/a	26	2 starch, 3 medium-fat meat, 2 fat
Chicken Fillet Sandwich	1	480	18	34	3	55	1280	54	n/a	26	3 1/2 starch, 2 lean meat, 2 fat

Item	Amount										Exchanges/Choices
Fisherman's Fillet Sandwich	1	560	27	43	7	65	1330	54	n/a	26	3 1/2 starch, 2 lean meat, 4 fat
✔Grilled Chicken Sandwich	1	350	11	28	2	65	950	38	n/a	25	2 1/2 starch, 3 lean meat
Hot Dog	1	450	32	64	12	55	1240	25	n/a	15	1 1/2 starch, 2 medium-fat meat, 4 fat
Hot Ham 'N' Cheese	1	310	12	35	6	50	1410	34	n/a	16	2 starch, 1 medium-fat meat, 1 fat
✔Regular Roast Beef	1	320	16	45	6	43	820	26	n/a	17	2 starch, 2 medium-fat meat, 1 fat

SHAKES

Item	Amount										Exchanges/Choices
Chocolate	12 oz	370	5	12	3	30	270	67	n/a	13	4 1/2 carb., 1 fat
Vanilla	12 oz	350	5	13	3	20	300	65	n/a	12	4 carb., 1 fat

✔ = Healthiest Bets; n/a = not available

(Continued)

SIDES

	Amount	Cal.	Fat (g)	% Cal. Fat	Sat. Fat (g)	Chol. (mg)	Sod. (mg)	Carb. (g)	Fiber (g)	Pro. (g)	Servings/Exchanges
Cole Slaw	4 oz	240	20	75	3	10	340	13	n/a	2	1 veg., 1/2 carb., 4 fat
Crispy Curls (medium)	1 order	340	18	48	4	0	950	41	n/a	5	3 starch, 3 1/2 fat
Crispy Curls (large)	1 order	520	28	48	5	0	1450	62	n/a	7	4 starch, 5 1/2 fat
Crispy Curls (jumbo)	1 order	590	31	47	6	0	1640	70	n/a	8	4 1/2 starch, 6 fat
French Fries (regular)	1 order	340	16	42	2	0	390	45	n/a	4	3 starch, 3 fat
French Fries (large)	1 order	440	21	43	3	0	520	59	n/a	5	4 starch, 4 fat
French Fries (jumbo)	1 order	510	24	42	3	0	590	67	n/a	6	4 1/2 starch, 5 fat
✔Gravy	1.5 oz	20	0	0	0	0	260	3	n/a	0	free
✔Mashed Potatoes	4 oz	70	0	0	0	0	330	14	n/a	2	1 starch

✔ = Healthiest Bets; n/a = not available

Jack in the Box

❖Jack in the Box provides nutrition information for all its menu items in a brochure.

Light 'n Lean Choice

Garden Chicken Salad
French Fries (*regular*)

Calories......................550	Sodium (mg)..........1,130
Fat (g) 25	Carbohydrate (g).........54
% calories from fat..41	Fiber (g) 6
Saturated fat (g)........8	Protein (g) 27
Cholesterol (mg) 65	

Exchanges: 3 starch, 1 veg., 3 lean meat, 3 fat

Healthy 'n Hearty Choice

Chicken Teriyaki Bowl
Milk (2%)

Calories......................800	Sodium (mg)..........1,815
Fat (g) 9	Carbohydrate (g).......142
% calories from fat..18	Fiber (g) 3
Saturated fat (g)........4	Protein (g) 35
Cholesterol (mg) 40	

Exchanges: 7 starch, 2 veg., 1 low-fat milk, 1 lean meat

(*Continued*)

Jack in the Box

	Amount	Cal.	Fat (g)	% Cal. Fat	Sat. Fat (g)	Chol. (mg)	Sod. (mg)	Carb. (g)	Fiber (g)	Pro. (g)	Servings/Exchanges
BEVERAGES											
✓Milk (2%)	8 oz	130	5	35	3	25	85	14	0	9	1 low-fat milk
✓Orange Juice	10 oz	150	0	0	0	0	20	34	1	2	2 fruit
BREAKFAST											
✓Breakfast Jack	1	280	12	39	5	195	920	30	1	17	2 starch, 2 medium-fat meat
Hash Brown	1	170	12	64	3	0	250	14	1	1	1 starch, 2 fat
✓Pancakes with Bacon	1 order	370	9	22	2	30	1020	59	3	12	4 starch, 2 fat
Sausage Croissant	1	690	51	67	20	240	1000	37	1	21	2 1/2 starch, 2 medium-fat meat, 8 fat
Sourdough Breakfast Sandwich	1	440	24	49	8	355	1120	36	1	20	2 1/2 starch, 2 medium-fat meat, 3 fat

Supreme Croissant	1	520	32	55	13	235	1240	39	1	21	2 1/2 starch, 2 medium-fat meat, 4 fat
Ultimate Breakfast Sandwich	1	620	36	52	15	455	1800	40	2	34	2 1/2 starch, 4 medium-fat meat, 3 fat

BURGERS

Bacon Ultimate Cheeseburger	1	1150	89	70	30	230	1770	41	4	53	3 starch, 6 medium-fat meat, 12 fat
Double Cheeseburger	1	460	27	53	12	80	920	31	2	23	2 starch, 2 medium-fat meat, 3 fat
✔Hamburger	1	280	12	39	4	45	560	30	2	12	2 starch, 1 medium-fat meat, 1 fat
✔Hamburger with Cheese	1	320	16	45	6	60	760	30	2	14	2 starch, 1 medium-fat meat, 2 fat

✔ = Healthiest Bets; n/a = not available

(Continued)

BURGERS (Continued)	Amount	Cal.	Fat (g)	% Cal. Fat	Sat. Fat (g)	Chol. (mg)	Sod. (mg)	Carb. (g)	Fiber (g)	Pro. (g)	Servings/Exchanges
Jumbo Jack	1	590	36	55	11	80	720	42	4	25	3 starch, 2 medium-fat meat, 5 fat
Jumbo Jack with Cheese	1	680	44	58	15	105	1180	43	4	29	3 starch, 3 medium-fat meat, 6 fat
Sourdough Jack	1	690	46	60	15	110	1180	38	3	31	2 1/2 starch, 3 medium-fat meat, 6 fat
Ultimate Cheeseburger	1	1030	79	69	26	205	1370	40	4	47	2 1/2 starch, 5 medium-fat meat, 11 fat

CONDIMENTS

	Amount	Cal.	Fat (g)	% Cal. Fat	Sat. Fat (g)	Chol. (mg)	Sod. (mg)	Carb. (g)	Fiber (g)	Pro. (g)	Servings/Exchanges
✔ Barbeque Dipping Sauce	1 oz/2 Tbsp	45	0	0	0	0	310	11	0	1	1 carb.
Buttermilk House Dipping Sauce	1 oz/2 Tbsp	130	13	90	5	10	240	3	0	0	2 1/2 fat

✔ Country Crock Spread	1 tsp	25	3	108	0.5	0	45	0	0	0	1/2 fat
✔ Grape Jelly	1/2 oz/1 Tbsp	40	0	0	0	0	5	10	0	0	1/2 carb.
✔ Pancake Syrup	1.5 oz/3 Tbsp	130	0	0	0	0	5	30	0	0	2 starch
✔ Salsa	1 oz/2 Tbsp	10	0	0	0	0	200	2	0	0	free
✔ Sour Cream	1 oz/2 Tbsp	60	6	90	4	20	30	1	0	1	1 fat
✔ Sweet & Sour Dipping Sauce	1 oz/2 Tbsp	45	0	0	0	0	160	11	0	0	1 carb.
Tartar Sauce	1.5 oz/3 Tbsp	210	22	94	3	30	340	2	0	1	4 fat
DESSERTS											
Carrot Cake	1	370	16	39	3	40	340	54	2	3	3 carb., 3 fat
Cheesecake	1	320	18	51	10	65	220	32	0	7	2 carb., 3 1/2 fat
✔ Double Fudge Cake	1	300	10	30	2	50	320	50	1	3	3 carb., 2 fat
Hot Apple Turnover	1	340	18	48	4	0	510	41	2	4	3 carb., 3 1/2 fat

✔ = Healthiest Bets; n/a = not available

(*Continued*)

FINGER FOODS

	Amount	Cal.	Fat (g)	% Cal. Fat	Sat. Fat (g)	Chol. (mg)	Sod. (mg)	Carb. (g)	Fiber (g)	Pro. (g)	Servings/Exchanges
Bacon & Cheddar Potato Wedges	1 order	800	58	65	16	55	1470	49	4	20	3 starch, 2 medium-fat meat, 10 fat
Chicken & Fries	1 order	730	34	42	7	65	1690	79	5	26	5 starch, 2 lean meat, 5 1/2 fat
✔Chicken Breast Pieces (breaded and fried)	5 pieces	360	17	43	3	80	970	24	1	27	1 1/2 starch, 3 lean meat, 2 fat
Egg Rolls-3 piece	1 order	440	24	49	6	35	1020	40	4	15	1 veg., 2 starch, 1 medium-fat meat, 4 fat
Egg Rolls-5 piece	1 order	730	41	51	10	60	1700	67	7	25	1 veg., 4 starch, 2 medium-fat meat, 6 fat

Fish & Chips	1 order	780	39	45	9	45	1740	86	6	19	4 starch, 1 veg., 1 lean meat, 7 fat
Stuffed Jalapeños-10 piece	1 order	750	44	53	17	80	2470	65	5	20	3 1/2 starch, 1 veg., 1 high-fat meat, 7 fat
Stuffed Jalapeños-7 piece	1 order	530	31	53	12	60	1730	46	3	14	3 starch, 1 high-fat meat, 4 fat

OTHER ENTREES

Chicken Teriyaki Bowl	1	670	4	5	1	15	1730	128	3	26	7 starch, 2 veg., 1 lean meat
✔Monster Taco	1	270	17	57	6	30	670	19	4	12	1 starch, 1 medium-fat meat, 2 fat
✔Taco	1	170	10	53	4	20	460	12	2	7	1 starch, 1 medium-fat meat, 1 fat

(Continued)

✔ = Healthiest Bets; n/a = not available

	Amount	Cal.	Fat (g)	% Cal. Fat	Sat. Fat (g)	Chol. (mg)	Sod. (mg)	Carb. (g)	Fiber (g)	Pro. (g)	Servings/Exchanges
SALAD DRESSINGS											
Blue Cheese	2 oz/4 Tbsp	210	15	64	2.5	25	750	11	0	1	1 carb., 3 fat
Buttermilk House	1 oz/2 Tbsp	290	30	93	11	20	560	6	0	1	1/2 carb., 6 fat
✔Low Calorie Italian	1 oz/2 Tbsp	25	2	72	0	0	670	2	0	0	free
Thousand Island	2 oz/4 Tbsp	250	24	86	4	35	570	10	0	1	1/2 carb., 5 fat
SALADS											
✔Croutons	1 pkg.	50	2	36	0.5	0	105	8	0	1	1/2 starch
✔Garden Chicken	1	200	9	41	4	65	420	8	3	23	1 veg., 3 lean meat
✔Side	1	50	3	54	1.5	10	75	3	1	2	1 veg. 1/2 fat
SANDWICHES											
Chicken	1	450	26	52	5	45	1030	39	2	16	2 1/2 starch, 1 lean meat, 4 1/2 fat

Chicken Caesar	1	490	26	48	6	55	1050	41	3	24	3 starch, 2 lean meat, 4 fat
✔ Chicken Fajita Pita	1	280	9	29	4	75	840	25	3	24	1 1/2 starch, 3 lean meat
Chicken Supreme	1	680	45	60	11	85	1500	46	4	23	3 starch, 2 lean meat, 8 fat
Grilled Chicken Fillet	1	520	26	45	6	140	1240	42	4	27	2 1/2 starch, 3 lean meat, 4 fat
Philly Cheesesteak	1	520	25	43	9	155	1980	41	4	33	3 starch, 3 medium-fat meat, 2 fat
Spicy Crispy Chicken	1	560	27	43	5	50	1140	55	-2	25	3 1/2 starch, 2 lean meat, 4 fat

SHAKES

Cappuccino Classic	16 oz	630	29	41	17	90	320	80	0	11	5 carb., 6 fat
Chocolate Ice Cream Shake	16 oz	630	27	39	16	85	330	85	0	11	5 1/2 carb., 5 fat
Oreo Cookie Ice Cream Shake	1E oz	740	36	44	19	95	490	91	2	13	6 carb., 7 fat

(*Continued*)

✔ = Healthiest Bets; n/a = not available

SHAKES (*Continued*)	Amount	Cal.	Fat (g)	% Cal. Fat	Sat. Fat (g)	Chol. (mg)	Sod. (mg)	Carb. (g)	Fiber (g)	Pro. (g)	Servings/Exchanges
Strawberry Ice Cream Shake	16 oz	640	28	39	15	85	300	85	0	10	5 1/2 carb., 5 1/2 fat
Vanilla Ice Cream Shake	16 oz	610	31	46	18	95	320	73	0	12	5 carb., 6 fat
SIDES											
Chili Cheese Curly Fries	1 order	650	41	57	12	25	1760	60	4	14	4 starch, 8 fat
French Fries (regular)	1 order	350	16	41	4	0	710	46	3	4	3 starch, 3 fat
French Fries (jumbo)	1 order	430	20	42	5	0	890	58	4	4	4 starch, 4 fat
Onion Rings	1 order	460	25	49	5	0	780	50	3	7	3 starch, 5 fat
Seasoned Curly Fries	1 order	410	23	50	5	0	1010	45	4	6	3 starch, 4 1/2 fat
Super Scoop French Fries	1 order	610	28	41	6	0	1250	82	5	6	5 starch, 5 1/2 fat

✓ = Healthiest Bets; n/a = not available

McDonald's

❖McDonald's provides nutrition information for all its menu items in a brochure. McDonald's nutrition facts are used with permission from McDonald's Corporation.

Light 'n Lean Choice

Hamburger
Garden Salad
Fat Free Herb Vinaigrette (*2 Tbsp*)
Vanilla Reduced Fat Ice Cream Cone

Calories	495	Sodium (mg)	1,005
Fat (g)	4	Carbohydrate (g)	75
% calories from fat	25	Fiber (g)	5
Saturated fat (g)	6.5	Protein (g)	19
Cholesterol (mg)	50		

Exchanges: 2 starch, 1 veg., 2 carb., 2 medium-fat meat, 2 fat

Healthy 'n Hearty Choice

Grilled Chicken Deluxe (*without mayonnaise*)
French Fries (*small*)
Garden Salad with Ranch Salad Dressing (*2 Tbsp*)

Calories	660	Sodium (mg)	1,360
Fat (g)	26	Carbohydrate (g)	76
% calories from fat	35	Fiber (g)	9
Saturated fat (g)	4	Protein (g)	33
Cholesterol (mg)	60		

Exchanges: 4 starch, 1 veg., 3 lean meat, 4 fat

(*Continued*)

McDonald's

	Amount	Cal.	Fat (g)	% Cal. Fat	Sat. Fat (g)	Chol. (mg)	Sod. (mg)	Carb. (g)	Fiber (g)	Pro. (g)	Servings/Exchanges
BEVERAGES											
✓Milk, lowfat 1%	8 oz	100	3	20	1.5	10	115	13	0	8	1 low-fat milk
✓Orange Juice	6 oz	80	0	0	0	0	20	20	0	1	1 fruit
BREAKFAST											
Bacon, Egg & Cheese Biscuit	1	470	28	54	8	235	1250	36	1	18	2 1/2 starch, 2 medium-fat meat, 3 1/2 fat
Biscuit	1	290	15	47	3	0	780	34	1	5	2 starch, 3 fat
✓Breakfast Burrito	1	320	20	53	7	195	600	23	2	13	1 1/2 starch, 1 medium-fat meat, 3 fat
✓Egg McMuffin	1	290	12	37	4.5	235	790	27	1	17	2 starch, 2 medium-fat meat

Item	Amount	Calories	Fat (g)	% Fat Cal.	Sat. Fat (g)	Chol. (mg)	Sodium (mg)	Carb. (g)	Fiber (g)	Protein (g)	Servings/Exchanges
✔English Muffin	1	140	2	13	0	0	210	25	1	4	1 1/2 starch
✔Hash Browns	1 order	130	8	55	1.5	0	330	14	1	1	1 starch, 1 1/2 fat
✔Hotcakes (2 pats margarine and syrup)	1 order	570	16	25	3	15	750	100	2	9	4 1/2 starch, 2 carb., 3 fat
✔Hotcakes (plain)	1 order	310	7	20	1.5	15	610	53	2	9	3 1/2 starch, 1 fat
Sausage	1 order	170	16	85	5	35	290	0	0	6	1 high-fat meat, 1 fat
Sausage Biscuit	1	470	31	59	9	35	1080	35	1	11	2 starch, 1 high-fat meat, 4 fat
Sausage Biscuit with Egg	1	550	37	61	10	245	1160	35	1	18	2 starch, 2 high-fat meat, 3 fat
Sausage McMuffin	1	360	23	58	8	45	740	26	1	13	2 starch, 1 medium-fat meat, 3 1/2 fat

(Continued)

✔ = Healthiest Bets; n/a = not available

BREAKFAST (*Continued*)	Amount	Cal.	Fat (g)	% Cal. Fat	Sat. Fat (g)	Chol. (mg)	Sod. (mg)	Carb. (g)	Fiber (g)	Pro. (g)	Servings/Exchanges
Sausage McMuffin with Egg	1	440	28	57	10	255	890	27	1	19	2 starch, 2 medium-fat meat, 3 1/2 fat
✓Scrambled Eggs (2)	1 order	160	11	62	3.5	425	170	1	0	13	2 medium-fat meat
BURGERS											
Arch Deluxe	1	550	31	51	11	90	1010	39	4	28	2 1/2 starch, 3 medium-fat meat, 3 fat
Arch Deluxe with Bacon	1	590	34	52	12	100	1150	39	4	32	2 1/2 starch, 3 medium-fat meat, 4 fat
Big Mac	1	560	31	50	10	85	1070	45	3	26	3 starch, 2 medium-fat meat, 4 fat
✓Cheeseburger	1	320	13	37	6	40	820	35	2	15	2 starch, 1 medium-fat meat, 1 1/2 fat

✔Hamburger	1	260	9	31	3.5	30	580	34	2	13	2 starch, 1 medium-fat meat, 1 fat
✔Quarter Pounder	1	420	21	45	8	70	820	37	2	23	2 1/2 starch, 2 medium-fat meat, 2 fat
Quarter Pounder with Cheese	1	530	30	51	13	95	1290	38	2	28	2 1/2 starch, 3 medium-fat meat, 3 fat

CONDIMENTS

✔Barbeque Sauce	1 oz/2 Tbsp	45	0	10	0	0	250	10	0	0	1/2 carb.
✔Honey Mustard	1/2 oz/1 Tbsp	50	5	5	0.5	10	85	3	0	0	1 fat
✔Hot Mustard	1 oz/2 Tbsp	60	4	7	0	5	240	7	0	1	1/2 carb, 1 fat
✔Light Mayonnaise	1/2 oz/1 Tbsp	40	4	1	0.5	5	85	1	0	0	1 fat
✔Sweet'N Sour Sauce	1 oz/2 Tbsp	50	0	11	0	0	140	11	0	1	1 carb.

✔ = Healthiest Bets; n/a = not available

(Continued)

	Amount	Cal.	Fat (g)	% Cal. Fat	Sat. Fat (g)	Chol. (mg)	Sod. (mg)	Carb. (g)	Fiber (g)	Pro. (g)	Servings/Exchanges
DANISHES/MUFFINS											
Apple Danish	1	360	16	40	5	40	290	51	1	5	3 1/2 carb., 3 fat
Cheese Danish	1	410	22	48	8	70	340	47	0	7	3 carb., 4 fat
Cinnamon Roll	1	390	18	42	5	65	310	50	2	6	3 carb., 3 1/2 fat
✔Lowfat Apple Bran Muffin	1	300	3	9	0.5	0	380	61	3	6	4 starch, 1/2 fat
DESSERTS											
Baked Apple Pie	1	260	13	45	3.5	0	200	34	0	3	2 carb., 3 1/2 fat
✔Chocolate Chip Cookie	1	170	10	53	6	20	120	22	1	2	1 1/2 carb., 2 fat
Hot Caramel Sundae	1	360	10	25	6	35	180	61	0	7	4 carb., 2 fat
Hot Fudge Sundae	1	340	12	32	9	30	170	52	1	8	3 carb., 2 fat
✔McDonaldland Cookies	1 pkg.	180	5	25	1	0	190	32	0	3	2 carb., 1 fat
✔Nuts (on sundaes)	7 g	40	4	90	0	0	55	2	0	2	1 fat

Strawberry Sundae	1	290	7	22	5	30	95	50	0	7	3 carb, 1 fat
✔ Vanilla Reduced Fat Ice Cream Cone	1	150	5	27	3	20	75	23	0	4	1 1/2 carb., 1 fat

OTHER ENTREES

✔ Chicken McNuggets (4 piece)	1 order	190	11	52	2.5	40	340	10	0	12	1/2 starch, 2 lean meat, 1 fat
✔ Chicken McNuggets (6 piece)	1 order	290	17	53	3.5	60	510	15	0	18	1 starch, 1 lean meat, 3 fat
Chicken McNuggets (9 piece)	1 order	430	26	54	5	90	770	23	0	27	1 1/2 starch, 3 lean meat, 3 fat

SALAD DRESSINGS

✔ Caesar (1 pkg.)	2 oz/4 Tbsp	160	14	79	3	20	450	7	0	2	1/2 carb, 3 fat
✔ Fat Free Herb Vinaigrette (1 pkg.)	2 oz/4 Tbsp	50	0	0	0	0	330	11	0	0	1 carb.
Ranch (1 pkg.)	2 oz/4 Tbsp	230	21	82	3	20	550	10	0	1	1/2 carb, 4 fat

✔ = Healthiest Bets; n/a = not available

(Continued)

SALAD DRESSINGS (*Continued*)	Amount	Cal.	Fat (g)	% Cal. Fat	Sat. Fat (g)	Chol. (mg)	Sod. (mg)	Carb. (g)	Fiber (g)	Pro. (g)	Servings/Exchanges
✓Red French Reduced Calorie (1 pkg.)	2 oz/4 Tbsp	160	8	45	1	0	490	23	0	0	1 1/2 carb., 1 1/2 fat
SALADS											
✓Croutons	1 pkg.	50	2	36	0	0	80	7	1	2	1/2 starch
✓Garden Salad	1	35	0	0	0	0	20	7	3	2	1 veg.
✓Grilled Chicken Salad Deluxe	1	120	2	15	0	45	240	7	3	21	1 veg, 3 very lean meat
SANDWICHES											
Crispy Chicken Deluxe (fried)	1	500	25	45	4	55	1100	43	4	26	3 starch, 2 lean meat, 4 fat
Filet-o-Fish	1	450	25	50	4.5	50	870	42	2	16	3 starch, 1 lean meat, 4 fat
Fish Filet Deluxe	1	560	28	45	6	60	1060	54	4	23	3 1/2 starch, 2 lean meat, 4 fat
Grilled Chicken Deluxe	1	440	20	41	3	60	1040	38	4	27	2 1/2 carb, 3 lean meat, 2 fat

	Serving										Exchanges
✓Grilled Chicken Deluxe (w/o mayonnaise)	1	300	5	15	1	50	930	38	4	27	2 1/2 starch, 3 very lean meat

SHAKES

	Serving										Exchanges
Chocolate Shake (small)	1	360	9	23	6	40	250	60	1	11	4 carb., 2 fat
Strawberry Shake (small)	1	360	9	23	6	40	180	60	0	11	4 carb., 2 fat
Vanilla Shake (small)	1	360	9	23	6	40	250	59	0	11	4 carb., 2 fat

SIDES

	Serving										Exchanges
✓French Fries (small)	1 order	210	10	43	1.5	0	135	26	2	3	2 starch, 2 fat
French Fries (large)	1 order	450	22	44	4	0	290	57	5	6	4 starch, 4 fat
French Fries (super size)	1 order	540	26	43	4.5	0	350	68	6	8	4 1/2 starch, 5 fat

✓ = Healthiest Bets; n/a = not available

Notes

Rally's Hamburgers

❖Rally's Hamburgers provided nutrition
information for all its menu items.

Light 'n Lean Choice

Spicy Chicken Sandwich (*fried*)
French Fries (*1/2 of regular order*)

Calories......................543
Fat (g) 24
  % calories from fat..40
  Saturated fat (g) ....n/a
Cholesterol (mg) 44

Sodium (mg) 1,034
Carbohydrate (g).........63
  Fiber (g) ....n/a
Protein 20

Exchanges: 5 starch, 1 lean meat, 4 fat

Healthy 'n Hearty Choice

Rallyburger
Onion Rings

Calories......................643
Fat (g) 24
  % calories from fat..34
  Saturated fat (g) ....n/a
Cholesterol (mg) 63

Sodium (mg) 2,031
Carbohydrate (g).........80
  Fiber (g) ....n/a
Protein (g) 26

Exchanges: 5 starch, 2 medium-fat meat, 2 fat

Rally's Hamburgers

	Amount	Cal.	Fat (g)	% Cal. Fat	Sat. Fat (g)	Chol. (mg)	Sod. (mg)	Carb. (g)	Fiber (g)	Pro. (g)	Servings/Exchanges
BURGERS											
Big Bufford	1	743	46	56	n/a	151	1860	35	n/a	41	2 starch, 5 medium-fat meat, 4 fat
Classic Burger	1	500	29	52	n/a	81	1351	35	n/a	23	2 starch, 2 medium-fat meat, 4 fat
Rallyburger	1	433	22	46	n/a	63	1176	35	n/a	20	2 starch, 2 medium-fat meat, 2 fat
Rallyburger with Cheese	1	488	27	50	n/a	78	1376	35	n/a	23	2 starch, 2 medium-fat meat, 3 fat

(Continued)

✔ = Healthiest Bets; n/a = not available

BURGERS *(Continued)*	Amount	Cal.	Fat (g)	% Cal. Fat	Sat. Fat (g)	Chol. (mg)	Sod. (mg)	Carb. (g)	Fiber (g)	Pro. (g)	Servings/Exchanges
Super Barbecue Bacon	1	583	31	48	n/a	88	1709	49	n/a	28	3 starch, 3 medium-fat meat, 3 fat
Super Double Cheeseburger	1	762	48	57	n/a	154	1734	37	n/a	41	2 1/2 starch, 5 medium-fat meat, 4 1/2 fat
OTHER ENTREES											
Chili with Cheese and Onion	7 oz	360	22	55	n/a	74	1144	20	n/a	23	1 starch, 3 medium-fat meat, 1 fat
Chili with Cheese and Onion	13 oz	669	41	55	n/a	137	2125	37	n/a	43	2 1/2 starch, 5 medium-fat meat, 3 fat
SANDWICHES											
✔Chicken Fillet Sandwich (fried)	1	389	15	35	n/a	42	790	43	n/a	21	3 starch, 2 lean meat, 2 fat
✔Spicy Chicken Sandwich (fried)	1	437	18	37	n/a	40	887	50	n/a	18	3 starch, 1 lean meat, 3 fat

SIDES

French Fries (regular)	1 order	211	11	47	n/a	7	293	26	n/a	3	2 starch, 2 fat
French Fries (large)	1 order	317	16	45	n/a	10	439	39	n/a	5	2 1/2 starch, 3 fat
French Fries (X-large)	1 order	423	21	45	n/a	13	585	52	n/a	7	3 1/2 starch, 4 fat
✔ Onion Rings	1 order	210	2	9	n/a	0	855	45	n/a	6	3 starch

✔ = Healthiest Bets; n/a = not available

Notes

Wendy's

❖Wendy's provides nutrition information for all its menu items in a brochure.

Light 'n Lean Choice

Plain Baked Potato
Chili (*small*)
Side Salad
Hidden Valley Ranch Salad Dressing
(*reduced fat and calories; 1 Tbsp*)

Calories......................610	Sodium (mg)..........1,125
Fat (g) 13	Carbohydrate (g).........98
% calories from fat..19	Fiber (g) 14
Saturated fat (g).....3.5	Protein (g) 26
Cholesterol (mg) 35	

Exchanges: 6 1/2 starch, 1 veg., 1 medium-fat meat, 1 1/2 fat

Healthy 'n Hearty Choice

Garden Ranch Chicken Fresh Stuffed Pita
French Fries (*small*)

Calories......................750	Sodium (mg) 1,265
Fat (g) 31	Carbohydrate (g).........86
% calories from fat..37	Fiber (g) 8
Saturated fat (g)........6	Protein (g) 34
Cholesterol (mg) 70	

Exchanges: 5 1/2 starch, 3 lean meat, 3 fat

Wendy's

	Amount	Cal.	Fat (g)	% Cal. Fat	Sat. Fat (g)	Chol. (mg)	Sod. (mg)	Carb. (g)	Fiber (g)	Pro. (g)	Servings/Exchanges
BAKED POTATOES											
Bacon & Cheese	1	530	18	31	4	20	1390	78	7	17	5 starch, 3 1/2 fat
✔Broccoli & Cheese	1	470	14	31	2.5	5	470	80	9	9	5 starch, 3 fat
Cheese	1	570	23	36	8	30	640	78	7	14	5 starch, 1 medium-fat meat, 4 fat
Chili & Cheese	1	630	24	34	9	40	770	83	9	20	5 1/2 starch, 1 medium-fat meat, 4 fat
✔Sour Cream & Chives	1	380	6	14	4	15	40	74	8	8	5 starch, 1 fat
✔Plain	1	310	0	0	0	0	25	71	7	7	5 starch

(Continued)

✔ = Healthiest Bets; n/a = not available

	Amount	Cal.	Fat (g)	% Cal. Fat	Sat. Fat (g)	Chol. (mg)	Sod. (mg)	Carb. (g)	Fiber (g)	Pro. (g)	Servings/Exchanges
BEVERAGES											
✔ Hot Chocolate	6 oz	80	3	34	0	0	135	15	0	1	1 carb.
Lemonade	11 oz	130	0	0	0	0	0	37	0	0	2 1/2 carb.
✔ Milk, Reduced Fat	8 oz	110	4	33	2.5	15	115	11	0	8	1 low-fat milk
BURGERS											
Big Bacon Classic	1	580	30	47	12	100	1460	46	3	34	3 starch, 3 medium-fat meat, 3 fat
✔ Jr. Bacon Cheeseburger	1	380	19	45	7	60	850	34	2	20	2 starch, 2 medium-fat meat, 2 fat
✔ Jr. Cheeseburger	1	320	13	37	6	45	830	34	2	17	2 starch, 2 medium-fat meat, 1/2 fat
✔ Jr. Cheeseburger Deluxe	1	360	17	43	6	50	890	36	3	18	2 1/2 starch, 2 medium-fat meat, 1 fat

✔Jr. Hamburger	1	270	10	33	3.5	30	610	34	2	15	2 starch, 1 medium-fat meat, 1 fat
✔Plain Single Hamburger	1	360	16	40	6	65	580	31	2	24	2 starch, 2 medium-fat meat, 1 fat
✔Single Hamburger with Everything	1	420	20	43	7	70	920	37	3	25	2 1/2 starch, 3 medium-fat meat, 1 fat

CHICKEN NUGGET SAUCE

✔Barbecue	1 pkt/2 Tbsp	45	0	0	0	0	160	10	0	1	1 carb.
Honey Mustard	1 pkt/2 Tbsp	130	12	83	2	10	220	6	0	0	1/2 carb., 2 fat
✔Sweet & Sour	1 pkt/2 Tbsp	50	0	0	0	0	120	12	0	0	1 carb.

CONDIMENTS

✔Cheddar Cheese (shredded)	1 oz/2 Tbsp	70	6	77	3.5	15	110	1	0	4	1/2 high-fat meat
Salad Oil	1/2 oz/1 Tbsp	120	14	105	2	0	0	0	0	0	3 fat

✔ = Healthiest Bets; n/a = not available

(Continued)

CONDIMENTS (*Continued*)	Amount	Cal.	Fat (g)	% Cal. Fat	Sat. Fat (g)	Chol. (mg)	Sod. (mg)	Carb. (g)	Fiber (g)	Pro. (g)	Servings/Exchanges
✓Sour Cream	1 pkt./2 Tbsp	60	6	90	3.5	10	15	1	0	1	1 fat
Whipped Margarine	1 pkt/1 Tbsp	60	7	100	1.5	0	115	0	0	0	1 fat
✓Wine Vinegar	1/2 oz/1 Tbsp	0	0	0	0	0	0	0	0	0	free
DESSERTS											
Chocolate Chip Cookie	1	270	13	43	6	30	120	36	1	3	2 1/2 carb., 2 1/2 fat
Frosty (small)	12 oz	330	8	22	5	35	200	56	0	8	4 carb., 1 1/2 fat
Frosty (medium)	16 oz	440	11	23	7	50	260	73	0	11	5 carb., 2 fat
Frosty (large)	20 oz	540	14	23	9	60	320	91	0	14	6 carb., 3 fat
KIDS' MEALS											
✓Cheeseburger	1	320	13	37	6	45	830	33	2	17	2 starch, 2 medium-fat meat, 1/2 fat
✓Chicken Nuggets	4 pieces	190	13	62	2.5	25	380	9	0	9	1/2 starch, 1 lean meat, 2 fat

✔Hamburger		1	270	10	33	3.5	30	610	33	2	15	2 starch, 2 medium-fat meat

OTHER ENTREES

✔Chicken Nuggets	5 pieces	230	16	63	3	30	470	11	0	11	1 starch, 1 very lean meat, 3 fat
✔Chili (small)	8 oz	210	7	30	2.5	30	800	21	5	15	1 1/2 starch, 1 medium-fat meat
Chili (large)	12 oz	310	10	29	3.5	45	1190	32	7	23	2 starch, 2 medium-fat meat

PITA DRESSINGS

Caesar Vinaigrette	1/2 oz/1 Tbsp	70	7	90	1	0	170	1	0	0	1 fat
✔Garden Ranch Sauce	1/2 oz/1 Tbsp	50	5	80	1	10	125	1	0	0	1 fat

(Continued)

✔ = Healthiest Bets; n/a = not available

SALAD BAR ITEMS

	Amount	Cal.	Fat (g)	% Cal. Fat	Sat. Fat (g)	Chol. (mg)	Sod. (mg)	Carb. (g)	Fiber (g)	Pro. (g)	Servings/Exchanges
✓Applesauce	2 Tbsp	30	0	0	0	0	0	7	0	0	1/2 fruit
✓Bacon Bits	2 Tbsp	45	2	40	1	10	550	0	0	6	1 lean meat
✓Bananas & Strawberry Glaze	1/4 cup	30	0	0	0	0	0	8	1	0	1/2 carb.
✓Broccoli	1/4 cup	0	0	0	0	0	0	1	0	0	free
✓Cantaloupe, sliced	1 piece	15	0	0	0	0	0	4	0	0	free
✓Carrots	1/4 cup	5	0	0	0	0	5	2	0	0	free
✓Cauliflower	1/4 cup	0	0	0	0	0	0	1	0	0	free
✓Cheese, shredded (imitation)	1 oz/2 Tbsp	50	4	72	0.5	0	260	1	0	3	1 fat
✓Chicken Salad	2 Tbsp	70	5	64	1	0	135	2	0	4	1 lean meat
✓Chocolate Pudding	1/4 cup	70	3	39	0.5	0	60	10	0	0	1/2 carb., 1/2 fat
✓Cottage Cheese	2 Tbsp	30	2	60	1	5	125	1	0	4	1 lean meat

✓ Croutons	2 Tbsp	25	1	36	0	0	65	4	0	1	free
✓ Cucumbers	2 slices	0	0	0	0	0	0	0	0	0	free
✓ Eggs, hard cooked	2 Tbsp	40	3	104	1	110	30	0	0	3	1/2 medium-fat meat
✓ Green Peas	2 Tbsp	15	0	0	0	0	25	3	1	1	free
✓ Green Peppers	2 pieces	0	0	0	0	0	0	0	0	0	free
✓ Lettuce (Iceberg/Romaine)	1 cup	10	0	0	0	0	5	2	1	0	free
✓ Mushrooms	1/4 cup	0	0	0	0	0	0	1	0	0	free
✓ Orange, sliced	2 slices	15	0	0	0	0	0	4	1	0	free
✓ Parmesan Blend, grated	2 Tbsp	70	4	51	2	10	290	5	0	4	1 medium-fat meat
✓ Pasta Salad	2 Tbsp	35	2	51	0	0	180	4	1	1	free
✓ Peaches, sliced	1 piece	15	0	0	0	0	0	4	0	0	free
✓ Pepperoni, sliced	6 slices	30	3	90	1	5	70	0	0	1	1/2 fat
Potato Salad	2 Tbsp	80	7	79	2.5	5	180	5	0	0	1 fat

✓ = Healthiest Bets; n/a = not available

(Continued)

SALAD BAR ITEMS (Continued)	Amount	Cal.	Fat (g)	% Cal. Fat	Sat. Fat (g)	Chol. (mg)	Sod. (mg)	Carb. (g)	Fiber (g)	Pro. (g)	Servings/Exchanges
✓Red Onions	3 rings	0	0	0	0	0	0	1	0	0	free
✓Sunflower Seeds & Raisins	2 Tbsp	80	5	56	0.5	0	0	5	1	0	1 fat
Tomato, wedged	1 piece	5	0	0	0	0	0	1	0	0	free
✓Turkey Ham, diced	2 Tbsp	50	4	72	1	25	280	0	0	3	1/2 lean meat, 1/2 fat
✓Watermelon, wedged	1 piece	20	0	0	0	0	0	4	0	0	free
SALAD DRESSINGS											
Blue Cheese	1 oz/2 Tbsp	180	19	95	3.5	15	180	0	0	1	4 fat
French	1 oz/2 Tbsp	120	10	75	1.5	0	330	6	0	0	1/2 starch, 2 fat
✓French, Fat Free	1 oz/2 Tbsp	35	0	0	0	0	150	8	0	0	1/2 carb.
✓Hidden Valley Ranch	1 oz/2 Tbsp	100	10	90	1.5	10	220	1	0	1	2 fat
✓Hidden Valley Ranch (reduced fat and calories)	1 oz/2 Tbsp	60	5	75	1	10	240	2	0	1	1 fat

✔ Italian (reduced fat and calories)	1 oz/2 Tbsp	40	3	68	0	0	340	2	0	0	1/2 fat
Italian Caesar	1 oz/2 Tbsp	150	16	96	2.5	20	240	1	0	1	3 fat
✔ Thousand Island	1 oz/2 Tbsp	90	8	80	1.5	10	125	2	0	0	1 1/2 fat

SALADS-TO-GO

✔ Caesar Side (without dressing)	1	100	5	36	2.5	15	650	7	1	10	1 veg., 1 medium-fat meat
✔ Deluxe Garden (without dressing)	1	110	6	49	1	0	350	9	3	7	2 veg., 1 medium-fat meat
✔ Grilled Chicken (without dressing)	1	200	8	36	1.5	50	720	9	3	25	2 veg., 3 lean meat
✔ Side (without dressing)	1	60	3	45	0	0	180	5	2	4	1 veg., 1/2 fat
Taco (without dressing)	1	380	19	45	10	65	1040	28	7	26	2 starch, 3 medium-fat meat, 1 fat

SANDWICHES

✔ Breaded Chicken Sandwich	1	440	18	37	3.5	60	840	44	2	28	3 starch, 3 lean meat, 2 fat

(Continued)

✔ = Healthiest Bets; n/a = not available

SANDWICHES (Continued)	Amount	Cal.	Fat (g)	% Cal. Fat	Sat. Fat (g)	Chol. (mg)	Sod. (mg)	Carb. (g)	Fiber (g)	Pro. (g)	Servings/Exchanges
✓Chicken Club Sandwich	1	470	20	37	4	70	970	44	2	31	3 starch, 3 lean meat, 2 fat
✓Grilled Chicken Sandwich	1	310	8	23	1.5	65	790	35	2	27	2 starch, 3 lean meat
Spicy Chicken Sandwich	1	410	15	33	2.5	65	1280	43	2	28	3 starch, 3 lean meat, 1 fat
SIDES											
French Fries (small)	1	270	13	43	2	0	85	35	3	4	2 starch, 2 1/2 fat
French Fries (medium)	1	390	19	44	3	0	120	50	5	5	3 starch, 4 fat
French Fries (Biggie)	1	470	23	44	3.5	0	150	61	6	7	4 starch, 4 1/2 fat
French Fries (Great Biggie)	1	570	27	43	4	0	180	73	7	8	5 starch, 5 fat
✓Saltine Crackers	2	25	1	36	0	0	80	4	0	1	free
✓Soft Breadstick	1	130	3	21	0.5	5	250	23	1	4	1 1/2 starch, 1/2 fat
Taco Chips	15	210	11	47	1.5	0	180	24	2	3	1 1/2 starch, 2 fat

STUFFED PITAS

Chicken Caesar Pita (with dressing)	1	490	18	33	5	65	1320	48	4	34	3 starch, 3 lean meat, 2 fat
Classic Greek Pita (with dressing)	1	440	20	41	8	35	1050	50	4	15	3 starch, 1 veg, 1 high-fat meat, 2 fat
✔Garden Ranch Chicken Pita (with dressing)	1	480	18	38	4	70	1180	51	5	30	3 starch, 1 veg., 3 lean meat, 2 fat
✔Garden Veggie Pita (with dressing)	1	400	17	38	3.5	20	760	52	5	11	3 starch, 1 veg, 3 fat

✔ = Healthiest Bets; n/a = not available

Notes

Whataburger

❖Whataburger provided nutrition information for all of its menu items.

Light 'n Lean Choice

Beef Fajita
Garden Salad
Lite Ranch Dressing (*1 Tbsp*)

Calories......................448	Sodium (mg)..........1,309
Fat (g) 16	Carbohydrate (g).........54
% calories from fat..32	Fiber (g).................n/a
Saturated fat (g) ....n/a	Protein (g) 26
Cholesterol (mg) 43	

Exchanges: 2 starch, 2 veg., 1/2 carb., 2 medium-fat meat, 1/2 fat

Healthy 'n Hearty Choice

Whataburger, Jr.
French Fries (*junior size*)
Garden Salad
Low Fat Vinaigrette Dressing (*1 packet*)

Calories......................636	Sodium (mg)..........1,670
Fat (g) 28	Carbohydrate (g).........77
% calories from fat..39	Fiber (g).................n/a
Saturated fat (g) ....n/a	Protein (g) 23
Cholesterol (mg) 42	

Exchanges: 3 1/2 starch, 2 veg., 1/2 carb., 1 medium-fat meat, 3 fat

Whataburger

	Amount	Cal.	Fat (g)	% Cal. Fat	Sat. Fat (g)	Chol. (mg)	Sod. (mg)	Carb. (g)	Fiber (g)	Pro. (g)	Servings/Exchanges
BEVERAGES											
✔Milk, 2%	8 oz	113	4	32	n/a	18	113	11	n/a	8	1 low-fat milk
✔Orange Juice	10 oz	140	0	0	n/a	0	2	33	n/a	2	2 fruit
BREAKFAST											
Biscuit with Bacon	1	359	20	50	n/a	15	730	37	n/a	10	2 1/2 starch, 4 fat
Biscuit with Egg and Cheese	1	434	26	54	n/a	202	797	38	n/a	14	2 1/2 starch, 1 high-fat meat, 3 fat
Biscuit with Egg, Cheese & Bacon	1	511	33	58	n/a	213	1010	38	n/a	18	2 1/2 starch, 2 high-fat meat, 2 1/2 fat

(Continued)

✔ = Healthiest Bets; n/a = not available

BREAKFAST (Continued)	Amount	Cal.	Fat (g)	% Cal. Fat	Sat. Fat (g)	Chol. (mg)	Sod. (mg)	Carb. (g)	Fiber (g)	Pro. (g)	Servings/Exchanges
Biscuit with Egg, Cheese & Sausage	1	601	42	63	n/a	236	1081	38	n/a	21	2 1/2 starch, 2 high-fat meat, 4 fat
Biscuit with Gravy	1	479	27	51	n/a	20	1253	48	n/a	9	3 starch, 5 fat
Biscuit with Sausage	1	446	29	59	n/a	37	794	37	n/a	12	2 1/2 starch, 1 high-fat meat, 4 fat
Biscuit, plain	1	280	13	42	n/a	3	509	37	n/a	5	2 1/2 starch, 2 1/2 fat
✔Blueberry Muffin	1	239	8	30	n/a	0	538	36	n/a	6	2 1/2 starch, 1 1/2 fat
Breakfast on the Bun	1	455	28	55	n/a	232	886	30	n/a	20	2 starch, 2 high-fat meat, 3 1/2 fat
✔Breakfast on the Bun with Bacon	1	365	19	5	n/a	210	815	29	n/a	18	2 starch, 2 high-fat meat
Breakfast Platter with Bacon	1	695	44	57	n/a	389	1162	54	n/a	22	3 1/2 starch, 2 high-fat meat, 5 fat

Breakfast Platter with Sausage	1	785	53	61	n/a	412	1234	54	n/a	25	3 1/2 starch, 2 high-fat meat, 6 1/2 fat
✔Egg Omelette Sandwich	1	288	13	41	n/a	198	602	29	n/a	13	2 starch, 1 medium-fat meat, 1 1/2 fat
✔Hashbrown	1 order	150	9	54	n/a	0	228	16	n/a	1	1 starch, 2 fat
✔Pancakes (3)	1 order	259	6	21	n/a	0	842	40	n/a	11	2 1/2 starch, 1 fat
Pancakes with Sausage (3)	1 order	426	21	44	n/a	34	1127	40	n/a	18	3 starch, 1 high-fat meat, 2 fat
✔Scrambled Eggs (2)	1 order	189	15	71	n/a	374	211	2	n/a	11	2 medium-fat meat, 1 fat

BURGERS

✔Justaburger	1	298	13	36	n/a	42	598	30	n/a	15	2 starch, 1 medium fat meat, 1 1/2 fat

✔ = Healthiest Bets; n/a = not available

(Continued)

BURGERS *(Continued)*	Amount	Cal.	Fat (g)	% Cal. Fat	Sat. Fat (g)	Chol. (mg)	Sod. (mg)	Carb. (g)	Fiber (g)	Pro. (g)	Servings/Exchanges
Whataburger	1	598	26	39	n/a	84	1096	61	n/a	30	4 starch, 2 medium-fat meat, 3 fat
Whataburger, double meat	1	823	42	46	n/a	168	1298	62	n/a	49	4 starch, 5 medium-fat meat, 3 fat
✔Whataburger, Jr.	1	322	13	36	n/a	42	603	35	n/a	16	2 starch, 1 medium-fat meat, 1 1/2 fat
✔Whataburger, small bun w/o bun oil	1	407	19	42	n/a	84	839	34	n/a	25	2 starch, 3 medium-fat meat, 1 fat
CONDIMENTS											
✔Club Crackers	1 packet	30	2	29	n/a	0	75	4	n/a	1	free
✔Croutons	1 packet	30	1	31	n/a	0	75	5	n/a	1	free
✔Grape Jelly	1 packet	45	0	0	n/a	0	15	10	n/a	0	1/2 carb.

✔Jalapeno Pepper	1 piece	3	0	0	n/a	0	190	1	n/a	0	free
Pancake Syrup	1 packet	180	0	0	n/a	0	50	42	n/a	0	3 carb.
✔Peppered Gravy	3 oz	75	5	60	n/a	0	375	8	n/a	0	1/2 starch, 1 fat
✔Picante Sauce	1 packet	5	0	0	n/a	0	130	1	n/a	0	free
✔Strawberry Jam	1 packet	40	0	0	n/a	0	15	9	n/a	0	1/2 carb.

DESSERTS

✔Apple Turnover	1	215	11	46	n/a	0	241	27	n/a	2	2 carb., 2 fat
Chocolate Chunk Cookie	1	247	16	58	n/a	36	75	28	n/a	4	2 carb., 3 fat
Macadamia Nut Cookie	1	269	16	54	n/a	34	80	31	n/a	3	2 carb., 3 fat

OTHER ENTREES

✔Beef Fajita	1	326	12	33	n/a	28	670	34	n/a	22	2 starch, 2 medium-fat meat
✔Chicken Fajita	1	272	7	23	n/a	33	691	35	n/a	18	2 starch, 2 lean meat

(Continued)

✔ = Healthiest Bets; n/a = not available

OTHER ENTREES *(Continued)*	Amount	Cal.	Fat (g)	% Cal. Fat	Sat. Fat (g)	Chol. (mg)	Sod. (mg)	Carb. (g)	Fiber (g)	Pro. (g)	Servings/Exchanges
✓Taquito, Bacon	1	335	16	43	n/a	286	761	32	n/a	15	2 starch, 1 medium-fat meat, 2 fat
Taquito, Potato	1	446	22	44	n/a	281	883	48	n/a	14	3 starch, 1 medium-fat meat, 3 fat
Taquito, Sausage	1	443	26	53	n/a	315	790	32	n/a	20	2 starch, 2 high-fat meat, 1 fat
SALAD DRESSINGS											
✓Low fat Ranch	1 packet	66	3	41	n/a	15	607	9	n/a	1	1/2 carb., 1/2 fat
✓Low fat Vinaigrette	1 packet	37	2	49	n/a	0	896	6	n/a	0	1/2 carb.
Ranch	1 packet	320	33	93	n/a	50	750	4	n/a	0	6 1/2 fat
Thousand Island	1 packet	160	12	68	n/a	15	470	12	n/a	0	1 carb., 2 fat

SALADS

✓Garden Salad	1	56	1	16	n/a	0	32	11	n/a	3	2 veg.
✓Grilled Chicken Salad	1	150	1	6	n/a	49	434	14	n/a	23	2 veg., 2 very lean meat

SANDWICHES

Grilled Chicken	1	442	14	29	n/a	66	1103	48	n/a	34	3 starch, 4 very lean meat, 3 fat
✓Grilled Chicken, w/o bun oil or salad dressing	1	358	6	9	n/a	66	989	46	n/a	34	3 starch, 4 very lean meat
✓Grilled Chicken, w/o bun oil, mustard, no dressing	1	300	3	9	n/a	66	994	35	n/a	33	2 starch, 4 very lean meat
✓Grilled Chicken, w/o salad dressing	1	385	9	21	n/a	66	989	46	n/a	34	3 starch, 4 very lean meat, 1 fat
Whatacatch	1	467	25	48	n/a	33	636	43	n/a	18	3 starch, 1 lean meat, 4 fat

(*Continued*)

✓ = Healthiest Bets; n/a = not available

SANDWICHES (*Continued*)	Amount	Cal.	Fat (g)	% Cal. Fat	Sat. Fat (g)	Chol. (mg)	Sod. (mg)	Carb. (g)	Fiber (g)	Pro. (g)	Servings/Exchanges
Whatachick'n	1	501	23	41	n/a	40	1122	51	n/a	27	3 starch, 3 lean meat, 3 fat
SHAKES											
Chocolate	12 oz	364	9	22	n/a	36	172	61	n/a	9	4 carb., 2 fat
Strawberry	12 oz	352	9	23	n/a	35	168	60	n/a	9	4 carb., 2 fat
Vanilla	12 oz	325	10	28	n/a	37	172	51	n/a	9	3 1/2 carb., 2 fat
SIDES											
✓Chicken Strips	2 pieces	120	5	38	n/a	14	420	10	n/a	7	1/2 starch, 1 medium-fat meat
French Fries (junior)	1 order	221	12	49	n/a	0	139	25	n/a	4	1 1/2 starch, 2 fat
French Fries (regular)	1 order	332	18	49	n/a	0	208	37	n/a	5	2 1/2 starch, 3 1/2 fat
French Fries (large)	1 order	442	24	49	n/a	0	227	49	n/a	7	3 starch, 5 fat
Onion Rings (regular)	1 order	329	19	52	n/a	0	596	34	n/a	5	2 starch, 4 fat

Onion Rings (large)	1 order	493	29	53	n/a	0	893	51	n/a	8	3 starch, 6 fat
✔ Texas Toast	1 slice	147	5	31	n/a	0	250	22	n/a	4	1 1/2 starch, 1 fat

✔ = Healthiest Bets; n/a = not available

Notes

Chicken—Fried, Roasted, or Grilled

RESTAURANTS

Boston Market

Chick-fil-A

Churchs Chicken

El Pollo Loco

Kenny Rogers Roasters

KFC

Koo Koo Roo

Popeye's Chicken & Biscuits

NUTRITION PROS

- No foods greet you at the table. What you order is what you eat. This puts you in the driver's seat.
- There's no waiting for food. You order, then eat.
- You can be in the know. Most large chicken chains provide full disclosure of nutrition information.
- In several of the chains, you see the food and the server right in front of you as you order. This makes it easy for you to ask them to hold or lighten up on the gravy, or to request less salad dressing or a serving on the side. You can also cast a glance at the starches or vegetables to see if they glisten. If they shine, you know that fat grams are lurking there.
- If you pick and choose carefully, a quick and healthy meal can be ready and waiting.
- A cup of broth-based (not cream) soup, when available, can be a good filler or a good match for a salad or side item.

Healthy Tips

★ You are better off skinless. If the chicken is served with skin, take the skin off and save some fat grams. You'll also lighten up on cholesterol and saturated fat.

★ If there's enough for two meals, ask for a take-out tray and split the meal into two before you dig in.

★ To keep fat grams and calories down, go with the quarter white meat. Wings and thighs have the most fat.

★ If you will eat the meal at home, a better buy (price and healthwise) is a whole chicken and several sides. That way you— rather than the server—can decide on your portions.

★ Split a quarter of a chicken meal and add an extra side or two. This keeps the protein portion where it should be, about 2–3 ounces.

■ You know the menu well, so you can have your order in mind before you cross the threshold.

■ Order à la carte. That makes it easier for you to order and eat smaller quantities.

■ Fried is not the only option in most chicken chains. They've mastered roasting and/or grilling. A few chicken chains never even learned to fry.

■ Healthier side items can fill your plate— corn, green beans, baked beans, rice, potatoes—

but make sure they're not dowsed in butter or gravy.

■ You can find a salad once in a while. But take control: You pour the dressing.

NUTRITION CONS

■ Portions are often enough for two mouths or two meals.

■ Some chicken chains stick to their one and only, tried and true, high-fat battered and fried chicken.

■ Some side items are sure candidates for the high-fat column: french fries, fried okra, potato salad, coleslaw, and biscuits.

■ Some side items hide their fat grams: baked beans, mashed potatoes, chicken salad, pasta salad, and butternut squash.

■ Unadulterated cooked vegetables don't appear often.

■ Fruit is virtually nowhere to be found unless it is hidden in sugar and/or fat.

Get It Your Way

★ Ask to hold the gravy from chicken, stuffing, or potatoes.

★ Ask to have the skin removed if you'll not be able to muster the courage.

★ Ask the server to take the wing off the breast.

★ Ask for the gravy, butter, or salad dressing on the side.

Boston Market

❖Boston Market provides nutrition information for all its menu items in a brochure.

Light 'n Lean Choice

1/4 White Meat Chicken No Skin or Wing
Whole Kernel Corn
Fruit Salad
Corn Bread

Calories	645	Sodium (mg)	1,050
Fat (g)	15	Carbohydrate (g)	82
% calories from fat	21	Fiber (g)	5
Saturated fat (g)	3	Protein (g)	42
Cholesterol (mg)	110		

Exchanges: 4 starch, 1 fruit, 5 very lean meat, 2 fat

Healthy 'n Hearty Choice

Ham with Cinnamon Apples
New Potatoes
Steamed Vegetables
Honey Wheat Roll (*1/2 roll*)

Calories	635	Sodium (mg)	1,975
Fat (g)	17	Carbohydrate (g)	96
% calories from fat	24	Fiber (g)	9
Saturated fat (g)	4	Protein (g)	35
Cholesterol (mg)	75		

Exchanges: 3 1/2 starch, 1 veg., 1 fruit, 1 carb., 4 lean meat

Boston Market

	Amount	Cal.	Fat (g)	% Cal. Fat	Sat. Fat (g)	Chol. (mg)	Sod. (mg)	Carb. (g)	Fiber (g)	Pro. (g)	Servings/Exchanges
BREADS											
✔Corn Bread	1 piece	200	6	27	1.5	25	390	33	1	3	2 starch, 1 fat
✔Honey Wheat Roll	1/2 roll	150	2	12	0	0	280	29	2	5	2 starch
COLD SIDES											
Cole Slaw	3/4 cup	280	16	51	2.5	25	520	32	3	2	1 veg., 1 1/2 carb., 2 fat
✔Cranberry Relish	3/4 cup	370	5	12	0.5	0	5	84	5	2	1 fruit, 4 carb., 1 fat
✔Fruit Salad	3/4 cup	70	1	7	0	0	10	17	2	1	1 fruit
Mediterranean Pasta Salad	3/4 cup	170	10	53	2.5	10	490	16	2	4	1 starch, 2 fat
Tortellini Salad	3/4 cup	380	24	57	4.5	90	530	29	2	14	2 starch, 1 medium-fat meat, 4 fat

(Continued)

✔ = Healthiest Bets; n/a = not available

	Amount	Cal.	Fat (g)	% Cal. Fat	Sat. Fat (g)	Chol. (mg)	Sod. (mg)	Carb. (g)	Fiber (g)	Pro. (g)	Servings/Exchanges
DESSERTS											
Brownie	1	450	27	54	7	80	190	47	3	6	3 carb., 5 fat
Chocolate Chip Cookie	1	340	17	45	6	25	240	48	1	4	3 carb., 3 fat
Oatmeal Raisin Cookie	1	320	13	37	2.5	25	260	48	1	4	3 carb., 2 fat
ENTREES											
1/2 Chicken with Skin	1	590	33	50	10	290	1010	4	0	70	10 lean meat, 1/2 fat
✓1/4 Dark Meat Chicken No Skin	1	190	10	47	3	115	440	1	0	22	3 lean meat
1/4 Dark Meat Chicken with Skin	1	320	21	59	6	155	500	2	0	30	4 lean meat, 2 fat
✓1/4 White Meat Chicken No Skin or Wing	1	170	4	21	1	85	480	2	0	33	5 very lean meat
✓1/4 White Meat Chicken with Skin	1	280	12	39	3.5	135	510	2	0	40	6 very lean meat, 1 fat
Ham with Cinnamon Apples	1 order	320	11	31	4.0	75	1510	35	2	25	1 fruit, 1 carb, 4 lean meat

Meat Loaf & Brown Gravy	1 order	390	22	51	8	120	1040	19	1	30	1 starch, 4 medium-fat meat
Meat Loaf & Chunky Tomato Sauce	1 order	370	18	44	8	120	1170	22	2	30	1 1/2 carb., 4 medium-fat meat
Original Chicken Pot Pie	1	750	34	41	9	115	2380	78	6	34	5 starch, 3 lean meat, 5 fat
✔Skinless Rotisserie Turkey Breast	1 order	170	1	5	0.5	100	850	1	0	36	5 very lean meat

HOT SIDES

BBQ Baked Beans	3/4 cup	270	5	17	2	0	540	48	12	8	3 starch, 1 fat
✔Butternut Squash	3/4 cup	160	6	34	4	15	580	25	3	2	1 1/2 starch, 1 fat
✔Chicken Gravy	1 oz/2 Tbsp	15	1	60	0	0	170	2	0	0	free
✔Cinnamon Apples	3/4 cup	250	5	16	0.5	0	45	56	3	0	1 fruit, 2 1/2 carb., 1 fat
Creamed Spinach	3/4 cup	260	20	68	13	55	740	11	2	9	2 veg, 4 fat

✔ = Healthiest Bets; n/a = not available

(Continued)

HOT SIDES (*Continued*)	Amount	Cal.	Fat (g)	% Cal. Fat	Sat. Fat (g)	Chol. (mg)	Sod. (mg)	Carb. (g)	Fiber (g)	Pro. (g)	Servings/Exchanges
Homestyle Mashed Potatoes & Gravy	3/4 cup	210	10	41	6	25	740	26	1	4	2 starch, 2 fat
Macaroni & Cheese	3/4 cup	280	11	32	6	30	830	32	1	13	2 starch, 1 high-fat meat
Mashed Potatoes	2/3 cup	190	9	40	6	25	570	24	1	3	1 1/2 starch, 2 fat
✔New Potatoes	3/4 cup	130	3	15	0	0	150	25	2	3	1 1/2 starch, 1/2 fat
Penne Marinara	1 order	190	9	43	3.5	5	460	20	2	7	1 starch, 1 veg, 2 fat
Rice Pilaf	2/3 cup	180	5	25	1	0	600	32	2	5	2 starch, 1 fat
✔Steamed Vegetables	2/3 cup	35	1	14	0	0	35	7	3	2	1 veg.
Stuffing	3/4 cup	310	12	35	2	0	1140	44	3	6	3 starch, 2 fat
✔Whole Kernel Corn	3/4 cup	180	4	20	0.5	0	170	30	2	5	2 starch, 1 fat
SALADS											
Caesar Salad Entree	1	510	42	74	11	35	1130	17	3	17	3 veg, 2 medium-fat meat, 6 fat

	Amount	Calories	Fat (g)	% Cal. Fat	Sat. Fat (g)	Chol. (mg)	Sodium (mg)	Carb. (g)	Fiber (g)	Prot. (g)	Servings/Exchanges
Caesar Salad without Dressing	1	230	12	49	6	20	500	14	3	16	3 veg., 1 medium-fat meat, 1 fat
Caesar Side Salad	1	200	17	73	4.5	15	450	7	1	7	1 veg., 3 fat
Chicken Caesar Salad	1	650	45	63	12	105	1580	17	3	43	3 veg., 2 medium-fat meat, 7 fat

SANDWICHES

	Amount	Calories	Fat (g)	% Cal. Fat	Sat. Fat (g)	Chol. (mg)	Sodium (mg)	Carb. (g)	Fiber (g)	Prot. (g)	Servings/Exchanges
✓Chicken No Sauce or Cheese	1	430	5	10	1	65	910	62	5	34	4 starch, 3 very lean meat
Chicken w/ Cheese & Sauce	1	750	33	40	12	135	1860	72	5	41	5 starch, 4 lean meat, 4 fat
Ham and Turkey Club No Cheese or Sauce	1	420	6	13	2	50	1260	64	4	29	4 starch, 3 lean meat
Ham and Turkey Club w/ Cheese & Sauce	1	890	43	44	20	150	2280	76	4	48	5 starch, 5 lean meat, 5 1/2 fat

(Continued)

✔ = Healthiest Bets; n/a = not available

SANDWICHES (*Continued*)	Amount	Cal.	Fat (g)	% Cal. Fat	Sat. Fat (g)	Chol. (mg)	Sod. (mg)	Carb. (g)	Fiber (g)	Pro. (g)	Servings/Exchanges
Ham No Cheese or Sauce	1	440	8	18	2.5	45	1450	66	4	25	4 1/2 starch, 2 lean meat
Ham w/ Cheese & Sauce	1	750	34	41	12	100	1730	72	5	38	4 1/2 starch, 4 medium-fat meat, 3 fat
Meat Loaf No Cheese	1	690	21	27	7	120	1610	86	6	40	5 1/2 starch, 4 medium-fat meat
Meat Loaf w/ Cheese	1	860	33	35	16	165	2270	95	6	46	6 starch, 4 medium-fat meat, 2 1/2 fat
✓Turkey No Cheese or Sauce	1	400	4	9	1	60	1070	61	4	32	4 starch, 4 very lean meat
Turkey w/ Cheese & Sauce	1	710	28	35	10	110	1390	68	4	45	4 1/2 starch, 5 lean meat, 2 1/2 fat
SOUPS											
✓Chicken Noodle Soup	3/4 cup	100	3	34	1	30	990	9	1	9	1/2 carb., 1 lean meat

| Chicken Tortilla Soup | 1 cup | 220 | 11 | 45 | 4 | 35 | 1410 | 19 | 2 | 10 | 1 carb., 2 fat |

✔ = Healthiest Bets; n/a = not available

*Notes*_____

Chick-fil-A

❖Chick-fil-A provides nutrition information for all its menu items in a brochure.

Light 'n Lean Choice

Hearty Breast of Chicken Soup
Chick-fil-A Chargrilled Chicken Garden Salad
Icedream (*small cone*)

Calories......................420	Sodium (mg)..........1,650
Fat (g) 8	Carbohydrate (g).........36
% calories from fat..17	Fiber (g) 6
Saturated fat (g)........2	Protein (g) 53
Cholesterol (mg) 110	

Exchanges: 1 starch, 2 veg., 1 carb., 5 very lean meat, 1 fat

Healthy 'n Hearty Choice

Chargrilled Chicken Deluxe Sandwich
Carrot & Raisin Salad
Chick-fil-A Waffle Potato Fries (*split small order*)

Calories......................585	Sodium (mg)..........1,770
Fat (g) 10	Carbohydrate (g).........91
% calories from fat..15	Fiber (g) 4
Saturated fat (g)........3	Protein (g) 34
Cholesterol (mg) 49	

Exchanges: 3 1/2 starch, 2 veg., 1 carb., 3 very lean meat, 1 fat

Chick-fil-A

	Amount	Cal.	Fat (g)	% Cal. Fat	Sat. Fat (g)	Chol. (mg)	Sod. (mg)	Carb. (g)	Fiber (g)	Pro. (g)	Servings/Exchanges
BEVERAGES											
✔ Diet Lemonade	9 oz	5	0	0	0	0	4	2	0	0	free
CHICKEN ITEMS											
✔ Chargrilled Chicken (no bun, no pickles)	1	130	3	21	1	30	630	0	0	27	3 very lean meat
✔ Chicken (no bun, no pickles)	1	160	8	45	2	45	690	1	0	21	3 lean meat
✔ Chick-fil-A Chick-n-Strips (4 count)	1 order	230	8	31	2	20	380	10	0	29	1/2 starch, 4 very lean meat, 1 fat
✔ Chick-fil-A Nuggets (8 pack)	1 order	290	14	43	3	60	770	12	0	28	1 starch, 3 lean meat, 1 fat
DESSERTS											
Cheesecake	1 slice	270	21	70	9	10	510	7	0	13	1/2 carb., 2 high-fat meat

(Continued)

✔ = Healthiest Bets; n/a = not available

DESSERTS (Continued)	Amount	Cal.	Fat (g)	% Cal. Fat	Sat. Fat (g)	Chol. (mg)	Sod. (mg)	Carb. (g)	Fiber (g)	Pro. (g)	Servings/Exchanges
Cheesecake with Blueberry Topping	1 slice	290	23	71	10	10	550	9	0	14	1/2 carb., 2 high-fat meat, 1/2 fat
Cheesecake with Strawberry Topping	1 slice	290	23	71	10	10	580	8	0	14	1/2 carb., 2 high-fat meat, 1/2 fat
Fudge Nut Brownie	1	350	16	41	3	30	650	41	0	10	3 carb., 3 fat
✓Icedream (small cone)	1	140	4	26	1	40	240	16	0	11	1 carb., 1 fat
Icedream (small cup)	1	350	10	26	3	70	390	50	0	16	3 carb., 2 fat
Lemon Pie	1 slice	320	16	45	5	135	280	40	1	7	2 1/2 carb., 3 fat
SALADS											
✓Chick-fil-A Chargrilled Chicken Garden Salad	1	170	3	16	1	25	650	10	5	26	2 veg., 3 very lean meat
✓Chick-fil-A Chicken Salad Plate	1	290	5	16	0	35	570	40	6	21	2 starch, 2 veg., 2 lean meat

✔Chick-fil-A Chick-n-Strips Salad	1	290	9	28	2	20	430	21	5	32	1 starch, 1 veg., 4 very lean meat, 1 fat
✔Tossed Salad	1	70	0	0	0	0	0	13	1	5	2 veg.
SANDWICHES											
✔Chargrilled Chicken Club (no dressing)	1	390	12	28	5	70	980	38	2	33	2 starch, 1 veg., 3 lean meat
✔Chargrilled Chicken Deluxe	1	290	3	9	1	40	640	38	2	28	2 1/2 starch, 3 very lean meat
✔Chicken Deluxe	1	300	9	27	2	50	870	31	2	25	2 starch, 3 lean meat, 1/2 fat
✔Chick-fil-A Chargrilled Chicken Sandwich	1	280	3	10	1	40	640	36	1	27	2 1/2 starch, 3 very lean meat
✔Chick-fil-A Chicken Salad Sandwich (on whole wheat)	1	320	5	14	2	10	810	42	1	25	3 starch, 2 lean meat

(Continued)

✔ = Healthiest Bets; n/a = not available

	Amount	Cal.	Fat (g)	% Cal. Fat	Sat. Fat (g)	Chol. (mg)	Sod. (mg)	Carb. (g)	Fiber (g)	Pro. (g)	Servings/Exchanges
SANDWICHES (*Continued*)											
✔ Chick-fil-A Chicken Sandwich	1	290	9	28	2	50	870	29	1	24	2 starch, 2 lean meat, 1/2 fat
SIDES											
✔ Carrot & Raisin Salad (small)	1	150	2	12	0	6	650	28	2	5	1 carb., 2 veg.
✔ Chick-fil-A Waffle Potato Fries (small/salted)	1 order	290	10	31	4	5	960	49	0	1	3 starch, 2 fat
✔ Chick-fil-A Waffle Potato Fries (small/unsalted)	1 order	290	10	31	4	5	80	49	0	1	3 starch, 2 fat
✔ Cole Slaw (small)	1	130	6	42	1	15	430	11	1	6	1 carb., 1 veg., 1 fat
✔ Hearty Breast of Chicken Soup (cup)	7.6 oz	110	1	8	0	45	760	10	1	16	1 starch, 2 very lean meat

✔ = Healthiest Bets; n/a = not available

Churchs Chicken

❖Churchs Chicken provided nutrition information for all of its menu items.

Light 'n Lean Choice

2 Tender Strips (*fried chicken*)
Corn on the Cob
Cajun Rice
Cole Slaw

Calories	521	Sodium (mg)	785
Fat (g)	24	Carbohydrate (g)	56
% calories from fat	41	Fiber (g)	12
Saturated fat (g)	n/a	Protein (g)	21
Cholesterol (mg)	35		

Exchanges: 3 starch, 1 veg., 2 medium-fat meat, 2 fat

Healthy 'n Hearty Choice

Chicken Breast (*fried*)
Potatoes & Gravy (*2 orders*)
Corn on the Cob
Cole Slaw

Calories	611	Sodium (mg)	1,795
Fat (g)	27	Carbohydrate (g)	64
% calories from fat	40	Fiber (g)	13
Saturated fat (g)	n/a	Protein (g)	29
Cholesterol (mg)	65		

Exchanges: 3 starch, 1 veg., 3 lean meat, 1 1/2 fat

Churchs Chicken

	Amount	Cal.	Fat (g)	% Cal. Fat	Sat. Fat (g)	Chol. (mg)	Sod. (mg)	Carb. (g)	Fiber (g)	Pro. (g)	Servings/Exchanges
DESSERTS											
Apple Pie	1 slice	280	12	39	n/a	5	340	41	1	2	2 1/2 carb., 2 fat
FRIED CHICKEN											
✓Breast	1	200	12	54	n/a	65	510	4	0	19	3 lean meat, 1/2 fat
✓Leg	1	140	9	58	n/a	45	160	2	0	13	2 lean meat, 1/2 fat
✓Tender Strip	1 strip	80	4	45	n/a	15	140	5	0	6	1 medium-fat meat
✓Thigh	1	230	16	63	n/a	80	520	5	0	16	2 lean meat, 2 fat
✓Wing	1	250	16	58	n/a	60	540	8	0	19	1/2 starch, 3 medium-fat meat
SIDES											
Biscuit	1	250	16	58	n/a	5	640	26	1	2	2 starch, 3 fat

	Amount	Cal.	Fat (g)	% Cal. Fat	Sat. Fat (g)	Chol. (mg)	Sod. (mg)	Carb (g)	Pro. (g)	Exchanges
Cajun Rice		130	7	48	n/a	5	260	16	1	1	1 starch, 1 fat
Cole Slaw	1	92	6	59	n/a	0	230	8	2	4	1 veg., 1 fat
✔Corn on the Cob	1	139	3	19	n/a	0	15	24	9	4	1 1/2 starch, 1/2 fat
✔French Fries	1 order	210	11	45	n/a	0	60	29	2	3	1 1/2 starch, 2 fat
Okra (fried)	1 order	210	16	69	n/a	0	520	19	4	3	1 starch, 1 veg., 3 fat
✔Potatoes & Gravy	1 order	90	3	30	n/a	0	520	14	1	1	1 starch

✔ = Healthiest Bets; n/a = not available

Notes _____

El Pollo Loco

❖ El Pollo Loco provides nutrition information for all its menu items in a brochure.

Light 'n Lean Choice

Tostada Salad, Chicken
Pinto Beans

Calories......................517	Sodium (mg) 2,024
Fat (g) 18	Carbohydrate (g).........55
% calories from fat..31	Fiber (g) 12
Saturated fat (g)........5	Protein (g) 46
Cholesterol (mg) 80	

Exchanges: 3 starch, 5 lean meat

Healthy 'n Hearty Choice

Taco al Carbon, Chicken
Corn on the Cob
Spanish Rice
Pico de Gallo *(2 servings)*

Calories......................563	Sodium (mg) 900
Fat (g) 19	Carbohydrate (g).........91
% calories from fat..30	Fiber (g) 6
Saturated fat (g)........3	Protein (g) 17
Cholesterol (mg) 28	

Exchanges: 5 1/2 starch, 1 lean meat, 1 fat

El Pollo Loco

BURRITOS

	Amount	Cal.	Fat (g)	% Cal. Fat	Sat. Fat (g)	Chol. (mg)	Sod. (mg)	Carb. (g)	Fiber (g)	Pro. (g)	Servings/Exchanges
BRC Burrito	1	482	15	28	5	15	1250	72	9	16	5 starch, 3 fat
Classic Chicken Burrito	1	556	22	36	7	117	1499	61	8	30	4 starch, 2 lean meat, 3 fat
Grilled Steak Burrito	1	705	32	41	13	77	1689	68	10	39	4 1/2 starch, 4 medium-fat meat, 2 fat
Loco Grande Burrito	1	632	26	37	7	129	1649	67	8	33	4 1/2 starch, 3 medium-fat meat, 2 fat
Smokey Black Bean Burrito	1	566	22	35	8	22	1337	78	9	16	5 starch, 4 fat
Spicy Hot Chicken Burrito	1	559	22	35	7	117	1503	61	8	30	4 starch, 3 lean meat, 2 fat

(Continued)

✔ = Healthiest Bets; n/a = not available

BURRITOS (*Continued*)	Amount	Cal.	Fat (g)	% Cal. Fat	Sat. Fat (g)	Chol. (mg)	Sod. (mg)	Carb. (g)	Fiber (g)	Pro. (g)	Servings/Exchanges
Whole Wheat Chicken Burrito	1	592	26	40	9	146	1199	60	8	31	4 starch, 3 lean meat, 3 1/2 fat
CONDIMENTS											
✔Chipotle Salsa	1 oz/2 Tbsp	8	0	0	0	0	156	2	0	0	free
✔Guacamole	1.8 oz/3 1/2 Tbsp	52	3	52	0	0	280	5	0	0	1 veg., 1/2 fat
✔House Salsa	1 oz/2 Tbsp	6	0	0	0	0	96	1	0	0	free
✔Jalapeno Hot Sauce	1 oz/2 Tbsp	5	0	0	0	0	110	1	0	0	free
✔Light Sour Cream	1 oz/2 Tbsp	45	3	60	0	12	25	2	0	2	1 fat
✔Picante Salsa	1 oz/2 Tbsp	5	0	0	0	0	66	2	0	0	free
✔Pico de Gallo	1 oz/2 Tbsp	11	1	82	0	0	131	2	0	0	free
✔Verde Salsa	1 oz/2 Tbsp	6	0	0	0	0	90	1	0	0	free

DESSERTS

	Amount										Exchanges
✔Churro	1	149	8	48	2	4	160	18	1	2	1 carb., 1 1/2 fat
✔Flan	1	220	2	8	2	5	140	46	0	6	3 carb.
✔Fosters Freeze	1 oz	38	1	24	n/a	n/a	n/a	n/a	n/a	n/a	free

GRILLED CHICKEN

	Amount										Exchanges
✔Breast	1	160	6	34	2	110	390	0	0	26	4 very lean meat
✔Leg	1	90	5	50	1.5	75	150	0	0	11	2 lean meat
✔Thigh	1	180	12	60	4	130	230	0	0	16	2 lean meat, 1 fat
✔Wing	1	110	6	49	2	80	220	0	0	12	2 medium-fat meat

OTHER ENTREES

	Amount										Exchanges
✔Chicken Soft Taco	1	224	12	48	4	66	585	15	0	16	1 starch, 2 lean meat, 1 fat
Pollo Bowl	1	504	13	23	2	56	2068	69	9	37	4 starch, 2 veg., 3 lean meat, 1 fat

(*Continued*)

✔ = Healthiest Bets; n/a = not available

OTHER ENTREES (*Continued*)	Amount	Cal.	Fat (g)	% Cal. Fat	Sat. Fat (g)	Chol. (mg)	Sod. (mg)	Carb. (g)	Fiber (g)	Pro. (g)	Servings/Exchanges
Steak Bowl	1	616	26	38	10	68	1743	62	8	37	3 1/2 starch, 2 veg., 3 medium-fat meat, 2 fat
✔Taco al Carbon, Chicken	1	265	12	41	2	28	223	30	3	10	2 starch, 1 lean meat, 2 fat
Taco al Carbon, Steak	1	394	22	50	7	46	473	30	3	20	2 starch, 2 medium-fat meat, 2 fat
✔Taquito	1	370	17	41	4	25	690	43	3	15	3 starch, 1 medium-fat meat, 2 fat
Tortilla Wrap, Chicken Caesar	1	518	19	33	3	48	1709	59	3	28	3 starch, 2 veg., 2 lean meat, 3 fat
Tortilla Wrap, Southwest	1	632	27	38	4	61	1792	69	5	30	4 starch, 2 veg., 2 lean meat, 4 fat

SALADS

	Amount										
✔ Flame-Broiled Chicken Salad	1	167	5	27	0	56	765	11	4	27	2 veg., 3 very lean meat
✔ Garden Salad	1	29	0	0	0	0	20	6	2	3	1 veg.
Garden Salad, w/ 1,000 Island Dressing	1	299	27	90	4	30	480	15	2	4	2 veg., 5 fat
Garden Salad, w/ Blue Cheese Dressing	1	329	32	96	6	50	610	8	2	5	1 veg., 6 fat
✔ Garden Salad, w/ Light Italian Dressing	1	54	1	36	1	0	1110	9	2	3	1 veg.
Garden Salad, w/ Ranch Dressing	1	379	39	100	6	5	520	8	2	4	1 veg., 8 fat
Tostada Salad, Chicken	1	332	14	38	5	80	1280	26	4	35	2 starch, 4 lean meat
Tostada Salad, Steak	1	525	31	53	14	100	1206	26	4	40	2 starch, 5 medium-fat meat, 1 fat

(Continued)

✔ = Healthiest Bets; n/a = not available

	Amount	Cal.	Fat (g)	% Cal. Fat	Sat. Fat (g)	Chol. (mg)	Sod. (mg)	Carb. (g)	Fiber (g)	Pro. (g)	Servings/Exchanges
S I D E S											
Broccoli Slaw	5 oz	203	17	75	0	0	365	14	3	3	1 veg, 1/2 carb., 3 fat
✔Chicken Tamale	1	190	8	38	2	10	480	23	2	6	1 1/2 starch, 1 lean meat, 1 fat
Cole Slaw	5 oz	206	16	70	3	11	358	12	2	2	2 veg, 3 fat
Cornbread Stuffing	6 oz	281	12	38	2	0	832	40	6	6	2 1/2 starch, 2 fat
✔Corn on the Cob, 5 1/2"	1	146	2	12	0	0	18	33	2	5	2 starch
✔Crispy Green Beans	5 oz	41	2	44	1	0	667	6	3	1	1 veg.
✔Cucumber Salad	4.2 oz	34	0	0	0	0	11	7	1	2	1 veg.
✔Fiesta Corn	5 oz	152	6	36	1	0	397	25	6	4	1 1/2 starch, 1 fat
French Fries	1 order	323	14	39	3	0	330	44	0	5	3 starch, 3 fat
✔Gravy	1 oz/2 Tbsp	14	0	0	2	0	139	2	0	0	free

✔Honey Glazed Carrots	5 oz	104	6	52	1	0	403	14	3	1	1 veg., 1/2 carb., 1 fat
✔Lime Parfait	1	125	3	22	3	0	107	25	0	1	1 1/2 carb., 1 fat
Macaroni & Cheese	6 oz	238	12	45	5	31	919	22	1	10	1 1/2 starch, 1 high-fat meat
✔Mashed Potatoes	5 oz	97	1	9	0	0	369	21	2	3	1 starch
✔Pinto Beans	6 oz	185	4	19	0	0	744	29	8	11	1 starch, 1 lean meat
Potato Salad	6 oz	256	14	49	2	15	527	30	3	3	2 starch, 2 fat
✔Rainbow Pasta Salad	5 oz	157	1	6	0	0	533	30	2	6	2 starch
Smokey Black Beans	5 oz	255	13	46	5	11	609	29	4	6	2 starch, 2 1/2 fat
Southwest Cole Slaw	5 oz	178	13	66	2	8	267	15	3	2	1 veg., 1/2 carb., 2 1/2 fat
✔Spanish Rice	4 oz	130	3	21	1	0	397	24	1	2	1 1/2 starch, 1/2 fat
✔Spiced Apples	5 oz	146	0	0	0	0	139	39	0	0	2 1/2 carb.

✔ = Healthiest Bets; n/a = not available

Kenny Rogers Roasters

❖Kenny Rogers Roasters provides nutrition
information for all its menu items in a brochure.

Light 'n Lean Choice

BBQ Chicken Pita
Corn on the Cob
Steamed Vegetables

Calories	517	Sodium (mg)	1,377
Fat (g)	8	Carbohydrate (g)	73
% calories from fat	14	Fiber (g)	n/a
Saturated fat (g)	1.4	Protein (g)	38
Cholesterol (mg)	112		

Exchanges: 4 starch, 3 veg., 3 lean meat

Healthy 'n Hearty Choice

1/4 Chicken (*white meat, no skin*)
Tomato Cucumber Salad
Baked Sweet Potato
Corn Muffin

Calories	705	Sodium (mg)	1,452
Fat (g)	12	Carbohydrate (g)	96
% calories from fat	15	Fiber (g)	n/a
Saturated fat (g)	3.3	Protein (g)	38
Cholesterol (mg)	92		

Exchanges: 5 1/2 starch, 2 veg., 4 very lean meat,
1 1/2 fat

Kenny Rogers Roasters

	Amount	Cal.	Fat (g)	% Cal. Fat	Sat. Fat (g)	Chol. (mg)	Sod. (mg)	Carb. (g)	Fiber (g)	Pro. (g)	Servings/Exchanges
OTHER ENTREES											
Chicken Pot Pie	1	708	33	42	10.5	69	1500	78	0	26	5 starch, 1 veg., 1 lean meat, 5 fat
✓ Sliced Turkey Breast	1	158	2	11	1	78	586	0	0	34	5 very lean meat
ROAST CHICKEN											
1/2 Chicken, no skin	1	313	10	29	2.5	221	876	1	0	56	8 very lean meat
1/2 Chicken, with skin	1	515	28	49	7.3	301	1129	2	0	65	9 very lean meat, 4 fat
✓ 1/4 Chicken, dark, no skin	1	169	7	37	2	130	454	1	0	25	4 lean meat
1/4 Chicken, dark, with skin	1	271	17	56	4.3	165	524	1	0	29	4 lean meat, 1 fat

(Continued)

✓ = Healthiest Bets; n/a = not available

ROAST CHICKEN *(Continued)*	Amount	Cal.	Fat (g)	% Cal. Fat	Sat. Fat (g)	Chol. (mg)	Sod. (mg)	Carb. (g)	Fiber (g)	Pro. (g)	Servings/Exchanges
✔1/4 Chicken, white, no skin	1	144	2	13	0.6	92	422	0	0	31	4 very lean meat
✔1/4 Chicken, white, with skin	1	244	11	41	3	136	604	1	0	35	5 lean meat
SALAD DRESSINGS											
Blue Cheese	2.47 oz	370	39	95	7	65	720	3	0	3	8 fat
Buttermilk Ranch	2.47 oz	430	48	100	7	10	620	2	0	1	9 fat
Caesar	2.47 oz	340	36	95	5	15	780	3	0	1	7 fat
✔Fat Free Italian	2.47 oz	35	0	0	0	0	1040	8	0	0	1/2 carb.
Honey French	2.47 oz	350	29	75	4	0	490	22	0	0	1 1/2 carb., 6 fat
Honey Mustard	2.47 oz	320	28	79	4	40	410	18	0	1	1 carb., 5 1/2 fat
Thousand Island	2.47 oz	330	33	90	5	40	550	8	0	1	1/2 carb., 6 1/2 fat
SALADS											
✔Chicken Caesar	1	285	9	28	3.2	122	704	18	2	34	1/2 starch, 2 veg, 4 lean meat

✔Roasted Chicken	1	292	10	31	2.4	218	573	19	6	35	1/2 starch, 2 veg., 4 lean meat
✔Side	1	23	0	0	0	0	16	5	0	2	1 veg.
S A N D W I C H E S											
BBQ Chicken Pita	1	401	7	16	1.4	112	1307	51	0	33	3 starch, 1 veg., 3 lean meat
Chicken Caesar Pita	1	606	35	52	3	122	829	34	0	36	2 starch, 4 lean meat, 5 fat
Roasted Chicken Pita	1	685	35	46	2.8	159	1620	42	0	47	3 starch, 5 lean meat, 4 fat
✔Turkey	1	385	12	28	2.2	88	923	30	0	39	2 starch, 5 very lean meat, 1 fat
S I D E S											
✔Baked Sweet Potato	1	263	0	0	0	0	26	62	1	4	4 starch
Cornbread Stuffing	7.1 oz	326	19	52	3.4	5	765	34	0	7	2 starch, 4 fat

✔ = Healthiest Bets; n/a = not available

(*Continued*)

	Amount	Cal.	Fat (g)	% Cal. Fat	Sat. Fat (g)	Chol. (mg)	Sod. (mg)	Carb. (g)	Fiber (g)	Pro. (g)	Servings/Exchanges
SIDES (*Continued*)											
✔Corn Muffin	2 oz	175	8	41	1.4	0	210	24	1	2	1 1/2 starch, 1 1/2 fat
✔Corn on the Cob	1	68	1	13	0	0	11	14	0	2	1 starch
✔Honey Baked Beans	5 oz	148	1	6	0.3	0	787	32	0	6	1 starch, 1 carb.
✔Rice Pilaf	5 oz	173	5	26	1	0	146	43	0	3	3 starch, 1 fat
✔Steamed Vegetables	4.25 oz	48	0	0	0	0	59	8	4	3	2 veg.
✔Sweet Corn Niblets	5 oz	112	1	8	0	0	385	28	1	3	2 starch
✔Tomato Cucumber Salad	6 oz	123	2	15	1.3	0	794	10	1	1	2 veg.
SOUPS											
✔Chicken Noodle (bowl)	10 oz	91	2	20	0.3	22	931	12	0	7	1 starch, 1 very lean meat
✔Chicken Noodle (cup)	6 oz	55	1	16	0.2	13	559	7	0	4	1/2 starch

✔ = Healthiest Bets; n/a = not available

KFC

❖ KFC provides nutrition information for all its menu items in a brochure.

Light 'n Lean Choice

Tender Roast Chicken Breast (*without skin*)
Mashed Potatoes with Gravy
Green Beans
Cornbread

Calories......................562	Sodium (mg)..........2,161
Fat (g) 25	Carbohydrate (g).........50
% calories from fat..40	Fiber (g) 6
Saturated fat (g).....4.7	Protein (g) 36
Cholesterol (mg) 160	

Exchanges: 2 1/2 starch, 1 veg., 4 very lean meat, 3 1/2 fat

Healthy 'n Hearty Choice

Original Recipe Drumsticks (*2*)
Corn on the Cob
Mean Greens
BBQ Baked Beans

Calories......................690	Sodium (mg)..........2,274
Fat (g) 26	Carbohydrate (g).........87
% calories from fat..34	Fiber (g) 13
Saturated fat (g)........6	Protein (g) 41
Cholesterol (mg) 165	

Exchanges: 3 starch, 2 veg., 1 carb., 4 lean meat, 2 fat

KFC

	Amount	Cal.	Fat (g)	% Cal. Fat	Sat. Fat (g)	Chol. (mg)	Sod. (mg)	Carb. (g)	Fiber (g)	Pro. (g)	Servings/Exchanges
CRISPY STRIPS											
✓Colonel's Crispy Strips (3)	1 order	261	16	55	3.7	40	658	10	3	20	1/2 starch, 2 lean meat, 2 fat
✓Spicy Buffalo Crispy Strips (3)	1 order	350	19	49	4	35	1110	22	2	22	1 1/2 starch, 3 medium-fat meat, 1 fat
EXTRA TASTY CRISPY FRIED CHICKEN											
Breast	1	470	28	54	7	80	930	25	1	31	1 1/2 starch, 4 lean meat, 3 fat
✓Drumstick	1	190	11	52	3	60	260	8	1	13	1/2 starch, 2 medium-fat meat

Item	Amount									Exchanges
Thigh	1	370	25	61	6	70	540	18	2	19	1 starch, 2 lean meat, 4 fat
✔Whole Wing	1	200	13	59	4	45	290	10	1	10	1/2 starch, 1 medium-fat meat, 1 1/2 fat

HOT & SPICY FRIED CHICKEN

Item	Amount									Exchanges
Breast	1	530	35	59	8	110	1110	23	2	32	1 1/2 starch, 4 lean meat, 4 1/2 fat
✔Drumstick	1	190	11	52	3	50	300	10	1	13	1/2 carb., 2 lean meat, 1 fat
Thigh	1	370	27	66	7	90	570	13	1	18	1 starch, 2 lean meat, 4 fat
✔Whole Wing	1	210	15	64	4	50	340	9	1	10	1/2 starch, 1 medium-fat meat, 2 fat

ORIGINAL RECIPE FRIED CHICKEN

Item	Amount									Exchanges
Breast	1	400	24	54	6	135	1116	16	1	29	1 starch, 3 lean meat, 3 fat
✔Drumstick	1	140	9	58	2	75	422	4	0	13	2 lean meat, 1/2 fat

✔ = Healthiest Bets; n/a = not available

(Continued)

ORIGINAL RECIPE FRIED CHICKEN (*Continued*)	Amount	Cal.	Fat (g)	% Cal. Fat	Sat. Fat (g)	Chol. (mg)	Sod. (mg)	Carb. (g)	Fiber (g)	Pro. (g)	Servings/Exchanges
✔Thigh	1	250	18	65	4.5	95	747	6	1	16	1/2 starch, 2 lean meat, 2 fat
✔Whole Wing	1	140	10	64	2.5	55	414	5	0	9	1 medium-fat meat, 1 fat
OTHER ENTREES											
Chunky Chicken Pot Pie (seasonal entree)	1	770	42	49	13	70	2160	69	5	29	4 starch, 1 veg., 2 lean meat, 7 fat
Hot Wings (6)	1 order	471	33	63	8	150	1230	18	2	27	1 carb, 3 medium-fat meat, 3 1/2 fat
Original Recipe Chicken Sandwich	1	497	22	40	4.8	52	1213	46	3	29	3 starch, 3 lean meat, 2 1/2 fat
✔Value BBQ Flavored Chicken Sandwich	1	256	8	28	1	57	782	28	2	17	2 carb, 2 lean meat

SIDES

	Amount	Calories									Exchanges/Choices
✔ BBQ Baked Beans	5.5 oz	190	3	14	1	5	760	33	6	6	1 starch, 1 carb., 1/2 fat
✔ Biscuit	1	180	10	50	2.5	0	560	20	0	4	1 starch, 2 fat
Cole Slaw	5.0 oz	180	9	45	1.5	5	280	21	3	2	1 carb., 1 veg., 2 fat
Cornbread	1 piece	228	13	51	2	42	194	25	1	3	1 1/2 starch, 2 1/2 fat
✔ Corn on the Cob (1)	5.7 oz	150	2	12	0	0	20	35	2	5	2 starch
✔ Green Beans	4.7 oz	45	2	40	0.5	5	730	7	3	1	1 veg.
Macaroni & Cheese	5.4 oz	180	8	40	3	10	860	21	2	7	1 1/2 starch, 1 1/2 fat
Mashed Potatoes with Gravy	4.8 oz	120	6	45	1	1	440	17	2	1	1 starch, 1 fat
✔ Mean Greens	5.4 oz	70	3	39	1	10	650	11	5	4	2 veg., 1/2 fat
Potato Salad	5.6 oz	230	14	55	2	15	540	23	3	4	1 1/2 starch, 3 fat
Potato Wedges	4.8 oz	280	13	42	4	5	750	28	5	5	2 starch, 2 1/2 fat

(Continued)

✔ = Healthiest Bets; n/a = not available

TENDER ROAST CHICKEN

	Amount	Cal.	Fat (g)	% Cal. Fat	Sat. Fat (g)	Chol. (mg)	Sod. (mg)	Carb. (g)	Fiber (g)	Pro. (g)	Servings/Exchanges
✔ Breast, with skin	1	251	11	39	3	151	830	1	0	37	5 lean meat
✔ Breast, without skin	1	169	4	21	1.2	112	797	1	0	31	5 very lean meat
✔ Drumstick, with skin	1	97	4	37	1.2	85	271	1	0	15	2 lean meat
✔ Drumstick, without skin	1	67	2	27	0.7	63	259	1	0	11	2 very lean meat
✔ Thigh, with skin	1	207	12	52	3.8	120	504	2	0	18	3 lean meat, 1/2 fat
✔ Thigh, without skin	1	106	6	51	1.7	84	312	1	0	13	2 lean meat
✔ Wing, with skin	1	121	8	60	2.1	74	331	1	0	12	2 lean meat

✔ = Healthiest Bets; n/a = not available

Notes

Koo Koo Roo

❖Koo Koo Roo provides nutrition information for all its menu items in a brochure.

Light 'n Lean Choice

Chicken Chili
Cucumber Salad
Santa Fe Pasta
Lahvash

Calories......................428	Sodium (mg).............913
Fat (g) 8	Carbohydrate (g)........ 67
% calories from fat..17	Fiber (g).................n/a
Saturated fat (g)........1	Protein (g) 25
Cholesterol (mg) 30	

Exchanges: 4 starch, 1 veg., 2 lean meat

Healthy 'n Hearty Choice

Original Leg & Thigh
Homemade Stuffing
Butternut Squash
Koo Koo Slaw
Cranberry Sauce
Gravy (*4 Tbsp*)

Calories......................573	Sodium (mg)..........1,228
Fat (g) 20	Carbohydrate (g)........ 73
% calories from fat..31	Fiber (g).................n/a
Saturated fat (g)........7	Protein (g) 31
Cholesterol (mg) 81	

Exchanges: 3 starch, 2 veg., 1 carb., 3 very lean meat, 3 fat

(*Continued*)

Koo Koo Roo

	Amount	Cal.	Fat (g)	% Cal. Fat	Sat. Fat (g)	Chol. (mg)	Sod. (mg)	Carb. (g)	Fiber (g)	Pro. (g)	Servings/Exchanges
COLD SIDE DISHES											
✔Cucumber Salad	4.5 oz	30	0	0	0	0	109	7	n/a	1	1 veg.
✔Koo Koo Slaw	4 oz	55	2	33	0	0	230	10	n/a	1	2 veg.
✔Lentil Salad	4.5 oz	175	5	26	1	16	273	24	n/a	11	1 1/2 starch, 1 lean meat
✔Tangy Tomato Salad	5.5 oz	56	3	48	0	0	425	7	n/a	1	1 veg. 1/2 fat
EXTRAS											
✔Cranberry Sauce	1 oz	45	0	0	0	0	14	11	n/a	0	1 carb.
✔Gravy	2 oz	24	1	38	0	0	312	3	n/a	1	free
✔Lahvash (flatbread)	1 piece	94	0	0	0	0	143	20	n/a	4	1 starch
✔Roll	1/2	107	1	8	0	0	191	21	n/a	4	1 1/2 starch

FRESH ROASTED CARVED TURKEY

	Amount	Cal.	Fat (g)	% Fat Cal.	Sat. Fat (g)	Chol. (mg)	Sod. (mg)	Carb. (g)	Fiber (g)	Pro. (g)	Choices/Exchanges
✓1/2 Turkey Breast Sandwich	1	269	4	13	0	58	400	34	n/a	25	2 starch, 3 very lean meat
✓1/4-lb. Sliced Dark Meat	4 oz	212	8	34	3	96	89	0	n/a	32	5 very lean meat, 1/2 fat
✓1/4-lb. Sliced White Meat	4 oz	153	1	6	0	95	59	0	n/a	34	5 very lean meat
Hand Carved Turkey Dinner*	1	705	21	27	10	161	1421	76	n/a	53	5 starch, 5 lean meat, 1 fat
Open Faced Turkey Sandwich*	1	672	21	28	10	161	1394	69	n/a	51	4 1/2 starch, 5 lean meat, 1 fat
✓Turkey Breast Sandwich	1	538	7	12	0	118	800	68	n/a	49	4 1/2 starch, 5 very lean meat

HOT SIDE DISHES

	Amount	Cal.	Fat (g)	% Fat Cal.	Sat. Fat (g)	Chol. (mg)	Sod. (mg)	Carb. (g)	Fiber (g)	Pro. (g)	Choices/Exchanges
✓Artichokes	1/2	33	0	0	0	0	250	8	n/a	2	1 veg.
✓Asparagus	8 spears	24	0	0	0	0	5	4	n/a	3	1 veg.

✓ = Healthiest Bets; n/a = not available

(Continued)

HOT SIDE DISHES (*Continued*)	Amount	Cal.	Fat (g)	% Cal. Fat	Sat. Fat (g)	Chol. (mg)	Sod. (mg)	Carb. (g)	Fiber (g)	Pro. (g)	Servings/Exchanges
✔Baby Carrots	4.25 oz	73	0	0	0.5	0	173	18	n/a	1	3 veg.
Baked Yams	11 oz	362	0	0	0	0	25	86	n/a	5	5 1/2 starch
BBQ Beans	4.6 oz	139	2	13	0	0	505	28	n/a	5	2 starch
Black Beans	4 oz	139	2	13	0	0	567	23	n/a	8	1 1/2 starch
✔Brussels Sprouts	5 pieces	49	0	0	0	0	177	10	n/a	4	2 veg.
✔Butternut Squash	5.5 oz	87	0	0	0	0	7	23	n/a	2	1 1/2 starch
✔Confetti Rice	4.5 oz	131	0	0	0	0	166	29	n/a	3	2 starch
✔Cracked Wheat Rice	3.5 oz	97	1	9	0	0	140	21	n/a	3	1 1/2 starch
Creamed Spinach	4.5 oz	141	12	77	6	38	396	9	n/a	3	2 veg., 2 fat
✔Green Beans	3.5 oz	50	2	36	1	6	130	7	n/a	2	1 veg.
✔Hand-Mashed Potatoes	6.5 oz	185	5	24	3	15	362	32	n/a	3	2 starch, 1 fat
Homemade Stuffing	4 oz	189	9	43	5	27	613	23	n/a	6	1 1/2 starch, 2 fat

✔Hot Potatoes	4 oz	115	3	23	1	3	118	21	n/a	2	1 1/2 starch, 1/2 fat
✔Italian Vegetables	4.25 oz	36	2	50	1	5	123	4	n/a	1	1 veg.
✔Kernel Corn	4.25 oz	97	0	0	0	0	200	25	n/a	4	1 1/2 starch
Macaroni & Cheese	5.7 oz	270	11	37	6	31	243	28	n/a	11	2 starch, 2 fat
✔Roasted Garlic Potatoes	4 oz	116	2	16	1	3	163	22	n/a	2	1 1/2 starch
✔Steamed Vegetables	3.75 oz	33	0	0	0	0	27	7	n/a	2	1 veg.
ORIGINAL SKINLESS FLAME BROILED CHICKEN											
✔Original Breast Meat	3.4 oz	159	4	23	1	23	400	2	n/a	28	4 very lean meat
Half Original Chicken (wing has skin)	1	391	16	37	4	81	859	6	n/a	55	8 very lean meat, 1 1/2 fat
✔Original Breast & Wing (wing has skin)	1	218	8	33	2	27	495	3	n/a	34	5 very lean meat, 1/2 fat

(Continued)

✔ = Healthiest Bets; n/a = not available

ORIGINAL SKINLESS FLAME BROILED CHICKEN (Continued)	Amount	Cal.	Fat (g)	% Cal. Fat	Sat. Fat (g)	Chol. (mg)	Sod. (mg)	Carb. (g)	Fiber (g)	Pro. (g)	Servings/Exchanges
✓Original Leg & Thigh	1	173	8	45	2	54	364	3	n/a	21	3 very lean meat, 1 fat
PASTA SALADS											
✓Pesto Pasta	4 oz	168	5	27	1	16	251	21	n/a	10	1 1/2 starch, 1 fat
Santa Fe Pasta	5 oz	206	6	26	1	19	327	27	n/a	12	2 starch, 1 medium-fat meat
✓Tomato Basil Pasta	4 oz	108	2	17	0	0	223	19	n/a	3	1 starch
ROTISSERIE CHICKEN											
Half Rotisserie Chicken	1	655	34	47	9	254	1188	2	n/a	80	9 lean meat, 1 fat
✓Rotisserie Breast & Wing	1	355	16	41	4	140	675	1	n/a	49	7 very lean meat, 2 fat
✓Rotisserie Leg & Thigh	1	300	18	54	5	114	513	1	n/a	31	4 lean meat, 1 fat
SALAD DRESSING											
✓Chopped Salad Dressing	2 Tbsp	100	7	63	5	0	350	8	n/a	0	1 veg, 1 fat

	Amount	Cal.	Fat (g)	% Fat Cal.	Sat. Fat (g)	Chol. (mg)	Sod. (mg)	Carb. (g)	Fiber (g)	Prot. (g)	Exchanges/Choices
✓ Balsamic Vinaigrette	2 Tbsp	90	9	90	1	0	240	3	n/a	0	2 fat
✓ BBQ Dressing	2 Tbsp	40	0	0	0	0	280	10	n/a	0	1/2 carb.
Caesar Dressing	2 Tbsp	160	18	100	4	14	180	1	n/a	0	3 1/2 fat
✓ Chinese Chicken Salad Dressing	2 Tbsp	110	8	65	2	0	110	8	n/a	0	1/2 carb., 1 1/2 fat

SALADS (REGULAR SIZE, NO DRESSING)

	Amount	Cal.	Fat (g)	% Fat Cal.	Sat. Fat (g)	Chol. (mg)	Sod. (mg)	Carb. (g)	Fiber (g)	Prot. (g)	Exchanges/Choices
✓ 12 Vegetable Chopped Salad	1	78	1	12	0	0	65	16	n/a	5	3 veg.
✓ BBQ Chicken Salad	1	466	21	41	8	121	738	30	n/a	40	6 veg., 4 lean meat, 2 fat
✓ Caesar Salad	1	170	8	42	4	11	483	16	n/a	10	3 veg., 1 1/2 fat
✓ Chicken Caesar Salad	1	310	11	32	4	83	545	16	n/a	36	3 veg., 4 lean meat
✓ Chinese Chicken Salad	1	296	8	24	2	71	169	23	n/a	31	4 veg., 3 lean meat
✓ Koo Koo Roo House Salad	1	164	6	33	2	7	360	21	n/a	9	4 veg., 1 fat

SANDWICHES

	Amount	Cal.	Fat (g)	% Fat Cal.	Sat. Fat (g)	Chol. (mg)	Sod. (mg)	Carb. (g)	Fiber (g)	Prot. (g)	Exchanges/Choices
BBQ Chicken Sandwich	1	568	14	22	7	115	1542	69	n/a	43	4 1/2 starch, 4 lean meat

(Continued)

✓ = Healthiest Bets; n/a = not available

SANDWICHES (*Continued*)	Amount	Cal.	Fat (g)	% Cal. Fat	Sat. Fat (g)	Chol. (mg)	Sod. (mg)	Carb. (g)	Fiber (g)	Pro. (g)	Servings/Exchanges
Chicken Caesar Sandwich	1	728	37	46	12	144	2137	49	n/a	51	3 starch, 6 lean meat, 4 fat
Original Chicken Breast Sandwich	1	752	47	56	9	128	1076	50	n/a	35	3 starch, 4 lean meat, 7 fat
SOUPS											
✔Chicken Chili	4 oz	98	2	18	0	11	334	13	n/a	8	1 starch, 1 very lean meat
✔Ten Vegetable Soup	8 oz	121	3	22	0	0	620	21	n/a	3	1 starch, 1 veg., 1/2 fat
✔Turkey Dumpling Soup	8 oz	166	4	22	1	54	890	14	n/a	19	1 starch, 2 lean meat

✔ = Healthiest Bets; n/a = not available

*Hand Carved Turkey Dinner includes mashed potatoes, stuffing, gravy, steamed vegetables, and cranberry sauce. Open Faced Turkey Sandwich includes mashed potatoes, stuffing, gravy, and cranberry sauce.

Notes

Popeye's Chicken & Biscuits

❖Popeye's Chicken & Biscuits provided nutrition information for all its menu items.

Light 'n Lean Choice

Spicy Leg (*fried*)
Cajun Rice
Corn on the Cob

Calories......................397	Sodium (mg)..........1,520
Fat (g) 15	Carbohydrate (g).........42
% calories from fat..34	Fiber (g) 12
Saturated fat (g) ....n/a	Protein (g) 24
Cholesterol (mg) 65	

Exchanges: 2 starch, 3 lean meat, 1/2 fat

Healthy 'n Hearty Choice

Mild Breast (*fried*)
Cajun Rice
Corn on the Cob
Apple Pie (*split*)

Calories......................692	Sodium (mg)..........2,280
Fat (g) 32	Carbohydrate (g).........65
% calories from fat..41	Fiber (g) 15
Saturated fat (g) ....n/a	Protein (g) 38
Cholesterol (mg) 90	

Exchanges: 3 starch, 1/2 carb., 3 medium-fat meat, 3 1/2 fat

(*Continued*)

Popeye's Chicken & Biscuits

	Amount	Cal.	Fat (g)	% Cal. Fat	Sat. Fat (g)	Chol. (mg)	Sod. (mg)	Carb. (g)	Fiber (g)	Pro. (g)	Servings/Exchanges
DESSERT											
Apple Pie	1 slice	290	16	50	n/a	10	820	37	2	3	2 1/2 carb., 3 fat
FRIED CHICKEN											
✔Mild Breast	1	270	16	53	n/a	60	660	9	2	23	1/2 carb, 3 lean meat, 1 fat
✔Mild Leg	1	120	7	53	n/a	40	240	4	0	10	1 medium-fat meat, 1 fat
Mild Thigh	1	300	23	69	n/a	70	620	9	0	15	1/2 starch, 2 medium-fat meat, 2 1/2 fat
✔Mild Wing	1	160	11	62	n/a	40	290	7	0	9	1/2 starch, 1 medium-fat meat, 1 fat
✔Spicy Breast	1	270	16	53	n/a	60	590	9	2	23	1/2 carb, 3 lean meat, 1 fat

✔Spicy Leg	1	120	7	53	n/a	40	240	4	0	10	1 lean meat, 1 fat
Spicy Thigh	1	300	23	69	n/a	70	450	9	0	15	1/2 carb., 2 medium-fat meat, 2 1/2 fat
✔Spicy Wing	1	160	11	62	n/a	40	290	7	0	9	1/2 carb., 1 medium-fat meat, 1 fat

OTHER ENTREE ITEMS

✔Mild Tender (fried chicken strip)	1 strip	110	7	57	n/a	15	160	6	0	6	1/2 starch, 1 lean meat, 1 fat
Nuggets (fried chicken)	1 order	410	32	70	n/a	55	660	18	3	17	1 starch, 2 lean meat, 5 fat
✔Shrimp (fried)	1 order	250	16	58	n/a	110	650	13	3	16	1 starch, 2 very lean meat, 3 fat
✔Spicy Tender (fried chicken strip)	1 strip	110	7	57	n/a	15	215	6	0	6	1/2 carb., 1 lean meat, 1 fat

✔ = Healthiest Bets; n/a = not available

(Continued)

SIDES

	Amount	Cal.	Fat (g)	% Cal. Fat	Sat. Fat (g)	Chol. (mg)	Sod. (mg)	Carb. (g)	Fiber (g)	Pro. (g)	Servings/Exchanges
Biscuits	1	250	15	54	n/a	5	430	26	1	4	1 1/2 starch, 3 fat
✓Cajun Rice	3.9 oz	150	5	30	n/a	25	1260	17	3	10	1 starch, 1 lean meat
Cole Slaw	4.0 oz	149	11	66	n/a	3	271	14	3	1	1/2 carb., 1 veg., 2 fat
✓Corn on the Cob	5.2 oz	127	3	21	n/a	0	20	21	9	4	1 1/2 starch, 1/2 fat
French Fries	3.0 oz	240	12	45	n/a	10	610	31	3	4	2 starch, 2 fat
Onion Rings	3.1 oz	310	19	55	n/a	25	210	31	2	5	2 starch, 4 fat
Potatoes & Gravy	3.8 oz	100	6	54	n/a	5	460	11	3	5	1/2 starch, 1 fat
Red Beans & Rice	5.9 oz	270	17	57	n/a	10	680	30	7	8	2 starch, 1 lean meat, 3 fat

✓ = Healthiest Bets; n/a = not available

Seafood Catches

RESTAURANTS

Captain D's

Long John Silver's

NUTRITION PROS

- When fish and seafood are prepared with little fat, fish is low in total and saturated fat and low in calories.
- During the years of nutrition and health consciousness, some fast-food restaurants learned how to bake, broil, or grill seafood.
- Some healthy sides are available: baked potatoes, rice, salad, and cooked vegetables.

NUTRITION CONS

- The nutritional virtues of fish and seafood are lost in most chain seafood restaurants because their favorite preparation method is frying.
- After fish and seafood has been battered and fried, you wonder what happened to the fish. When you read the nutrition numbers, there's not much fish to speak of.
- Fried fish is often surrounded by high-fat plate fillers—hush puppies, french fries, or creamy coleslaw. Thus, the once healthy seafood is now part of a fat- and calorie-dense meal.
- Seafood restaurants load their starches—hush puppies, biscuits, cornbread, french fries, etc.—with fat.
- Fruit is nowhere to be found.

Healthy Tips

★ If you order a baked potato, have butter and sour cream held or served on the side.
★ Lemon is plentiful. Use it to add flavor without calories.
★ Use low-fat, low-calorie cocktail sauce to add flavor without extra calories.
★ Not all coleslaw is created equal. Some is high in fat, and some is relatively low. Check the nutrition numbers to know the score in the restaurant you choose.

Get It Your Way

★ Hold the tartar sauce and opt for lemon or vinegar.
★ Substitute a baked potato or rice for french fries or hush puppies.
★ Substitute a cooked vegetable, such as green beans or corn, for french fries.
★ Substitute breadsticks or a yeast roll for biscuits or corn bread if you have an option.

Captain D's

❖Captain D's provides nutrition information for most of its menu items in a brochure. Additional nutrition information was provided for this book.

Light 'n Lean Choice

Broiled Fish & Chicken Lunch
(*with rice, vegetable medley, and breadstick*)

Calories......................478	Sodium (mg)..............n/a
Fat (g) 8	Carbohydrate (g) ....n/a
% calories from fat..15	Fiber (g) ....n/a
Saturated fat (g)........1	Protein (g) 34
Cholesterol (mg) 66	

Exchanges: insufficient information to calculate

Healthy 'n Hearty Choice

Broiled Shrimp Platter
(*with rice, vegetable medley, baked potato, salad with low-fat Italian dressing, and breadstick*)

Calories......................753	Sodium (mg)..............n/a
Fat (g) 8	Carbohydrate (g) ....n/a
% calories from fat..10	Fiber (g) ....n/a
Saturated fat (g)........1	Protein (g) 32
Cholesterol (mg) 155	

Exchanges: insufficient information to calculate

(*Continued*)

Captain D's

BROILED MEALS*

	Amount	Cal.	Fat (g)	% Cal. Fat	Sat. Fat (g)	Chol. (mg)	Sod. (mg)	Carb. (g)	Fiber (g)	Pro. (g)	Servings/Exchanges
Broiled Chicken Lunch	1	503	9	16	2	82	n/a	n/a	n/a	39	insufficient info. to calculate
Broiled Chicken Platter	1	802	10	11	2	82	n/a	n/a	n/a	46	insufficient info. to calculate
Broiled Fish & Chicken Lunch	1	478	8	15	1	66	n/a	n/a	n/a	34	insufficient info. to calculate
Broiled Fish & Chicken Platter	1	777	10	12	1	66	n/a	n/a	n/a	41	insufficient info. to calculate
Broiled Fish Lunch	1	435	7	14	1	49	n/a	n/a	n/a	28	insufficient info. to calculate
Broiled Fish Platter	1	734	7	9	1	49	n/a	n/a	n/a	36	insufficient info. to calculate
Broiled Shrimp Lunch	1	421	7	15	1	155	n/a	n/a	n/a	25	insufficient info. to calculate
Broiled Shrimp Platter	1	720	8	10	1	155	n/a	n/a	n/a	32	insufficient info. to calculate

CONDIMENTS

✓Cocktail Sauce	1 oz/2 Tbsp	34	0	0	n/a	0	252	8	0	1/2 carb.
Imitation Sour Cream	n/a	29	3	93	3	0	n/a	n/a	0	insufficient info. to calculate
✓Sweet & Sour Sauce	1.8 oz	52	0	0	n/a	0	5	13	0	1 carb.
✓Tartar Sauce	1 oz/2 Tbsp	75	7	84	n/a	10	158	3	0	1 fat

DESSERTS

Cheesecake	1 slice	420	31	66	n/a	141	480	30	7	2 carb, 6 fat
✓Chocolate Cake	1 slice	303	10	30	n/a	20	259	49	4	3 carb, 2 fat
Pecan Pie	1 slice	458	20	39	n/a	4	373	64	5	4 carb, 4 fat

SALAD DRESSINGS

French (fat free)	1 oz/2 Tbsp	111	11	89	n/a	7	187	4	0	2 fat
Italian (fat free)	1 oz/2 Tbsp	33	0	0	n/a	0	1579	6	1	1/2 carb.
✓Ranch	1 oz/2 Tbsp	92	10	98	n/a	15	230	0	0	2 fat

✓ = Healthiest Bets; n/a = not available

(Continued)

	Amount	Cal.	Fat (g)	% Cal. Fat	Sat. Fat (g)	Chol. (mg)	Sod. (mg)	Carb. (g)	Fiber (g)	Pro. (g)	Servings/Exchanges
SALADS											
Blackened Chicken Salad	1	314	9	26	n/a	n/a	n/a	n/a	n/a	n/a	insufficient info. to calculate
Seafood Salad	1	308	8	23	n/a	n/a	n/a	n/a	n/a	n/a	insufficient info. to calculate
SANDWICHES											
✔Broiled Chicken Sandwich	1	451	19	37	n/a	105	858	29	n/a	40	2 starch, 7 lean meat
SIDES											
Baked Potato	1	278	0	0	0	0	n/a	n/a	n/a	6	insufficient info. to calculate
Breadstick	1	113	4	32	0	0	n/a	n/a	n/a	3	insufficient info. to calculate
Cole Slaw	4 oz	158	12	68	n/a	16	246	12	2	3	1 veg., 1/2 carb., 2 fat
✔Corn on the Cob	1	251	2	7	n/a	0	13	60	n/a	9	4 starch
✔Crackers	4	50	1	18	n/a	3	147	8	0	1	1/2 starch
Cracklins	1 oz	218	17	70	n/a	0	741	16	0	1	1 starch, 3 fat

✓French Fried Potatoes	1 order	302	10	30	n/a	0	152	50	0	3	3 starch, 2 fat
Fried Okra	4 oz	300	16	48	n/a	0	445	34	0	7	2 starch, 3 fat
Green Beans (seasoned)	4 oz	46	2	39	n/a	4	752	5	1	2	1 veg.
Hushpuppies (6)	1 order	756	25	29	n/a	0	2790	119	1	13	8 starch, 5 fat
✓Rice	4 oz	124	0	0	n/a	0	9	28	1	3	2 starch
Rice (included w/ Broiled Meal)	n/a	184	0	0	0	0	n/a	n/a	n/a	1	insufficient info. to calculate
Salad	n/a	20	0	0	0	0	n/a	n/a	n/a	1	insufficient info. to calculate
Vegetable Medley (included w/ Broiled Meal)	n/a	36	1	25	0	0	n/a	n/a	n/a	1	insufficient info. to calculate

✓ = Healthiest Bets; n/a = not available

*Broiled Lunches include rice, vegetable medley, and breadstick. Broiled Platters include rice, vegetable medley, baked potato, salad, and breadstick.

Long John Silver's

❖Long John Silver's provides nutrition information for most of its menu items in a brochure. Additional nutrition information was provided for this book.

Light 'n Lean Choice

Flavorbaked Chicken (*1 piece*)
Rice Pilaf
Corn Cobbette (*without butter*), **Coleslaw**

Calories......................470	Sodium (mg)..........1,070
Fat (g) 13	Carbohydrate (g).........65
% calories from fat..25	Fiber (g) 3
Saturated fat (g)........2	Protein (g) 26
Cholesterol (mg).........55	

Exchanges: 3 starch, 3 veg., 1/2 carb., 4 very lean meat, 1 fat

Healthy 'n Hearty Choice

Flavorbaked Fish (*2 pieces*)
Baked Potato (*with 2 Tbsp sour cream*)
Green Beans, Coleslaw

Calories......................620	Sodium (mg)..........1,235
Fat (g) 18	Carbohydrate (g).........77
% calories from fat..26	Fiber (g) 8
Saturated fat (g).....5.5	Protein (g) 35
Cholesterol (mg).........85	

Exchanges: 3 starch, 2 veg., 1/2 carb., 3 very lean meat, 1 fat

Long John Silver's

	Amount	Cal.	Fat (g)	% Cal. Fat	Sat. Fat (g)	Chol. (mg)	Sod. (mg)	Carb. (g)	Fiber (g)	Pro. (g)	Servings/Exchanges
CHICKEN WRAPS											
Cajun (regular)	1	720	35	44	7	25	1860	83	5	18	5 1/2 starch, 1 lean meat, 6 fat
Classic (regular)	1	730	36	44	7	25	1780	83	5	18	5 1/2 starch, 1 lean meat, 6 1/2 fat
Ranch (regular)	1	730	36	44	7	25	1810	82	5	18	5 1/2 starch, 1 lean meat, 6 1/2 fat
CONDIMENTS											
✔Honey Mustard Sauce	0.42 oz	20	0	0	0	0	60	5	0	0	free
✔Shrimp Sauce	0.42 oz	15	0	0	0	0	180	3	0	0	free

(Continued)

✔ = Healthiest Bets; n/a = not available

CONDIMENTS (Continued)	Amount	Cal.	Fat (g)	% Cal. Fat	Sat. Fat (g)	Chol. (mg)	Sod. (mg)	Carb. (g)	Fiber (g)	Pro. (g)	Servings/Exchanges
✓Sour Cream	1 oz/2 Tbsp	60	6	90	3.5	15	15	1	0	0	1 fat
✓Sweet 'N' Sour Sauce	0.42 oz	20	0	0	0	0	45	5	0	0	free
✓Tartar Sauce	0.42 oz	35	2	51	n/a	0	35	5	0	0	free
DESSERTS											
Key Lime Cream Cheese Pie	1 slice	310	19	55	11	20	n/a	n/a	n/a	n/a	insufficient info. to calculate
FISH											
Lemon Crumb	1	195	2	9	n/a	145	635	10	n/a	35	1/2 starch, 5 very lean meat
FISH WRAPS											
Ranch (regular)	1	730	36	44	8	30	1760	85	5	18	5 1/2 starch, 1 lean meat, 6 1/2 fat
FLAVORBAKED ITEMS											
✓Chicken	1 piece	110	3	25	1	55	600	0	0	19	3 very lean meat

	Amount										Exchanges
✓Fish	1 piece	90	3	26	1	35	320	1	0	14	2 very lean meat

FRIED ITEMS

	Amount										Exchanges
✓Batter-Dipped Chicken	1 piece	120	6	45	1.5	15	400	11	3	8	1 starch, 1 lean meat, 1/2 fat
✓Batter-Dipped Fish	1 piece	170	11	58	2.5	30	470	12	5	11	1 starch, 1 lean meat, 1 1/2 fat
✓Batter-Dipped Shrimp	1 piece	35	3	57	0.5	10	95	2	0	1	1/2 fat
Clams	1 order	300	17	51	4	40	670	31	5	11	2 starch, 1 lean meat, 3 fat
Popcorn Chicken Munchers	1 order	380	23	54	4	35	1030	20	2	23	1 1/2 starch, 3 lean meat, 3 fat
Popcorn Shrimp Munchers	1 order	320	15	42	2.5	85	1440	33	1	15	2 starch, 1 lean meat, 2 fat

GRAB N GO SANDWICHES

	Amount										Exchanges
✓Battered Chicken	1	320	12	34	3	20	850	41	4	14	3 starch, 1 lean meat, 2 fat
Battered Chicken w/ Cheese	1	370	17	41	8	35	1090	41	4	17	3 starch, 1 lean meat, 2 1/2 fat
✓Battered Fish	1	300	11	33	2.5	20	770	39	2	11	2 1/2 starch, 1 lean meat, 1 1/2 fat

(Continued)

✓ = Healthiest Bets; n/a = not available

GRAB N GO SANDWICHES (Continued)	Amount	Cal.	Fat (g)	% Cal. Fat	Sat. Fat (g)	Chol. (mg)	Sod. (mg)	Carb. (g)	Fiber (g)	Pro. (g)	Servings/Exchanges
Battered Fish w/ Cheese	1	350	16	41	8	35	1010	39	2	14	2 1/2 starch, 1 lean meat, 2 1/2 fat
POPCORN SHRIMP WRAPS											
Cajun (regular)	1	720	35	44	9	50	1830	86	5	16	5 1/2 starch, 1 lean meat, 6 fat
Classic (regular)	1	730	36	44	9	45	1750	86	5	16	5 1/2 starch, 1 lean meat, 6 1/2 fat
Ranch (regular)	1	720	35	44	9	50	1830	86	5	16	5 1/2 starch, 1 lean meat, 6 1/2 fat
SALAD DRESSINGS											
✓Fat-Free French	1.5 oz/3 Tbsp	50	0	0	0	0	360	14	n/a	0	1 carb.
✓Fat-Free Ranch	1.5 oz/3 Tbsp	50	0	0	0	0	380	13	n/a	2	1 carb.
Italian	1 oz/2 Tbsp	130	14	97	2	0	280	2	n/a	0	3 fat
Ranch	1 oz/2 Tbsp	170	18	95	3	5	260	1	n/a	0	3 1/2 fat

Thousand Island	1 oz/2 Tbsp	110	10	82	2	15	280	5	n/a	0	2 fat

SALADS

Garden	1	45	0	0	0	0	25	9	4	3	2 veg.
Grilled Chicken	1	140	3	19	0.5	45	260	10	4	20	2 veg., 2 very lean meat
Ocean Chef	1	130	2	14	0	60	540	15	4	14	3 veg., 2 very lean meat

SANDWICHES

✔Battered Fish (w/o sauce)	1	320	13	37	3.5	30	800	40	6	17	2 1/2 starch, 1 very lean meat, 2 fat
Ultimate Fish	1	430	21	44	7	35	1340	44	3	18	3 starch, 1 very lean meat, 4 fat

SIDES

✔Baked Potato	1	210	0	0	0	0	10	49	3	4	3 starch
✔Cheese Sticks	1 order	160	9	51	4	10	360	12	0	6	1 starch, 2 fat

✔ = Healthiest Bets; n/a = not available

(Continued)

SIDES (Continued)	Amount	Cal.	Fat (g)	% Cal. Fat	Sat. Fat (g)	Chol. (mg)	Sod. (mg)	Carb. (g)	Fiber (g)	Pro. (g)	Servings/Exchanges
✔Coleslaw	3.4 oz	140	6	39	n/a	0	260	20	3	1	2 veg., 1/2 carb., 1 fat
Corn Cobbette	3.3 oz	140	8	51	2	0	0	19	0	3	1 starch, 1 1/2 fat
✔Corn Cobbette (w/o butter)	3.05 oz	80	1	6	0	0	0	19	0	3	1 starch
French Fries (regular)	1 order	250	15	54	2.5	0	500	28	3	3	2 starch, 3 fat
French Fries (large)	1 order	420	24	51	4	0	830	46	4	5	3 starch, 5 fat
✔Green Beans	3.5 oz	30	1	16	0	0	310	5	2	2	1 veg.
Hushpuppy	1 piece	60	3	33	0	0	25	9	0	1	1 starch, 1/2 fat
✔Rice Pilaf	3 oz	140	3	19	1	0	210	26	0	3	2 starch, 1/2 fat
✔Side Salad	1	25	0	0	0	0	15	4	0	1	1 veg.
SOUPS											
Broccoli Cheese	8 oz	180	12	60	4.5	15	1240	13	2	5	1 carb, 2 fat

✔ = Healthiest Bets; n/a = not available

Subs and Sandwiches

RESTAURANTS

Arby's
Au Bon Pain
Blimpie
Subway

NUTRITION PROS

- Healthier sub and sandwich condiments, such as mustard and vinegar, are available. They keep your sub or sandwich moist without adding a lot of calories and fat.
- Subs and sandwiches are often made to order. That's good because you can specify what you want on and off your order.
- Healthy breads, even whole wheat with extra fiber, can hold the contents of your sub or sandwich.
- Healthy sub and sandwich fillers are available— turkey, smoked turkey, ham, chicken breast, or roast beef.
- Healthy broth-based vegetable and grain soups are warm and ready in some sandwich shops.
- Sub shops offer smaller-sized sandwiches. No need to order the foot-long size.
- Salads with light or fat-free salad dressings are an option in most sub and sandwich shops.

NUTRITION CONS

- Large sandwiches and long subs can be stuffed with enough protein for the whole day.

- Common sub and sandwich condiments, such as mayonnaise and oil, are high in fat.
- Tuna fish, chicken, and seafood salads sound healthy, but they are chock full of fat and calories.
- Cheese is a frequent sub or sandwich addition. Some restaurants give their nutrition information minus the cheese. Make sure you read the numbers for the way you eat yours.
- Fruit and cooked vegetables are rarely available.

Healthy Tips

- ★ To keep your sodium meter on low, go light on or hold the pickles and olives.
- ★ Complement a sub or sandwich with a healthier side than a fried snack food (potato chips, tortilla chips, and the like). For some crunch, try a side salad, popcorn, or pretzels.
- ★ Order a large sub. Ask your sandwich maker to cut it in two. Pack one half for another day.
- ★ In sandwich shops, order a cup of broth-based vegetable or bean soup to fill you up and not out.
- ★ In a sub shop, try a Greek salad and piece of pita bread for a high-carbohydrate and light-on-protein meal.
- ★ Pack a piece of fruit from home to bring to the sub or sandwich shop.

Get It Your Way

* ★ Hold the mayonnaise and oil. Substitute mustard or vinegar.
* ★ Ask the sub maker to go light on the meat and heavy on the lettuce, onions, tomatoes, and peppers.
* ★ Hold the cheese.
* ★ Ask for the salad dressing on the side.

Arby's

❖Arby's provides nutrition information for all of its menu items in a brochure.

Light 'n Lean Choice

Light Roast Beef Deluxe
Garden Salad
Reduced Calorie Buttermilk Ranch Dressing
(*2 Tbsp*)
Curly Fries (*split order*)

Calories......................532	Sodium (mg) 1,648
Fat (g) 16	Carbohydrate (g).........70
% calories from fat..27	Fiber (g) 11
Saturated fat (g)........5	Protein (g) 23
Cholesterol (mg) 42	

Exchanges: 3 starch, 2 veg., 1/2 carb., 2 medium-fat meat, 1 fat

Healthy 'n Hearty Choice

Broccoli 'n Cheddar Baked Potato
Garden Salad
Honey French Salad Dressing (*2 Tbsp*)

Calories......................772	Sodium (mg) 805
Fat (g) 32	Carbohydrate (g).......110
% calories from fat..37	Fiber (g) 14
Saturated fat (g)........7	Protein (g) 17
Cholesterol (mg) 12	

Exchanges: 6 starch, 2 veg., 1/2 carb., 3 1/2 fat

Arby's

	Amount	Cal.	Fat (g)	% Cal. Fat	Sat. Fat (g)	Chol. (mg)	Sod. (mg)	Carb. (g)	Fiber (g)	Pro. (g)	Servings/Exchanges
ARBY'S SUPER STUFFED BAKED POTATOES											
Chicken Broccoli	1	841	56	60	6	49	350	56	n/a	29	4 starch, 2 lean meat, 10 fat
Cool Ranch	1	480	25	47	7	25	190	56	n/a	8	4 starch, 5 fat
Jalapeno	1	640	38	53	13	48	970	61	n/a	15	4 starch, 7 1/2 fat
Philly Chicken	1	860	54	57	10	69	1060	64	n/a	32	4 starch, 3 lean meat, 9 fat
BEVERAGES											
✔ Hot Chocolate	8 oz	110	1	8	0.7	0	120	23	0	2	1 1/2 carb.
✔ Milk, 2%	8 oz	120	4	30	2.5	15	110	11	0	8	1 low-fat milk
✔ Orange Juice	6 oz	82	0	0	0	0	2	20	0	0	1 fruit

✔ = Healthiest Bets; n/a = not available

(Continued)

BREAKFAST

	Amount	Cal.	Fat (g)	% Cal. Fat	Sat. Fat (g)	Chol. (mg)	Sod. (mg)	Carb. (g)	Fiber (g)	Pro. (g)	Servings/Exchanges
✔Bacon	1 order	90	7	70	3	15	220	0	0	5	1 high-fat meat
Biscuit, plain	1	280	15	48	3	0	730	34	1	6	2 starch, 3 fat
✔Blueberry Muffin	1	230	9	35	2	25	290	35	0	2	2 starch, 2 fat
Cinnamon Nut Danish	1	360	11	28	1	0	105	60	1	6	4 carb., 2 fat
Croissant, plain	1	220	12	49	7	25	230	25	0	4	1 1/2 starch, 2 fat
Egg Portion	1	95	8	76	2	180	54	1	0	5	1 medium-fat meat, 1/2 fat
French-Toastix	1 order	430	21	44	5	0	550	52	3	10	3 1/2 carb., 4 fat
✔Ham	1 order	45	1	20	0.5	20	405	0	0	7	1 very lean meat
Sausage	1 order	163	15	83	6	25	321	0	0	7	1 high-fat meat, 1 fat

CONDIMENTS

	Amount	Cal.	Fat (g)	% Cal. Fat	Sat. Fat (g)	Chol. (mg)	Sod. (mg)	Carb. (g)	Fiber (g)	Pro. (g)	Servings/Exchanges
✔Arby's Sauce	0.5 oz/1 Tbsp	15	0	0	0	0	113	4	0	0	free

Item	Serving Size	Cal.	Fat (g)	% Fat Cal.	Sat. Fat (g)	Chol. (mg)	Sod. (mg)	Carb. (g)	Fiber (g)	Pro. (g)	Exchanges/Choices
✔ Barbeque Sauce	0.5 oz/1 Tbsp	30	0	0	0	0	185	7	0	0	1/2 carb.
✔ Cheddar Cheese Sauce	3/4 oz	35	3	77	1	4	139	1	0	1	1/2 fat
Horsey Sauce	0.5 oz/1 Tbsp	60	5	75	1	5	150	2	0	0	1 fat
✔ Table Syrup	1 oz/2 Tbsp	100	0	0	0	0	30	25	0	0	1 1/2 carb.

DESSERTS

Item	Serving Size	Cal.	Fat (g)	% Fat Cal.	Sat. Fat (g)	Chol. (mg)	Sod. (mg)	Carb. (g)	Fiber (g)	Pro. (g)	Exchanges/Choices
Apple Turnover	3.2 oz	330	14	38	7	0	180	48	0	4	3 carb., 3 fat
Cheesecake, plain	1	320	23	65	14	95	240	23	0	5	1 1/2 carb., 4 1/2 fat
Cherry Turnover	1	320	13	37	5	0	190	46	0	4	3 carb., 2 1/2 fat

MISCELLANEOUS

Item	Serving Size	Cal.	Fat (g)	% Fat Cal.	Sat. Fat (g)	Chol. (mg)	Sod. (mg)	Carb. (g)	Fiber (g)	Pro. (g)	Exchanges/Choices
Chicken Finger Snack (2 pieces with Curly Fries)	1 order	290	16	50	2	32	677	20	1	16	1 1/2 starch, 2 medium-fat meat, 1 fat

SALAD DRESSINGS

Item	Serving Size	Cal.	Fat (g)	% Fat Cal.	Sat. Fat (g)	Chol. (mg)	Sod. (mg)	Carb. (g)	Fiber (g)	Pro. (g)	Exchanges/Choices
Blue Cheese	2 oz/4 Tbsp	290	31	96	6	50	580	2	0	2	6 fat

(Continued)

✔ = Healthiest Bets; n/a = not available

SALAD DRESSINGS (Continued)	Amount	Cal.	Fat (g)	% Cal. Fat	Sat. Fat (g)	Chol. (mg)	Sod. (mg)	Carb. (g)	Fiber (g)	Pro. (g)	Servings/Exchanges
Honey French	2 oz/4 Tbsp	280	23	74	3	0	400	18	0	0	1 carb., 4 1/2 fat
✔ Reduced Calorie Buttermilk Ranch	2 oz/4 Tbsp	50	0	0	0	0	710	12	0	0	1 carb.
✔ Reduced Calorie Italian	2 oz/4 Tbsp	20	1	45	0	0	1000	3	0	0	free
Thousand Island	2 oz/4 Tbsp	260	26	90	4	30	420	7	0	0	1/2 carb., 5 fat
SALADS											
✔ Garden	1	61	1	8	0	0	40	12	5	3	2 veg.
✔ Roast Chicken	1	149	2	12	0.5	29	418	12	5	20	2 veg., 3 very lean meat
✔ Side	1	23	0	0	0	0	15	4	2	1	1 veg.
SANDWICHES, CHICKEN & FISH											
Breaded Chicken Fillet	1	536	28	47	5	45	1016	46	5	28	3 starch, 3 medium-fat meat, 2 1/2 fat

Chicken Bacon and Swiss	1	590	29	44	8	60	1550	50	5	35	2 starch, 4 lean meat, 3 fat
Chicken Cordon Bleu	1	623	33	48	8	77	1594	46	5	38	3 starch, 4 lean meat, 4 fat
Fish Fillet (seasonal for Lent)	1	529	27	46	7	43	864	50	2	23	3 starch, 2 medium-fat meat, 3 fat
✔Grilled Chicken Deluxe	1	430	20	42	4	61	848	41	3	23	3 starch, 2 medium-fat meat, 2 fat
Roast Chicken Club	1	546	31	51	9	58	1103	37	2	31	2 1/2 starch, 3 medium-fat meat, 3 fat

SANDWICHES, LIGHT MENU

✔Roast Beef Deluxe	1	296	10	30	3	42	826	33	6	18	2 starch, 2 medium-fat meat
✔Roast Chicken Deluxe	1	276	6	20	2	33	777	33	4	20	2 starch, 2 lean meat

(Continued)

✔ = Healthiest Bets; n/a = not available

SANDWICHES, LIGHT MENU (*Continued*)	Amount	Cal.	Fat (g)	% Cal. Fat	Sat. Fat (g)	Chol. (mg)	Sod. (mg)	Carb. (g)	Fiber (g)	Pro. (g)	Servings/Exchanges
Roast Chicken Santa Fe	1	300	9	45	3	40	820	30	3	25	2 starch, 3 medium-fat meat
Roast Turkey Deluxe	1	260	7	24	2	33	1262	33	4	20	2 starch, 2 lean meat
SANDWICHES, ROAST BEEF											
Arby Q	1	431	18	38	6	37	1321	48	3	20	3 starch, 2 medium-fat meat, 2 fat
✔Arby's Melt	1	368	18	44	6	31	937	36	2	18	2 starch, 2 medium-fat meat, 2 fat
Bac'n Cheddar Deluxe	1	539	34	57	10	44	1140	38	3	22	2 1/2 starch, 2 medium-fat meat, 5 fat
Beef 'n Cheddar	1	507	28	52	9	50	1216	40	2	25	2 1/2 starch, 3 medium-fat meat, 3 fat

Giant Roast Beef	1	555	28	45	11	71	1561	43	5	35	3 starch, 4 medium-fat meat, 2 fat
✔ Junior Roast Beef	1	324	14	39	5	30	779	35	2	17	2 starch, 2 medium-fat meat, 1 fat
Regular Roast Beef	1	388	19	44	7	43	1009	33	3	23	2 starch, 2 medium-fat meat, 2 fat
Super Roast Beef	1	523	27	46	9	43	1189	50	5	25	3 starch, 2 medium-fat meat, 3 fat

SHAKES

Chocolate	12 oz	451	12	24	3	36	341	76	0	15	5 carb., 2 fat
Jamocha	12 oz	384	10	23	3	36	262	62	0	15	4 carb., 2 fat
Vanilla	12 oz	360	12	30	4	36	281	50	0	15	3 carb., 2 fat

(Continued)

✔ = Healthiest Bets; n/a = not available

	Amount	Cal.	Fat (g)	% Cal. Fat	Sat. Fat (g)	Chol. (mg)	Sod. (mg)	Carb. (g)	Fiber (g)	Pro. (g)	Servings/Exchanges
SIDES											
✔Baked Potato, plain	1	355	0	0	0	0	26	82	7	7	5 1/2 starch
Baked Potato, with margarine & sour cream	1	578	24	37	9	25	209	85	7	9	5 1/2 starch, 5 fat
✔Broccoli 'n Cheddar Baked Potato	1	571	20	32	5	12	565	89	9	14	6 starch, 4 fat
Cheddar Curly Fries	1 order	333	18	49	4	3	1016	40	0	5	2 1/2 starch, 3 1/2 fat
Curly Fries	1 order	300	10	45	3	0	853	38	0	4	2 1/2 starch, 2 fat
Deluxe Baked Potato	1	736	36	44	18	59	499	86	7	19	6 starch, 7 fat
Homestyle French Fries	1 order	212	10	48	3	0	414	29	2	2	2 starch, 2 fat
Potato Cakes	1 order	204	12	53	2	0	397	20	0	2	1 starch, 2 fat
SUB ROLL SANDWICHES											
Roast Beef Sub	1	700	42	54	14	84	2034	44	4	38	3 starch, 3 medium-fat meat, 5 fat

French Dip	1	475	22	42	8	55	1411	40	3	30	2 1/2 starch, 3 medium-fat meat, 1 fat
Hot Ham 'n Swiss	1	500	23	41	7	68	1664	43	2	30	3 starch, 3 medium-fat meat, 1 1/2 fat
Italian Sub	1	633	36	56	13	83	2089	46	2	30	3 starch, 2 medium-fat meat, 5 fat
Philly Beef 'n Swiss	1	755	47	56	15	91	2025	48	3	39	3 starch, 4 medium-fat meat, 5 fat
Turkey Sub	1	550	27	44	7	65	2084	47	2	31	3 starch, 2 lean meat, 4 fat

✔ = Healthiest Bets; n/a = not available

Notes

Au Bon Pain

❖Au Bon Pain provided nutrition information for all
its menu items. Healthier items are listed in a
brochure.

Light 'n Lean Choice

Thai Chicken Sandwich
Garden Salad (*small*)
Lite Honey Mustard Dressing (*2 Tbsp*)

Calories......................613	Sodium (mg)..........1,657
Fat (g) 13	Carbohydrate (g).......102
% calories from fat..19	Fiber (g) 7
Saturated fat (g)........2	Protein (g) 26
Cholesterol (mg) 33	

Exchanges: 5 1/2 starch, 2 veg., 1/2 carb., 2 lean meat,
1 fat

Healthy 'n Hearty Choice

Louisiana Beans & Rice Soup (*medium, 12 oz*)
Hearth Roll
Garden Salad (*large*)
Fat Free Tomato Basil Dressing (*4 Tbsp*)

Calories......................707	Sodium (mg)..........2,113
Fat (g) 11	Carbohydrate (g).......126
% calories from fat..14	Fiber (g) 10
Saturated fat (g).....1.5	Protein (g) 28
Cholesterol (mg) 15	

Exchanges: 4 starch, 2 1/2 carb., 1 lean meat, 1 fat

Au Bon Pain

BAGELS

	Amount	Cal.	Fat (g)	% Cal. Fat	Sat. Fat (g)	Chol. (mg)	Sod. (mg)	Carb. (g)	Fiber (g)	Pro. (g)	Servings/Exchanges
✔ Asiago Cheese Sourdough	1	380	6	14	3.5	15	690	66	3	17	4 1/2 starch, 1 medium-fat meat
✔ Chocolate Chip	1	380	7	17	3.5	5	480	69	3	12	4 1/2 starch, 1 fat
✔ Cinnamon Raisin Sourdough	1	390	1	2	0	0	550	83	4	14	5 1/2 starch
✔ Cranberry Walnut Sourdough	1	460	4	8	0.5	0	590	93	7	15	6 starch, 1 fat
✔ Dutch Apple with Walnut Streussel	1	350	5	13	0	0	480	77	4	11	5 starch, 1 fat
✔ Everything Sourdough	1	360	3	6	0	0	710	72	3	14	5 starch, 1/2 fat
✔ Honey 9 Grain Sourdough	1	360	2	5	0	0	580	72	6	14	5 starch

✔ = Healthiest Bets; n/a = not available

(Continued)

BAGELS (Continued)	Amount	Cal.	Fat (g)	% Cal. Fat	Sat. Fat (g)	Chol. (mg)	Sod. (mg)	Carb. (g)	Fiber (g)	Pro. (g)	Servings/Exchanges
✔Plain Sourdough	1	350	1	3	0	0	540	71	3	13	5 starch
✔Sesame Sourdough	1	380	4	9	0.5	0	540	71	3	15	4 1/2 starch, 1 fat
✔Wild Blueberry Sourdough	1	380	2	5	0	0	570	80	4	14	5 starch
BEVERAGES											
Frozen Mocha Blast	16 oz	320	3	8	2	10	150	64	2	9	1 low-fat milk, 3 carb.
Hot Hazelnut Blast	16 oz	310	6	17	3.5	25	180	57	0	11	1 low-fat milk, 2 carb.
✔Hot Mocha Blast (small)	9 oz	160	4	23	2.5	15	120	23	0	8	1 low-fat milk, 1 carb.
Hot Mocha Blast (medium)	13 oz	260	6	21	3.5	25	180	41	0	11	1 low-fat milk, 2 carb.
Hot Mocha Blast (large)	17 oz	310	8	23	5	30	230	45	0	14	1 1/2 low-fat milk, 1 1/2 carb.
Hot Strawberry Chocolate Blast	16 oz	330	6	16	3.5	25	180	57	0	11	1 low-fat milk, 2 carb.
Hot Vanilla Chocolate Blast	16 oz	310	6	17	3.5	25	180	57	0	11	1 low-fat milk, 2 1/2 carb.

Iced Caramel Mocha Blast	16 oz	310	6	17	3.5	25	180	54	0	11	1 low-fat milk, 2 carb.
Iced Hazelnut Blast	16 oz	310	6	17	3.5	25	180	54	0	11	1 low-fat milk, 2 carb.
✔ Iced Mocha Blast (small)	9 oz	180	5	25	3	20	135	25	0	9	1 low-fat milk, 1 carb.
Iced Mocha Blast (medium)	12 oz	260	6	21	3.5	25	180	41	0	11	1 low-fat milk, 2 carb.
Iced Mocha Blast (large)	20.5 oz	360	10	25	6	40	280	50	0	18	1 1/2 low-fat milk, 2 carb.
Iced Raspberry Mocha Blast	16 oz	310	6	17	3.5	25	180	54	0	11	1 low-fat milk, 2 carb.
Iced Strawberry Chocolate Blast	16 oz	310	6	17	3.5	25	180	54	0	11	1 low-fat milk, 2 carb.
Iced Vanilla Chocolate Blast	16 oz	310	6	17	3.5	25	180	54	0	11	1 1/2 low-fat milk, 2 carb.
✔ Peach Iced Tea (small)	8 oz	90	0	0	0	0	15	22	0	0	1 1/2 carb.
Peach Iced Tea (medium)	12 oz	130	0	0	0	0	20	33	0	0	2 carb.
Peach Iced Tea (large)	16 oz	170	0	0	0	0	30	44	0	0	3 carb.
✔ Raspberry Iced Tea (small)	8 oz	80	0	0	0	0	15	19	0	0	1 carb.
✔ Raspberry Iced Tea (medium)	12 oz	110	0	0	0	0	20	29	0	0	2 carb.

✔ = Healthiest Bets; n/a = not available

(Continued)

	Amount	Cal.	Fat (g)	% Cal. Fat	Sat. Fat (g)	Chol. (mg)	Sod. (mg)	Carb. (g)	Fiber (g)	Pro. (g)	Servings/Exchanges
BEVERAGES (*Continued*)											
Raspberry Iced Tea (large)	16 oz	150	0	0	0	0	30	38	0	0	2 1/2 carb.

COOKIES

	Amount	Cal.	Fat (g)	% Cal. Fat	Sat. Fat (g)	Chol. (mg)	Sod. (mg)	Carb. (g)	Fiber (g)	Pro. (g)	Servings/Exchanges
✔Biscotti	1	200	10	45	3.5	35	45	24	1	4	2 carb., 2 fat
Chocolate Biscotti	1	240	13	49	6	35	50	28	2	5	2 carb., 2 1/2 fat
Chocolate Chip	1	280	13	42	8	40	85	40	2	3	2 1/2 carb., 2 1/2 fat
Chocolate-Dipped Shortbread	1	410	27	59	19	55	160	41	2	4	3 carb., 5 fat
✔Cranberry Almond Macaroon	1	160	8	45	5	0	115	22	2	2	2 carb., 1 1/2 fat
Cranberry Almond Macaroon w/ Chocolate Coating	1	210	11	47	9	0	120	27	2	3	2 carb., 2 fat
English Toffee	1	220	12	49	7	45	110	28	0	2	2 carb., 2 fat
Ginger Pecan	1	260	15	52	6	40	115	30	1	5	2 carb., 3 fat
✔Oatmeal Raisin	1	250	10	36	3.5	30	240	40	2	3	2 1/2 carb., 2 fat

	Amount	Cal.	Fat (g)	% Cal. Fat	Sat. Fat (g)	Chol. (mg)	Sod. (mg)	Carb. (g)	Fiber (g)	Prot. (g)	Exchanges/Choices
Shortbread	1	390	25	58	15	65	190	39	1	3	2 1/2 carb, 5 fat

CROISSANTS

	Amount	Cal.	Fat (g)	% Cal. Fat	Sat. Fat (g)	Chol. (mg)	Sod. (mg)	Carb. (g)	Fiber (g)	Prot. (g)	Exchanges/Choices
Almond	1	560	37	59	15	105	260	50	4	12	3 starch, 7 fat
✓Apple	1	280	10	32	6	25	180	46	1	4	3 starch, 2 fat
Chocolate	1	440	23	47	15	30	230	53	4	7	3 1/2 starch, 4 1/2 fat
Cinnamon Raisin	1	380	13	31	8	35	290	61	2	7	4 starch, 2 1/2 fat
Ham and Cheese	1	380	20	47	12	70	690	36	1	16	2 1/2 starch, 1 medium-fat meat, 3 fat
Plain	1	270	15	50	9	40	240	30	1	6	2 starch, 3 fat
Raspberry Cheese	1	380	19	45	11	60	300	47	1	6	3 starch, 1/2 carb., 4 fat
Spinach and Cheese	1	270	16	53	9	40	330	27	2	9	2 starch, 3 fat
Sweet Cheese	1	390	22	51	12	75	330	42	1	7	3 starch, 4 fat

(Continued)

✓ = Healthiest Bets; n/a = not available

	Amount	Cal.	Fat (g)	% Cal. Fat	Sat. Fat (g)	Chol. (mg)	Sod. (mg)	Carb. (g)	Fiber (g)	Pro. (g)	Servings/Exchanges
DANISHES											
Cheese Swirl	1	450	28	56	14	95	410	46	1	7	3 carb., 5 1/2 fat
Cinnamon Roll	1	710	26	33	10	100	740	110	3	12	7 carb., 5 fat
Lemon Swirl	1	450	24	48	12	80	410	53	1	7	3 1/2 carb., 5 fat
Pecan Roll	1	900	48	48	16	50	480	111	4	11	7 carb., 9 fat
DESSERTS											
Apple Coffee Cake	1 piece	480	24	45	12	98	285	60	2	6	4 carb., 5 fat
Mochaccino Bar	1	404	24	53	10	37	294	44	1	5	3 carb., 5 fat
Pear Ginger Tea Cake	1 piece	380	20	47	2.8	0	202	47	1	3	3 carb., 4 fat
Walnut Fudge Brownie	1	380	18	43	11	100	150	56	4	5	3 1/2 carb., 3 1/2 fat
LOAF BREADS											
✔Baguette	1 slice	140	1	6	0	0	350	29	1	5	2 starch

✔Four Grain Loaf	1 slice	130	1	7	0	0	280	25	1	5	1 1/2 starch
✔Parisienne	1 slice	120	1	8	0	0	300	25	1	4	1 1/2 starch
MUFFINS											
Blueberry	1	410	15	33	2.5	85	380	64	1	8	4 starch, 3 fat
Carrot Pecan	1	480	23	43	5	55	650	61	3	8	4 starch, 4 1/2 fat
✔Chocolate Cake (low fat)	1	290	3	9	0.5	20	630	68	3	4	4 starch, 1/2 fat
Chocolate Chip	1	490	20	37	7	35	560	70	2	8	4 1/2 starch, 4 fat
Corn	1	470	18	34	2.5	65	570	70	2	8	4 1/2 carb., 3 1/2 fat
Pumpkin with Streusel Topping	1	470	18	34	3	60	550	74	2	8	4 starch, 1 carb., 3 1/2 fat
✔Triple Berry (low fat)	1	270	3	10	0.5	25	560	60	2	5	4 starch, 1/2 fat
ROLLS											
✔3 Seed-Pecan Raisin	1	250	6	22	1	0	240	43	3	9	3 starch, 1 fat
✔Hearth	1	220	2	8	0	0	410	43	2	9	3 starch

✔ = Healthiest Bets; n/a = not available

(Continued)

ROLLS *(Continued)*	Amount	Cal.	Fat (g)	% Cal. Fat	Sat. Fat (g)	Chol. (mg)	Sod. (mg)	Carb. (g)	Fiber (g)	Pro. (g)	Servings/Exchanges
✔Petit Pain	1	200	1	5	0	0	570	41	1	7	2 1/2 starch, 1 fat

SALAD DRESSINGS

	Amount	Cal.	Fat (g)	% Cal. Fat	Sat. Fat (g)	Chol. (mg)	Sod. (mg)	Carb. (g)	Fiber (g)	Pro. (g)	Servings/Exchanges
Bleu Cheese	3 oz/6 Tbsp	410	41	90	8	40	910	8	0	4	1/2 carb., 8 fat
Buttermilk Ranch	3 oz/6 Tbsp	310	32	93	4	35	270	4	0	3	6 fat
Caesar	3 oz/6 Tbsp	380	39	92	5	25	410	3	0	5	8 fat
Caribbean Balsamic Lime	3 oz/6 Tbsp	170	16	85	2.5	0	630	5	1	0	3 fat
✔Fat Free Tomato Basil	3 oz/6 Tbsp	70	0	0	0	0	650	17	1	1	1 carb.
Greek	3 oz/6 Tbsp	440	50	100	7	0	820	2	0	0	10 fat
Lemon Basil Vinaigrette	3 oz/6 Tbsp	330	32	87	2	0	460	15	0	0	1 carb., 6 fat
✔Lite Honey Mustard	3 oz/6 Tbsp	280	17	55	2.5	40	560	30	1	2	2 carb., 3 fat
✔Lite Italian	3 oz/6 Tbsp	230	20	78	1.5	0	570	15	0	0	1 carb., 4 fat
Sesame French	3 oz/6 Tbsp	370	30	73	4.5	0	1010	26	1	1	2 carb., 6 fat

SALADS

										Exchanges
Caesar Salad	1	270	10	6	20	800	27	5	19	2 veg., 1 carb., 1 medium-fat meat, 1 fat
✔ Chicken Caesar Salad	1	360	11	6	65	910	28	5	36	2 veg., 1 carb., 4 lean meat
Field Greens, Gorgonzola & Roasted Walnut Salad	1	400	34	13	50	800	9	3	20	2 veg., 2 high-fat meat, 3 fat
✔ Garden Salad (small)	1	100	1	0	0	150	20	4	5	2 veg., 1/2 carb.
✔ Garden Salad (large)	1	160	2	0	0	290	34	6	7	3 veg., 1 carb.
✔ Mozzarella & Roasted Red Pepper Salad	1	340	18	10	60	135	26	10	22	2 veg., 1 carb., 2 high-fat meat
✔ Pesto Chicken Salad	1	230	11	2	45	250	11	4	20	2 veg., 2 lean meat, 1 fat
Tuna Salad (w/ mayonnaise on greens)	1	490	27	4.5	45	750	40	7	26	2 veg., 2 carb., 3 lean meat, 3 fat

(Continued)

✔ = Healthiest Bets; n/a = not available

	Amount	Cal.	Fat (g)	% Cal. Fat	Sat. Fat (g)	Chol. (mg)	Sod. (mg)	Carb. (g)	Fiber (g)	Pro. (g)	Servings/Exchanges
SANDWICH BREADS											
✔Braided Roll	1 roll	170	5	26	15	0	320	26	1	5	2 starch, 1 fat
✔French Roll	1 roll	120	1	8	0	0	320	25	1	4	1 1/2 starch
✔Multigrain Loaf	1 slice	130	1	7	0	0	340	26	1	5	2 starch
✔Rye Loaf	1 slice	110	2	16	0	0	310	21	2	5	1 1/2 starch
SANDWICH FILLINGS											
✔Cheddar Cheese	43 g	170	14	74	9	45	260	1	0	11	2 medium-fat meat, 1 fat
✔Chicken Tarragon	113 g	240	17	64	3	65	170	1	0	20	3 lean meat, 2 fat
Country Ham	106 g	150	7	42	2.5	55	1370	1	0	21	3 lean meat
✔Cracked Pepper Chicken	112 g	140	2	13	0	72	184	2	0	27	4 very lean meat
✔Grilled Chicken	112 g	140	2	13	0	72	184	2	0	27	4 very lean meat
✔Provolone Cheese	43 g	150	11	66	7	30	370	1	0	11	2 medium-fat meat

											Exchanges
✔ Roast Beef	106 g	140	5	38	0	50	550	1	0	22	3 very lean meat
✔ Swiss Cheese	43 g	160	12	68	8	40	110	1	0	12	2 medium-fat meat
Tuna Salad	128 g	360	29	73	4.5	50	520	3	1	21	3 lean meat, 4 fat
Turkey Breast	106 g	120	1	8	0	20	1110	1	0	24	3 very lean meat
SANDWICHES											
Arizona Chicken	1	720	33	41	12	125	1190	57	4	49	4 starch, 5 lean meat, 3 1/2 fat
California Chicken	1	820	44	48	12	135	1200	55	4	51	3 1/2 starch, 6 lean meat, 5 fat
Chicken Foca-cha-cha	1	870	29	30	5.0	130	2280	80	10	74	1 veg., 5 starch, 8 lean meat, 1 fat
For the Love of Olive	1	570	13	21	1.5	40	2060	80	10	36	2 veg., 4 1/2 starch, 3 very lean meat, 2 fat

(Continued)

✔ = Healthiest Bets; n/a = not available

SANDWICHES (*Continued*)	Amount	Cal.	Fat (g)	% Cal. Fat	Sat. Fat (g)	Chol. (mg)	Sod. (mg)	Carb. (g)	Fiber (g)	Pro. (g)	Servings/Exchanges
Fresh Mozzarella, Tomato & Pesto	1	650	30	42	12	55	1090	69	4	30	4 1/2 starch, 3 medium-fat meat, 3 fat
Hot Roasted Turkey Club	1	950	50	47	16	135	2240	80	4	50	5 starch, 5 lean meat, 7 fat
Radically Roasted	1	620	10	15	4.5	30	1540	69	4	33	2 veg., 4 starch, 2 medium-fat meat
Thai Chicken	1	420	6	13	1	20	1320	72	3	20	5 starch, 2 lean meat
SCONES											
Cinnamon	1	520	28	48	14	145	230	60	1	10	4 starch, 5 fat
Orange	1	440	23	47	13	155	240	53	2	10	3 1/2 starch, 4 1/2 fat
SOUP IN A BREAD BOWL											
Beef Barley	21 oz	760	7	8	2	20	2940	147	8	36	9 starch, 1 medium-fat meat

Caribbean Black Bean	21 oz	830	5	5	1	10	3100	163	17	36	10 starch, 1 lean meat
Chicken Chili	21 oz	990	22	20	11	65	3970	162	12	48	10 starch, 3 lean meat, 2 fat
Chicken Noodle	21 oz	760	6	7	1	20	2950	146	7	39	9 starch, 2 lean meat
Clam Chowder	21 oz	1050	32	27	15	100	3040	155	5	43	10 starch, 2 lean meat, 5 fat
Cream of Broccoli	21 oz	970	31	29	15	60	3100	152	7	34	10 starch, 6 fat
French Onion	21 oz	760	8	9	2	0	3860	148	8	30	9 starch, 1 1/2 fat
New England Potato & Cheese with Ham	21 oz	860	15	16	9	40	3170	152	9	34	9 starch, 1 lean meat, 2 fat
Tomato Florentine	21 oz	760	5	6	2	10	3490	150	8	33	9 starch, 1 lean meat
Vegetarian Chili	21 oz	870	7	7	1	0	3550	171	8	36	11 starch, 1 fat

(Continued)

✔ = Healthiest Bets; n/a = not available

SOUPS

	Amount	Cal.	Fat (g)	% Cal. Fat	Sat. Fat (g)	Chol. (mg)	Sod. (mg)	Carb. (g)	Fiber (g)	Pro. (g)	Servings/Exchanges
✔Beef Barley (small)	8 oz	75	2	24	0.5	15	660	11	2	6	1 carb.
✔Beef Barley (medium)	12 oz	112	3	24	1	18	980	16	3	9	1 carb., 1 lean meat
Beef Barley (large)	16 oz	150	4	24	1.5	25	1310	22	5	12	1 carb., 1 lean meat
✔Caribbean Black Bean (small)	8 oz	120	1	8	0	5	770	22	8	7	1 carb., 1 lean meat
Caribbean Black Bean (medium)	12 oz	180	2	10	0	10	1150	32	12	10	2 carb., 1 lean mat
Caribbean Black Bean (large)	16 oz	250	2	7	0	10	1540	43	16	13	3 carb., 1 lean meat
Chicken Chili (small)	8 oz	240	12	45	7	45	1350	21	4	14	1 1/2 carb., 1 lean meat, 1 1/2 fat
Chicken Chili (medium)	12 oz	350	18	46	10	65	2030	31	6	21	2 carb., 2 lean meat, 2 fat
Chicken Chili (large)	16 oz	470	24	46	13	90	2700	41	8	28	3 carb., 3 lean meat, 3 fat
✔Chicken Noodle (small)	8 oz	80	2	23	0	15	670	10	1	8	1/2 carb., 1 very lean meat

											Exchanges
✔Chicken Noodle (medium)	12 oz	120	2	15	0.5	25	1000	14	2	12	1 carb., 1 very lean meat
Chicken Noodle (large)	16 oz	170	3	16	0.5	35	1340	19	2	16	1 carb., 2 lean meat
Clam Chowder (small)	8 oz	270	19	63	9	65	730	16	0	11	1 carb., 1 lean meat, 3 fat
Clam Chowder (medium)	12 oz	400	29	65	14	95	1090	24	1	16	1 1/2 carb., 2 lean meat, 4 fat
Clam Chowder (large)	16 oz	540	39	65	18	125	1460	32	1	22	2 carb., 2 lean meat, 6 fat
Cream of Broccolli (small)	8 oz	220	18	74	9	40	770	14	1	5	1 carb., 3 1/2 fat
Cream of Broccolli (medium)	12 oz	330	28	76	13	60	1160	21	2	8	1 1/2 carb., 5 1/2 fat
Cream of Broccolli (large)	16 oz	440	37	76	17	80	1550	28	3	10	2 carb., 7 fat
French Onion (small)	8 oz	80	4	45	0.5	0	1280	12	2	2	1 carb., 1 fat
French Onion (medium)	12 oz	120	5	38	1	0	1910	17	3	4	1 carb., 1 fat
French Onion (large)	16 oz	170	7	37	1	0	2550	23	4	5	1/12 carb., 1 fat
✔Louisiana Beans & Rice (small)	8 oz	180	5	25	1	10	660	25	1	9	1 1/2 carb., 1 lean meat

(Continued)

✔ = Healthiest Bets; n/a = not available

SOUPS (*Continued*)	Amount	Cal.	Fat (g)	% Cal. Fat	Sat. Fat (g)	Chol. (mg)	Sod. (mg)	Carb. (g)	Fiber (g)	Pro. (g)	Servings/Exchanges
✓Louisiana Beans & Rice (medium)	12 oz	280	7	23	1.5	15	980	37	2	13	2 1/2 carb., 1 lean meat, 1 fat
Louisiana Beans & Rice (large)	16 oz	360	9	23	2	20	1320	50	3	18	3 carb., 1 lean meat, 1 fat
✓New England Potato & Cheese with Ham (small)	8 oz	150	8	48	5	25	820	14	3	5	1 carb., 1 1/2 fat
New England Potato & Cheese with Ham (medium)	12 oz	220	12	49	8	40	1220	21	4	7	1 1/2 carb., 2 fat
New England Potato & Cheese with Ham (large)	16 oz	290	15	47	11	55	1630	28	5	10	2 carb., 3 fat
Potato Leek (small)	8 oz	200	13	59	8	45	1060	18	2	4	1 carb., 2 1/2 fat
Potato Leek (medium)	12 oz	320	20	56	12	70	1700	28	2	6	2 carb., 4 fat
Potato Leek (large)	16 oz	400	25	56	15	85	2120	35	3	7	2 carb., 5 fat
✓Santa Fe Chicken Tortilla (small)	8 oz	150	7	42	2	15	950	21	2	6	1 1/2 carb., 1 fat

Santa Fe Chicken Tortilla (medium)	12 oz	230	10	39	3	25	1430	32	3	9	2 carb., 2 fat
Santa Fe Chicken Tortilla (large)	16 oz	300	13	39	4	30	1900	42	4	12	3 carb., 1 lean meat, 1 1/2 fat
✔Tomato Florentine (small)	8 oz	61	1	15	0.5	5	1030	13	2	4	1 carb.
Tomato Florentine (medium)	12 oz	90	2	20	1	5	1550	20	2	6	1 carb.
Tomato Florentine (large)	16 oz	122	2	15	1	5	2070	27	3	8	2 carb.
✔Vegetarian Chili (small)	8 oz	139	3	13	0	0	1070	27	2	6	2 carb.
Vegetarian Chili (medium)	12 oz	210	4	17	0	0	1610	40	3	9	2 1/2 carb., 1 fat
Vegetarian Chili (large)	16 oz	278	5	16	0.5	0	2150	53	4	13	3 1/2 carb., 1 lean meat
Vegetarian Corn & Green Chile Bisque (small)	8 oz	190	10	47	6	30	1140	21	3	4	1 1/2 carb., 2 fat
Vegetarian Corn & Green Chile Bisque (medium)	12 oz	300	16	48	9	45	1830	33	4	7	2 carb., 3 fat

✔ = Healthiest Bets; n/a = not available

(Continued)

SOUPS *(Continued)*	Amount	Cal.	Fat (g)	% Cal. Fat	Sat. Fat (g)	Chol. (mg)	Sod. (mg)	Carb. (g)	Fiber (g)	Pro. (g)	Servings/Exchanges
Vegetarian Corn & Green Chile Bisque (large)	16 oz	380	20	47	12	60	2290	41	5	8	3 carb., 4 fat

SPREADS

	Amount	Cal.	Fat (g)	% Cal. Fat	Sat. Fat (g)	Chol. (mg)	Sod. (mg)	Carb. (g)	Fiber (g)	Pro. (g)	Servings/Exchanges
✔Lite Cream Cheese	2 oz/4 Tbsp	130	12	83	8	35	230	2	1	5	1 high-fat meat
✔Lite Honey Walnut Cream Cheese	2 oz/4 Tbsp	260	12	42	5	20	260	8	0	4	1 carb., 1 high-fat meat
✔Lite Raspberry Cream Cheese	2 oz/4 Tbsp	200	8	36	5	20	280	10	0	6	1/2 carb., 1 high-fat meat
✔Lite Strawberry Bagel Spread	2 oz/4 Tbsp	150	11	66	7	35	210	6	1	5	1/2 carb., 2 fat
✔Lite Sun-Dried Tomato Cream Cheese	2 oz/4 Tbsp	130	11	76	8	35	230	2	1	5	1 high-fat meat

	Amount	Cal.	Fat (g)	% Cal. Fat	Sat. Fat (g)	Chol. (mg)	Sod. (mg)	Carb. (g)	Fiber (g)	Pro. (g)	Exchanges
✓Lite Vanilla Hazelnut Bagel Spread	2 oz/4 Tbsp	150	11	66	7	35	210	6	1	5	1/2 carb., 1 high-fat meat
✓Plain Cream Cheese	2 oz/4 Tbsp	190	18	85	12	55	210	2	0	3	3 1/2 fat
✓Veggie Lite Cream Cheese	2 oz/4 Tbsp	100	10	90	5	20	300	6	0	6	1/2 carb., 1 high-fat meat
WRAP SANDWICH											
Chicken Caesar	1	630	31	44	8	80	1140	46	2	38	3 starch, 3 lean meat, 4 fat
Southwestern Tuna	1	950	64	61	17	110	1230	53	4	41	3 1/2 starch, 4 lean meat, 10 fat
Summer Turkey	1	340	9	24	1	35	1380	36	9	29	2 1/2 carb., 2 lean meat, 1/2 fat
Fields & Feta	1	560	17	27	4	10	850	89	13	20	2 veg., 5 starch, 3 fat

✓ = Healthiest Bets; n/a = not available

Blimpie

❖Blimpie provides nutrition information for only its 6-inch sub sandwiches in a brochure.

Light 'n Lean Choice

6" Roast Beef Sub

Calories......................340	Sodium (mg).............870
Fat (g) 5	Carbohydrate (g).........47
% calories from fat..12	Fiber (g) 2
Saturated fat (g)........1	Protein (g) 27
Cholesterol (mg).........20	

Exchanges: 3 starch, 3 very lean meat

Healthy 'n Hearty Choice

6" Ham & Swiss Sub

Calories......................400	Sodium (mg).............970
Fat (g) 13	Carbohydrate (g).........47
% calories from fat..29	Fiber (g) 5
Saturated fat (g)........7	Protein (g) 25
Cholesterol (mg).........35	

Exchanges: 3 starch, 2 medium-fat meat

Blimpie

	Amount	Cal.	Fat (g)	% Cal. Fat	Sat. Fat (g)	Chol. (mg)	Sod. (mg)	Carb. (g)	Fiber (g)	Pro. (g)	Servings/Exchanges
SALADS											
Grilled Chicken Salad	1	350	12	31	0	140	1190	13	0	47	2 veg., 6 very lean meat, 1 fat
SUBS											
5 Meatball	6" sub	500	22	40	8	25	970	52	2	23	3 1/2 starch, 2 medium-fat meat, 2 fat
Blimpie Best	6" sub	410	13	29	5	50	1480	47	4	26	3 starch, 2 medium-fat meat, 1/2 fat
Cheese Trio	6" sub	510	23	41	13	60	1060	51	2	26	3 starch, 2 high-fat meat, 1/2 fat

✔ = Healthiest Bets; n/a = not available

(*Continued*)

SUBS (*Continued*)	Amount	Cal.	Fat (g)	% Cal. Fat	Sat. Fat (g)	Chol. (mg)	Sod. (mg)	Carb. (g)	Fiber (g)	Pro. (g)	Servings/Exchanges
Club	6″ sub	450	13	26	6	40	1350	53	3	30	3 1/2 starch, 3 lean meat, 1 fat
✔ Grilled Chicken	6″ sub	400	9	20	2	30	950	52	2	28	3 1/2 starch, 3 lean meat
✔ Ham & Swiss	6″ sub	400	13	29	7	35	970	47	5	25	3 starch, 2 medium-fat meat, 1/2 fat
Ham, Salami, Provolone	6″ sub	590	28	43	11	70	1880	52	3	32	3 1/2 starch, 3 medium-fat meat, 2 1/2 fat
✔ Roast Beef	6″ sub	340	5	12	1	20	870	47	2	27	3 starch, 3 very lean meat
Steak & Cheese	6″ sub	550	26	43	4	70	1080	51	2	27	3 starch, 3 medium-fat meat, 2 fat
Tuna	6″ sub	570	32	51	4.5	50	790	50	2	21	3 starch, 2 lean meat, 5 fat
✔ Turkey	6″ sub	320	5	13	1	10	890	51	3	19	3 starch, 2 lean meat

✔ = Healthiest Bets; n/a = not available

Subway

❖Subway provides nutrition information for most of its healthier menu items in a brochure. The exchanges given here were not provided by Subway.

Light 'n Lean Choice

6" Roasted Chicken Breast Sub (*on wheat roll*)
Veggie Delite Salad
Fat Free Ranch Salad Dressing (*2 Tbsp, 1/2 packet*)

Calories	431	Sodium (mg)	1,556
Fat (g)	7	Carbohydrate (g)	65
% calories from fat	15	Fiber (g)	4
Saturated fat (g)	1	Protein (g)	29
Cholesterol (mg)	48		

Exchanges: 3 starch, 2 veg., 3 very lean meat

Healthy 'n Hearty Choice

6" Subway Club (*on wheat roll*)
Veggie Delite Salad
Fat Free Ranch Salad Dressing (*2 Tbsp, 1/2 packet*)
Oatmeal Raisin Cookie

Calories	597	Sodium (mg)	2,008
Fat (g)	14	Carbohydrate (g)	93
% calories from fat	21	Fiber (g)	5
Saturated fat (g)	3	Protein (g)	26
Cholesterol (mg)	41		

Exchanges: 3 starch, 2 1/2 carb., 2 lean meat, 1 1/2 fat

(*Continued*)

Subway

	Amount	Cal.	Fat (g)	% Cal. Fat	Sat. Fat (g)	Chol. (mg)	Sod. (mg)	Carb. (g)	Fiber (g)	Pro. (g)	Servings/Exchanges
COLD SUBS											
✓B.L.T. (wheat bread)	6″ sub	327	10	28	3	16	957	44	3	14	3 starch, 1 medium-fat meat, 1 fat
✓B.L.T. (white bread)	6″ sub	311	10	29	3	16	945	38	3	14	2 1/2 starch, 1 medium-fat meat, 1 fat
Classic Italian B.M.T. (wheat bread)	6″ sub	460	22	43	7	56	1664	45	3	21	3 starch, 2 lean meat, 3 fat
Classic Italian B.M.T. (white bread)	6″ sub	445	21	42	8	56	1652	39	3	21	2 1/2 starch, 2 lean meat, 3 fat
Cold Cut Trio (wheat bread)	6″ sub	378	13	31	4	64	1412	46	3	20	2 starch, 2 medium-fat meat, 1/2 fat

Cold Cut Trio (white bread)	6" sub	362	13	32	4	64	1401	39	3	19	2 1/2 starch, 2 medium-fat meat, 1/2 fat
Ham (wheat bread)	6" sub	302	5	15	1	28	1319	45	3	19	3 starch, 2 lean meat
Ham (white bread)	6" sub	287	5	16	1	28	1308	39	3	18	2 1/2 starch, 2 lean meat
✔Roast Beef (wheat bread)	6" sub	303	5	15	1	20	939	45	3	20	3 starch, 2 lean meat
✔Roast Beef (white bread)	6" sub	288	5	16	1	20	928	39	3	19	2 1/2 starch, 2 lean meat
Spicy Italian (wheat bread)	6" sub	482	25	47	9	57	1604	44	3	21	3 starch, 2 medium-fat meat, 3 fat
Spicy Italian (white bread)	6" sub	467	24	46	9	57	1592	38	3	20	2 1/2 starch, 2 medium-fat meat, 3 fat
Subway Club (wheat bread)	6" sub	312	5	14	1	26	1352	46	3	21	2 1/2 starch, 1 veg., 2 lean meat
Subway Club (white bread)	6" sub	297	5	15	1	26	1341	40	3	21	3 starch, 2 lean meat

✔ = Healthiest Bets; n/a = not available

(Continued)

270 *Subs and Sandwiches*

COLD SUBS (*Continued*)	Amount	Cal.	Fat (g)	% Cal. Fat	Sat. Fat (g)	Chol. (mg)	Sod. (mg)	Carb. (g)	Fiber (g)	Pro. (g)	Servings/Exchanges
✔Subway Seafood & Crab* (wheat bread, light mayonnaise)	6″ sub	347	10	26	2	32	884	45	3	20	3 starch, 2 lean meat
✔Subway Seafood & Crab* (white bread, light mayonnaise)	6″ sub	332	10	27	2	32	873	39	3	19	2 1/2 starch, 2 lean meat, 1 fat
✔Tuna (wheat bread, light mayonnaise))	6″ sub	391	15	35	2	32	940	46	3	19	3 starch, 2 lean meat, 2 fat
✔Tuna (white bread, light mayonnaise)	6″ sub	376	15	36	2	32	928	39	3	18	2 1/2 starch, 2 lean meat, 2 fat
Turkey Breast & Ham (wheat bread)	6″ sub	295	5	15	1	24	1361	46	3	18	3 starch, 2 lean meat
Turkey Breast & Ham (white bread)	6″ sub	280	5	16	1	24	1350	39	3	18	2 1/2 starch, 2 lean meat

Turkey Breast (wheat bread)	6" sub	289	4	12	1	19	1403	46	3	18	3 starch, 2 lean meat
Turkey Breast (white bread)	6" sub	273	4	13	1	19	1391	40	3	17	2 1/2 starch, 2 lean meat
✓Veggie Delite (wheat bread)	6" sub	237	3	11	0	0	593	44	3	9	3 starch, 1/2 fat
✓Veggie Delite (white bread)	6" sub	222	3	12	0	0	582	38	3	9	2 1/2 starch, 1/2 fat
COOKIES											
✓Chocolate Chip	1	210	10	43	3.5	10	140	29	1	2	2 carb., 2 fat
✓Chocolate Chip M&M	1	210	10	43	3	15	140	29	1	2	2 carb., 2 fat
✓Chocolate Chunk	1	210	10	43	3.5	10	140	29	1	2	2 carb., 2 fat
Double Chocolate Brazil Nut	1	230	12	47	3.5	10	115	27	1	3	2 carb., 2 fat
✓Oatmeal Raisin	1	200	8	36	2	15	160	29	1	3	2 carb., 1 1/2 fat
Peanut Butter	1	220	12	49	2.5	0	180	26	1	3	2 carb., 2 fat
Sugar	1	230	12	47	3	20	180	28	0	2	2 carb., 2 fat
✓White Chocolate Macademia Nut	1	230	12	39	2.5	10	140	28	1	2	2 carb., 2 fat

✓ = Healthiest Bets; n/a = not available

(Continued)

	Amount	Cal.	Fat (g)	% Cal. Fat	Sat. Fat (g)	Chol. (mg)	Sod. (mg)	Carb. (g)	Fiber (g)	Pro. (g)	Servings/Exchanges
DELI SANDWICHES											
✔Bologna	1	292	12	37	4	20	744	38	2	10	2 starch, 1 medium-fat meat
✔Ham	1	234	4	15	1	14	773	37	2	11	2 1/2 starch, 1 lean meat
✔Roast Beef	1	245	4	15	1	13	638	38	2	13	2 1/2 starch, 1 lean meat
✔Subway Seafood & Crab (light mayonnaise)	1	256	7	25	2	16	556	37	2	12	2 1/2 starch, 1 lean meat
✔Tuna (light mayonnaise)	1	279	9	29	2	16	583	38	2	11	2 1/2 starch, 1 lean meat, 1 fat
✔Turkey Breast	1	235	4	15	1	12	944	38	2	12	2 1/2 starch, 1 lean meat
HOT SUBS											
Meatball (wheat bread)	6" sub	419	16	34	6	33	1046	51	3	19	3 1/2 starch, 1 medium-fat meat, 2 fat

Meatball (white bread)	6" sub	404	16	36	6	33	1035	44	3	18	3 starch, 1 medium-fat meat, 2 fat
Pizza Sub (wheat bread, includes cheese)	6" sub	464	22	43	9	50	1621	48	3	19	3 starch, 1 medium-fat meat, 3 fat
Pizza Sub (white bread, includes cheese)	6" sub	448	22	44	9	50	1609	41	3	19	3 starch, 1 medium-fat meat, 3 fat
✔Roasted Chicken Breast (wheat bread)	6" sub	348	6	16	1	48	978	47	3	27	3 starch, 3 lean meat
✔Roasted Chicken Breast (white bread)	6" sub	332	6	16	1	48	967	41	3	26	3 starch, 2 lean meat
Steak & Cheese (wheat bread, includes cheese)	6" sub	398	10	23	6	70	1117	47	3	30	3 starch, 3 lean meat

(Continued)

✔ = Healthiest Bets; n/a = not available

HOT SUBS (*Continued*)	Amount	Cal.	Fat (g)	% Cal. Fat	Sat. Fat (g)	Chol. (mg)	Sod. (mg)	Carb. (g)	Fiber (g)	Pro. (g)	Servings/Exchanges
Steak & Cheese (white bread, includes cheese)	6" sub	383	10	23	6	70	1106	41	3	29	3 starch, 3 lean meat
Subway Melt (wheat bread, includes cheese)	6" sub	382	12	28	5	42	1746	46	3	23	3 starch, 2 medium-fat meat
Subway Melt (white bread, includes cheese)	6" sub	366	12	30	5	42	1735	40	3	22	2 1/2 starch, 2 medium-fat meat
SALAD DRESSINGS											
Creamy Italian	1 Tbsp	65	6	83	n/a	4	132	2	0	0	1 fat
Fat Free French	1 Tbsp	18	0	0	0	0	99	4	0	0	free
Fat Free Italian	1 Tbsp	6	0	0	0	0	142	1	0	0	free
Fat Free Ranch	1 Tbsp	16	0	0	0	0	135	4	0	0	free
French	1 Tbsp	64	5	69	1	0	85	5	0	0	1 fat

Ranch	1 Tbsp	74	7	85	1	6	108	2	0	0	1 fat
Thousand Island	1 Tbsp	51	5	83	1	5	156	3	0	0	1 fat

SALADS†

✔B.L.T. Salad	1	140	8	54	3	16	672	10	1	7	2 veg., 1/2 high-fat meat, 1/2 fat
Classic Italian B.M.T. Salad	1	274	20	66	7	56	1379	11	1	14	2 veg., 1 high-fat meat, 2 fat
✔Cold Cut Trio Salad	1	191	11	52	3	64	1127	11	1	13	2 veg., 1 medium-fat meat, 1 fat
✔Ham Salad	1	116	3	23	1	28	1034	11	1	12	2 veg., 1 lean meat
✔Meatball Salad	1	233	14	54	5	33	761	16	2	12	1/2 starch, 2 veg., 1 medium-fat meat, 2 fat

(Continued)

✔ = Healthiest Bets; n/a = not available

SALADS (Continued)	Amount	Cal.	Fat (g)	% Cal. Fat	Sat. Fat (g)	Chol. (mg)	Sod. (mg)	Carb. (g)	Fiber (g)	Pro. (g)	Servings/Exchanges
Pizza Salad (includes cheese)	1	277	20	65	8	50	1336	13	2	12	2 veg., 1 high-fat meat, 2 fat
✔Roast Beef Salad	1	117	3	23	1	20	654	11	1	12	2 veg., 1 lean meat
✔Roasted Chicken Breast Salad	1	162	4	22	1	48	693	13	1	20	2 veg., 2 lean meat
✔Steak & Cheese Salad (includes cheese)	1	212	8	34	5	70	832	13	1	22	2 veg., 2 lean meat
Subway Club Salad	1	126	3	21	1	26	1067	12	1	14	2 veg., 1 lean meat
Subway Melt Salad (includes cheese)	1	195	10	46	4	42	1461	12	1	16	2 veg., 2 medium-fat meat
✔Subway Seafood & Crab* Salad (light mayonnaise)	1	161	8	45	1	32	599	11	2	13	2 veg., 1 lean meat, 1 fat
✔Tuna Salad (light mayonnaise)	1	205	13	57	2	32	654	11	1	12	2 veg., 1 lean meat, 2 fat
✔Turkey Breast & Ham Salad	1	109	3	23	1	24	1076	11	1	11	2 veg., 1 lean meat

✔Turkey Breast Salad	1	102	2	18	1	19	1117	12	1	11	2 veg., 1 lean meat
✔Veggie Delite Salad	1	51	1	14	0	0	308	10	1	2	2 veg.

✔ = Healthiest Bets; n/a = not available

* A processed seafood & crab blend.

† Nutrition information for salads does not include salad dressing. Nutrition information for sandwiches does not include cheese or condiments such as oil or mayonnaise.

Notes

_____

_____

_____

_____

_____

_____

_____

_____

_____

Pizza, Pasta, and All Else Italian

RESTAURANTS

Domino's Pizza

Fazoli's

Godfather's Pizza

Little Caesars

Olive Garden

Papa John's Pizza

Pizza Hut

Romano's Macaroni Grill

Round Table Pizza

NUTRITION PROS

- Much to your surprise, pizza and pasta—as long as you top them wisely—are healthy restaurant choices.
- Pizza and pasta can hold the line on fat and calories better than some burger and french fry meals.
- Pizza and pasta meals match today's diabetes nutrition goals: low in fat, moderate in protein, and full of grains.
- You can eat vegetables, both raw and cooked, in most pizza and pasta restaurants. That's an accomplishment in a fast-food restaurant. Raw vegetables come as salads. Cooked vegetables come as pizza sauce and toppings, or as tomato-based sauces and toppings on pasta.

- You can design your own pizza with healthier toppings (see list on page 282). Pizza spots are used to made-for-you orders.
- Most pizza chains offer a veggie combination pizza.
- Pizza chains are slowly but surely divulging their nutrition information, so you can pick and choose with nutrition facts in hand.
- Several pizza chains have gone uptown. You might call them yuppie. That's good news for health-focused pizza lovers. They bake their pizzas in brick ovens, and they offer novel and healthy toppings. Pineapple, spinach, feta cheese, roasted red peppers, and grilled chicken are just a few.
- Pizza and pasta are served not only in pizza or Italian restaurants, but also in family-style and dinner house restaurants.

NUTRITION CONS

- It's hard to eat just two or three slices. There's always just one more piece of pizza begging you to eat it.
- High-fat pizza toppings—extra cheese, three kinds of cheese, pepperoni, and sausage—can quickly add fat and calories.
- The high-fat toppers—extra cheese, three kinds of cheese, pepperoni, and sausage—also add more sodium.
- Some pizza chains now promote more toppings, extra cheese, and bigger pizzas. That all adds up to more fat and calories.
- Restaurant combination pizzas often add high-fat and high-calorie toppers.

- Pasta with high-fat and high-calorie toppers—cream sauce, creamy cheese sauce, butter sauce—is easy to find.
- Pasta portions are often heavy-handed.
- Breadsticks and garlic bread sound healthy, but they are often doused in fat. Check their nutrition numbers.

Healthy Tips

★ If you count calories carefully, stick with the thin crust and load on the veggies.

★ If your favorite chain does not publish nutrition information, cast a glance at the nutrition information for like items from two other pizza chains. That gives you ballpark figures to base your choice on.

★ If your dining partner wants not-so-healthy pizza toppings, order healthier toppings on one half and let your partner handle the other.

★ Order just enough pieces for the mouths at the table to avoid that just-one-more-piece syndrome.

★ If you know a few extra pieces will be left over, package them up before you bite into your first piece.

★ Try an appetizer side portion of pasta, split an order with your dining partner, or stash a portion in a take-home container before you lift your fork to your mouth.

Continued

★ Along with pizza or pasta, crunch on a healthy garden salad to fill you up and not out.

★ Don't leave the crust for the birds; that's the healthy part. Eat it and count your grams of fiber.

★ The red pepper flakes you'll probably find sitting right on your table add zip to your pizza, pasta, or salad without adding calories.

HEALTHY PIZZA TOPPINGS

part-skim cheese	sliced tomatoes	chicken
green peppers	spinach	ham
onions	broccoli	Canadian bacon
mushrooms	pineapple	

NOT-SO-HEALTHY PIZZA TOPPINGS

extra cheese	pepperoni	anchovies
several types of cheese	sausage	bacon

Get It Your Way

★ Ask your pizza maker to go light on the cheese and heavy on the veggies.

★ Request a half-order of pasta if you don't have someone to split it with.

★ Remember to order your salad dressing on the side.

Domino's Pizza

❖Domino's provides nutrition information for most of its menu items in a brochure.

Light 'n Lean Choice

Small Garden Salad
Light Italian Dressing (*3 Tbsp*)
14″ Hand Tossed Crust Pizza with
Fresh Mushrooms (*3 slices*)

Calories	492	Sodium (mg)	1,799
Fat (g)	16	Carbohydrate (g)	74
% calories from fat	29	Fiber (g)	7
Saturated fat (g)	7.2	Protein (g)	22
Cholesterol (mg)	21		

Exchanges: 4 1/2 starch, 1 veg., 1/2 carb., 1 1/2 medium-fat meat, 1 1/2 fat

Healthy 'n Hearty Choice

Large Garden Salad
Fat-Free Ranch Dressing (*3 Tbsp*)
12″ Thin Crust Pizza with Pineapple Tidbits
(*1/2 pizza*)

Calories	631	Sodium (mg)	2,204
Fat (g)	24	Carbohydrate (g)	82
% calories from fat	34	Fiber (g)	8
Saturated fat (g)	10.4	Protein (g)	26
Cholesterol (mg)	38		

Exchanges: 4 starch, 2 veg., 1 carb., 2 medium-fat meat, 2 fat

(*Continued*)

Domino's Pizza

PIZZAS

	Amount	Cal.	Fat (g)	% Cal. Fat	Sat. Fat (g)	Chol. (mg)	Sod. (mg)	Carb. (g)	Fiber (g)	Pro. (g)	Servings/Exchanges
✔12" Medium Cheese Deep Dish	2 slices/ 1/4 pizza	477	22	42	8.5	19	1085	55	3	18	3 starch, 1 carb., 1 medium-fat meat, 3 fat
✔12" Medium Cheese Hand Tossed	2 slices/ 1/4 pizza	347	11	29	5	15	723	50	3	14	2 starch, 1 medium-fat meat, 1 fat
✔12" Medium Cheese Thin Crust	2 slices/ 1/4 pizza	271	12	40	5.2	15	809	31	2	12	2 starch, 1 medium-fat meat, 1 fat
✔14" Large Cheese Deep Dish	2 slices/ 1/6 pizza	455	20	40	7.8	18	1029	54	3	18	3 starch, 1 carb., 1 medium-fat meat, 3 fat
✔14" Large Cheese Hand Tossed	2 slices/ 1/6 pizza	317	10	28	4.8	14	669	45	3	13	3 starch, 1 medium-fat meat, 1 fat

	Amount										Exchanges/Choices
✓14" Large Cheese Thin Crust	2 slices/ 1/6 pizza	253	11	39	5	14	757	29	2	11	2 starch, 1 medium-fat meat, 1 fat
6" Cheese Deep Dish	1 whole	595	27	41	10.6	24	1300	68	4	23	4 starch, 1/2 carb., 2 medium-fat meat, 3 fat

SALAD DRESSINGS

	Amount										Exchanges/Choices
Blue Cheese	1.5 oz/3 Tbsp	220	24	98	4	40	440	2	0	0	5 fat
Creamy Caesar	1.5 oz/3 Tbsp	200	22	99	3	10	470	2	0	1	4 fat
✓Fat-Free Ranch	1.5 oz/3 Tbsp	40	0	0	0	0	560	10	1	0	1/2 carb.
Honey French	1.5 oz/3 Tbsp	210	18	77	2.5	0	300	14	0	0	1 carb., 3 1/2 fat
House Italian	1.5 oz/3 Tbsp	220	24	98	3	0	440	1	0	0	5 fat
✓Light Italian	1.5 oz/3 Tbsp	20	1	45	0	0	780	2	0	0	free
Ranch	1.5 oz/3 Tbsp	260	29	100	4	5	380	1	0	0	6 fat
Thousand Island	1.5 oz/3 Tbsp	200	20	90	3	25	320	5	0	0	4 fat

✓ = Healthiest Bets; n/a = not available

(Continued)

SALAD DRESSINGS (Continued)	Amount	Cal.	Fat (g)	% Cal. Fat	Sat. Fat (g)	Chol. (mg)	Sod. (mg)	Carb. (g)	Fiber (g)	Pro. (g)	Servings/Exchanges
SALADS											
✔ Garden Salad, Small	1	22	0	0	0	0	14	4	2	1	1 veg.
✔ Garden Salad, Large	1	39	0	0	0	0	26	8	3	2	1 veg.
SIDES											
✔ Barbeque Wings	1 piece	50	2	36	0.6	26	175	2	0	6	1 medium-fat meat
✔ Breadsticks	1 piece	78	3	35	0.6	0	158	11	0	2	1 starch, 1/2 fat
✔ Cheesy Bread	1 piece	103	5	44	2	5	187	11	0	3	1/2 starch, 1 medium-fat meat
✔ Hot Wings	1 piece	45	2	40	0.6	26	354	1	0	5	1 lean meat
TOPPINGS FOR 12" PIZZA											
✔ Anchovies	n/a	23	1	39	0	9	395	0	0	3	free
Bacon	n/a	82	7	77	2.5	12	226	0	0	4	1 high-fat meat
✔ Banana Peppers	n/a	3	0	0	0	0	92	1	n/a	0	free

Cheddar Cheese	n/a	57	5	79	3	15	88	0	0	4	1 medium-fat meat
Extra Cheese	n/a	48	4	75	2.3	7	150	1	0	3	1/2 high-fat meat
✔ Green Olives	n/a	12	1	75	0	0	255	0	0	0	free
✔ Green Peppers	n/a	3	0	0	0	0	0	1	0	0	free
✔ Ham	n/a	18	1	50	0.3	7	162	0	0	2	free
✔ Italian Sausage	n/a	55	4	65	1.7	11	171	2	0	2	1 fat
✔ Mushrooms, Canned	n/a	4	0	0	0	0	75	1	0	0	free
✔ Mushrooms, Fresh	n/a	4	0	0	0	0	1	1	0	0	free
✔ Onion	n/a	4	0	0	0	0	0	1	0	0	free
Pepperoni	n/a	62	6	87	2.2	13	198	0	0	3	1 fat
✔ Pineapple Tidbits	n/a	10	0	0	0	0	1	2	0	0	free
✔ Pre-Cooked Beef	n/a	56	5	80	2	11	154	0	0	3	1 medium-fat meat
✔ Ripe Olives	n/a	14	1	64	0	0	71	1	1	0	free

✔ = Healthiest Bets; n/a = not available

(Continued)

TOPPINGS FOR 14" PIZZA

	Amount	Cal.	Fat (g)	% Cal. Fat	Sat. Fat (g)	Chol. (mg)	Sod. (mg)	Carb. (g)	Fiber (g)	Pro. (g)	Servings/Exchanges
✔Anchovies	n/a	23	1	39	0	9	395	0	0	3	free
Bacon	n/a	75	6	72	2.3	11	207	0	0	4	1 medium-fat meat
✔Banana Peppers	n/a	3	0	0	0	0	81	1	n/a	0	free
Cheddar Cheese	n/a	48	4	75	2.5	12	73	0	0	3	1/2 high-fat meat
Extra Cheese	n/a	45	4	80	2.2	7	140	1	0	3	1/2 high-fat meat
✔Green Olives	n/a	11	1	82	0	0	227	0	0	0	free
✔Green Peppers	n/a	2	0	0	0	0	0	1	0	0	free
✔Ham	n/a	17	1	53	0	7	156	0	0	2	free
✔Italian Sausage	n/a	44	3	61	1.4	9	137	1	0	2	1/2 fat
✔Mushrooms, Canned	n/a	3	0	0	0	0	50	1	0	0	free
✔Mushrooms, Fresh	n/a	3	0	0	0	0	0	1	0	0	free

✓Onion	n/a	3	0	0	0	0	0	1	0	free
Pepperoni	n/a	55	5	82	2	12	177	0	2	1 fat
✓Pineapple Tidbits	n/a	8	0	0	0	0	1	2	0	free
✓Pre-Cooked Beef	n/a	44	4	82	1.6	8	123	0	2	1 fat
✓Ripe Olives	n/a	12	1	75	0	0	63	1	0	free

TOPPINGS FOR 6" PIZZA

✓Anchovies	n/a	45	2	40	0.5	18	790	0	6	1 lean meat
Bacon	n/a	82	7	77	2.5	12	226	0	4	1 high-fat meat
✓Banana Peppers	n/a	3	0	0	0	0	73	0	0	free
Cheddar Cheese	n/a	86	7	73	5	22	132	0	5	1 high-fat meat
Extra Cheese	n/a	57	5	79	3	9	180	1	4	1 medium-fat meat
✓Green Olives	n/a	10	1	90	0	0	204	0	0	free
✓Green Peppers	n/a	2	0	0	0	0	0	0	0	free

✓ = Healthiest Bets; n/a = not available

(*Continued*)

TOPPINGS FOR 6″ PIZZA (Continued)	Amount	Cal.	Fat (g)	% Cal. Fat	Sat. Fat (g)	Chol. (mg)	Sod. (mg)	Carb. (g)	Fiber (g)	Pro. (g)	Servings/Exchanges
✔Ham	n/a	17	1	53	0	7	156	0	0	2	free
✔Italian Sausage	n/a	44	3	61	1.4	9	137	1	0	2	1/2 fat
✔Mushrooms, Canned	n/a	2	0	0	0	0	36	0	0	0	free
✔Mushrooms, Fresh	n/a	2	0	0	0	0	0	0	0	0	free
✔Onion	n/a	3	0	0	0	0	0	1	0	0	free
Pepperoni	n/a	50	5	90	1.8	10	159	0	0	2	1 fat
✔Pineapple Tidbits	n/a	5	0	0	0	0	0	1	0	0	free
✔Pre-Cooked Beef	n/a	44	4	82	1.6	8	123	0	0	2	1 fat
✔Ripe Olives	n/a	11	1	82	0	0	57	0	0	0	free

✔ = Healthiest Bets; n/a = not available

Fazoli's

❖Fazoli's provides nutrition information for all of its menu items in a brochure.

Light 'n Lean Choice

Minestrone Soup
Spaghetti with Meat Sauce
Garden Salad
Reduced Calorie Italian Dressing (*2 Tbsp*)

Calories......................559	Sodium (mg)..........1,328
Fat (g) 13	Carbohydrate (g).........83
% calories from fat..21	Fiber (g)................n/a
Saturated fat (g) ....n/a	Protein (g)..................n/a
Cholesterol (mg) 20	

Exchanges: 3 starch, 1 veg., 2 carb., 3 medium-fat meat, 1 fat

Healthy 'n Hearty Choice

Bean and Pasta Soup
Chicken Parmesan (*served with pasta*)
Lemon Italian Ice

Calories......................797	Sodium (mg)..........1,456
Fat (g) 21	Carbohydrate (g).........90
% calories from fat..24	Fiber (g)................n/a
Saturated fat (g) ....n/a	Protein (g)..................n/a
Cholesterol (mg) 136	

Exchanges: 2 starch, 3 carb., 3 lean meat, 4 fat

(*Continued*)

Fazoli's

	Amount	Cal.	Fat (g)	% Cal. Fat	Sat. Fat (g)	Chol. (mg)	Sod. (mg)	Carb. (g)	Fiber (g)	Pro. (g)	Servings/Exchanges
BREADS											
✓Breadstick (dry)	1	99	1	9	n/a	0	204	20	n/a	n/a	insufficient info. to calculate
✓Breadstick (regular)	1	131	4	27	n/a	0	330	20	n/a	n/a	insufficient info. to calculate
DESSERTS											
Chesecake (plain)	1 slice	270	21	70	n/a	88	208	16	n/a	n/a	insufficient info. to calculate
Chocolate Cheesecake	1 slice	298	22	66	n/a	83	201	22	n/a	n/a	insufficient info. to calculate
Lemon Italian Ice	12 oz	142	0	0	n/a	0	9	36	n/a	n/a	insufficient info. to calculate
✓Strawberry Topping	1 oz/2 Tbsp	40	0	0	n/a	0	1	10	n/a	n/a	insufficient info. to calculate
OTHER ENTREES											
Broccoli Lasagna	1	571	27	43	n/a	120	1443	50	n/a	n/a	insufficient info. to calculate

✓Chicken Parmesan	1	481	14	26	n/a	132	368	34	n/a	insufficient info. to calculate
Lasagna	1	533	24	41	n/a	120	1148	47	n/a	insufficient info. to calculate
Meatball Sub	1	650	30	42	n/a	87	1534	62	n/a	insufficient info. to calculate
✓Sampler Platter	1	607	20	30	n/a	74	904	80	n/a	insufficient info. to calculate

PASTA ENTREES

✓Baked Spaghetti Parmesan	1	563	21	34	n/a	51	589	65	n/a	insufficient info. to calculate
✓Baked Ziti	1	331	13	35	n/a	30	347	38	n/a	insufficient info. to calculate
✓Baked Ziti (large)	1	573	21	33	n/a	109	519	68	n/a	insufficient info. to calculate
✓Broccoli Fettuccine	1	424	13	28	n/a	20	731	62	n/a	insufficient info. to calculate
Broccoli Fettuccine (large)	1	619	20	29	n/a	29	1068	91	n/a	insufficient info. to calculate
Cheese Ravioli with Meat Sauce	1	591	26	40	n/a	69	1200	60	n/a	insufficient info. to calculate
Cheese Ravioli with Tomato Sauce	1	562	25	40	n/a	51	1214	62	n/a	insufficient info. to calculate
✓Fettuccine Alfredo	1	400	13	29	n/a	20	711	58	n/a	insufficient info. to calculate

✓ = Healthiest Bets; n/a = not available

(Continued)

PASTA ENTREES (Continued)	Amount	Cal.	Fat (g)	% Cal. Fat	Sat. Fat (g)	Chol. (mg)	Sod. (mg)	Carb. (g)	Fiber (g)	Pro. (g)	Servings/Exchanges
Fettuccine Alfredo (large)	1	596	20	30	n/a	29	1048	87	n/a	n/a	insufficient info. to calculate
Shrimp & Scallop Fettuccine	1	522	14	24	n/a	181	1093	63	n/a	n/a	insufficient info. to calculate
✔ Spaghetti with Meat Sauce	1	372	8	19	n/a	20	161	60	n/a	n/a	insufficient info. to calculate
✔ Spaghetti with Meat Sauce (large)	1	553	12	20	n/a	30	223	90	n/a	n/a	insufficient info. to calculate
Spaghetti with Meatballs	1	582	25	39	n/a	59	864	67	n/a	n/a	insufficient info. to calculate
Spaghetti with Meatballs (large)	1	829	34	37	n/a	78	1163	100	n/a	n/a	insufficient info. to calculate
✔ Spaghetti with Tomato Sauce	1	343	7	18	n/a	2	175	62	n/a	n/a	insufficient info. to calculate
✔ Spaghetti with Tomato Sauce (large)	1	509	10	18	n/a	2	244	93	n/a	n/a	insufficient info. to calculate
PIZZAS											
✔ Cheese, Double Slice	1	360	11	28	n/a	33	622	45	n/a	n/a	insufficient info. to calculate
Combination, Double Slice	1	484	21	39	n/a	44	1042	47	n/a	n/a	insufficient info. to calculate
✔ Pepperoni, Double Slice	1	430	17	36	n/a	33	908	45	n/a	n/a	insufficient info. to calculate

SALAD DRESSINGS

Honey French	1 oz/2 Tbsp	160	14	79	n/a	0	230	11	n/a	n/a	insufficient info. to calculate
House Italian	1 oz/2 Tbsp	138	15	98	n/a	0	224	3	n/a	n/a	insufficient info. to calculate
Ranch	1 oz/2 Tbsp	180	20	100	n/a	0	250	1	n/a	n/a	insufficient info. to calculate
✔ Reduced Calorie Italian	1 oz/2 Tbsp	69	4	52	n/a	0	112	2	n/a	n/a	insufficient info. to calculate
Thousand Island	1 oz/2 Tbsp	140	14	90	n/a	15	230	4	n/a	n/a	insufficient info. to calculate

SALADS

✔ Garden	1	28	0	0	n/a	0	17	5	n/a	n/a	insufficient info. to calculate
Italian Chef	1	391	30	69	n/a	65	1307	10	n/a	n/a	insufficient info. to calculate
Pasta	1	397	20	45	n/a	14	1030	46	n/a	n/a	insufficient info. to calculate

SOUPS

Bean and Pasta	1	174	7	36	n/a	4	1079	20	n/a	n/a	insufficient info. to calculate
Minestrone	1	90	1	10	n/a	0	1038	16	n/a	n/a	insufficient info. to calculate

✔ = Healthiest Bets; n/a = not available

Godfather's Pizza

❖Godfather's Pizza provides nutrition information for several of its pizzas in a brochure and provided some additional nutrition information for this book.

Light 'n Lean Choice

Medium Cheese Pizza, Original Crust (*2 slices*)

Calories	462	Sodium (mg)	676
Fat (g)	10	Carbohydrate (g)	68
% calories from fat	19	Fiber (g)	n/a
Saturated fat (g)	n/a	Protein (g)	26
Cholesterol (mg)	28		

Exchanges: 4 starch, 2 medium-fat meat

Healthy 'n Hearty Choice

Medium Combo Pizza, Golden Crust (*3 slices*)

Calories	813	Sodium (mg)	1,686
Fat (g)	36	Carbohydrate (g)	84
% calories from fat	40	Fiber (g)	n/a
Saturated fat (g)	n/a	Protein (g)	39
Cholesterol (mg)	66		

Exchanges: 5 1/2 starch, 3 medium-fat meat, 3 fat

Godfather's Pizza

	Amount	Cal.	Fat (g)	% Cal. Fat	Sat. Fat (g)	Chol. (mg)	Sod. (mg)	Carb. (g)	Fiber (g)	Pro. (g)	Servings/Exchanges
GOLDEN CRUST											
✔Cheese Pizza (medium)	1/8 pizza	212	8	34	n/a	12	311	26	n/a	10	1 1/2 starch, 1 medium-fat meat, 1/2 fat
✔Cheese Pizza (large)	1/10 pizza	242	9	33	n/a	14	363	28	n/a	12	2 starch, 1 medium-fat meat, 1 fat
Combo Pizza (medium)	1/8 pizza	271	12	40	n/a	22	562	28	n/a	13	2 starch, 1 medium-fat meat, 1 1/2 fat
Combo Pizza (large)	1/10 pizza	305	14	41	n/a	25	674	31	n/a	16	2 starch, 1 medium-fat meat, 2 fat

(Continued)

✔ = Healthiest Bets; n/a = not available

	Amount	Cal.	Fat (g)	% Cal. Fat	Sat. Fat (g)	Chol. (mg)	Sod. (mg)	Carb. (g)	Fiber (g)	Pro. (g)	Servings/Exchanges
ORIGINAL CRUST											
✔ Beef and Onion Pizza (large)	1/10 pizza	306	9	26	4.6	30	660	37	1	19	2 1/2 starch, 2 medium-fat meat
✔ Beef Pizza (large)	1/10 pizza	304	9	27	4.6	30	660	37	1	19	2 1/2 starch, 2 medium-fat meat
✔ Cheese Pizza (mini)	1/4 pizza	131	3	21	n/a	8	183	19	n/a	7	1 starch, 1 lean meat
✔ Cheese Pizza (medium)	1/8 pizza	231	5	19	n/a	14	338	34	n/a	13	2 starch, 1 medium-fat meat
✔ Cheese Pizza (large)	1/10 pizza	258	6	21	n/a	18	396	36	n/a	15	2 starch, 1 medium-fat meat
✔ Cheese Pizza (jumbo)	1/10 pizza	382	9	21	n/a	27	580	53	n/a	22	3 1/2 starch, 2 medium-fat meat
✔ Combo Pizza (mini)	1/4 pizza	176	7	36	n/a	16	382	21	n/a	10	1 1/2 starch, 1 medium-fat meat

	Serving									
Combo Pizza (medium)	1/8 pizza	306	11	32	n/a	27	660	36	n/a	17	2 starch, 2 medium-fat meat
Combo Pizza (large)	1/10 pizza	338	12	32	n/a	31	740	38	n/a	19	2 1/2 starch, 2 medium-fat meat
Combo Pizza (jumbo)	1/10 pizza	503	18	32	n/a	47	1096	56	n/a	29	4 starch, 2 medium-fat meat, 1 1/2 fat
✔ Pepperoni & Black Olive Pizza (large)	1/10 pizza	300	10	30	4.7	25	577	36	0	16	2 1/2 starch, 1 medium-fat meat, 1 fat
✔ Pepperoni Pizza (large)	1/10 pizza	296	10	30	4.7	25	532	36	0	16	2 1/2 starch, 1 medium-fat meat, 1 fat
Sausage and Mushroom Pizza (large)	1/10 pizza	320	11	31	5	26	613	38	1	18	2 1/2 starch, 2 medium-fat meat
Sausage Pizza (large)	1/10 pizza	319	11	31	5	26	594	37	1	18	2 1/2 starch, 2 medium-fat meat

✔ = Healthiest Bets; n/a = not available

Little Caesars

❖Little Caesars provided nutrition information for most of its menu items.

Light 'n Lean Choice

14" **Veggie Pizza** (*2 slices*)

Calories......................500	Sodium (mg).............996
Fat (g) 18	Carbohydrate (g).........62
% calories from fat..32	Fiber (g) 4
Saturated fat (g)........8	Protein (g) 26
Cholesterol (mg).........40	

Exchanges: 4 starch, 2 medium-fat meat, 2 fat

Healthy 'n Hearty Choice

Deep Dish Pizza, Cheese Only (*3 slices*)

Calories......................630	Sodium (mg)..........1,317
Fat (g) 21	Carbohydrate (g).........81
% calories from fat..30	Fiber (g) 3
Saturated fat (g)...10.5	Protein (g) 30
Cholesterol (mg).........45	

Exchanges: 6 starch, 3 medium-fat meat

Little Caesars

	Amount	Cal.	Fat (g)	% Cal. Fat	Sat. Fat (g)	Chol. (mg)	Sod. (mg)	Carb. (g)	Fiber (g)	Pro. (g)	Servings/Exchanges
MISCELLANEOUS											
✔Crazy Bread (8 pieces)	1 order	110	3	25	0.5	0	114	16	1	3	1 starch, 1/2 fat
✔Crazy Sauce	3.5 oz/7 Tbsp	40	1	12	0	0	232	9	2	2	1/2 carb.
PIZZAS											
12″ Cheese	1 slice	180	6	30	3	15	240	22	1	10	1 1/2 starch, 1 medium-fat meat
12″ Pepperoni	1 slice	200	8	36	4	20	320	22	1	11	1 1/2 starch, 2 medium-fat meat
✔14″ Veggie	1 slice	250	9	32	4	20	498	31	2	13	2 starch, 1 medium-fat meat, 1 fat

✔ = Healthiest Bets; n/a = not available

(Continued)

Pizzas (Continued)	Amount	Cal.	Fat (g)	% Cal. Fat	Sat. Fat (g)	Chol. (mg)	Sod. (mg)	Carb. (g)	Fiber (g)	Pro. (g)	Servings/Exchanges
16" Pepperoni	1 slice	360	15	38	7	35	417	38	2	19	2 1/2 starch, 2 medium-fat meat, 1 fat
18" Pepperoni	1 slice	450	19	38	8.5	45	816	48	3	24	3 starch, 2 medium-fat meat, 1 fat
✔ Big! Big! Cheese (small)	1 slice	250	9	32	4.5	20	359	30	2	14	2 starch, 1 medium-fat meat, 1 fat
Big! Big! Cheese (medium)	1 slice	320	11	31	5.5	25	443	38	2	18	2 1/2 starch, 2 medium-fat meat
Big! Big! Cheese (large)	1 slice	400	14	32	7	30	552	48	3	22	3 starch, 2 medium-fat meat, 1 fat
Big! Big! Pepperoni (small)	1 slice	280	12	39	5.5	30	523	30	2	15	2 starch, 1 medium-fat meat, 1 fat

	Amount	Cal.	Fat (g)	% Cal. Fat	Sat. Fat (g)	Chol. (mg)	Sod. (mg)	Carb. (g)	Fiber (g)	Pro. (g)	Exchanges/Choices
Big! Big! Slice	1 slice	650	26	37	12	65	1162	66	4	33	4 1/2 starch, 3 medium-fat meat, 2 fat
Deep Dish	1 slice	280	13	42	5.5	30	630	27	2	14	2 starch, 1 medium-fat meat, 1/2 fat
✔ Deep Dish, Cheese Only (large)	1 slice	210	7	30	3.5	15	439	27	1	10	2 starch, 1 medium-fat meat
Stuffed Crust Cheese	1 slice	300	13	39	6	25	498	30	2	16	2 starch, 1 medium-fat meat, 1 1/2 fat
Stuffed Crust Pepperoni	1 slice	340	17	45	7.5	35	678	30	2	18	2 starch, 2 medium-fat meat, 1 fat

✔ = Healthiest Bets; n/a = not available

Notes

Olive Garden

❖Olive Garden provides nutrition information for its "Garden Fare" menu items in a brochure.

Light 'n Lean Choice

Minestrone Soup
Capellini Primavera (*dinner size*)

Calories.......................700	Sodium (mg)..........2,120
Fat (g) 13	Carbohydrate (g).......117
% calories from fat..17	Fiber (g).................n/a
Saturated fat (g)........4	Protein (g) 28
Cholesterol (mg).........10	

Exchanges: 7 starch, 2 veg., 2 fat

Healthy 'n Hearty Choice

Grilled Chicken Capri
Plain Breadstick
Apple Caramellina (*split*)

Calories.......................975	Sodium (mg)..........1,995
Fat (g) 16	Carbohydrate (g).......143
% calories from fat..15	Fiber (g).................n/a
Saturated fat (g)........5	Protein (g) 67
Cholesterol (mg).........75	

Exchanges: 5 starch, 4 carb., 6 very lean meat, 1 fat

Olive Garden

	Amount	Cal.	Fat (g)	% Cal. Fat	Sat. Fat (g)	Chol. (mg)	Sod. (mg)	Carb. (g)	Fiber (g)	Pro. (g)	Servings/Exchanges
DESSERTS											
Apple Caramellina	1	570	3	3	1.5	10	230	130	n/a	7	8 1/2 carb., 1/2 fat
DINNER ENTREES											
✔Capellini Pomodoro	1	620	16	24	4	10	1620	98	n/a	22	6 starch, 2 veg., 3 fat
✔Capellini Primavera	1	600	12	16	4	10	1450	99	n/a	23	6 starch, 2 veg., 2 fat
Capellini Primavera w/ Chicken	1	760	18	16	6	50	2190	101	n/a	48	6 starch, 2 veg., 3 lean meat, 2 fat
✔Chicken Giardino	1	550	11	18	4	85	1000	71	n/a	42	5 starch, 4 lean meat
Grilled Chicken Capri	1	550	12	20	3.5	70	1660	52	n/a	58	3 1/2 starch, 6 very lean meat, 1 fat

(Continued)

✔ = Healthiest Bets; n/a = not available

DINNER ENTREES (Continued)	Amount	Cal.	Fat (g)	% Cal. Fat	Sat. Fat (g)	Chol. (mg)	Sod. (mg)	Carb. (g)	Fiber (g)	Pro. (g)	Servings/Exchanges
✔Linguine Alla Marinara	1	530	9	16	1	0	1100	94	n/a	17	4 starch, 1 veg., 2 carb., 2 fat
Shrimp Primavera	1	730	12	18	4.5	255	1590	106	n/a	50	6 starch, 2 veg., 4 lean meat
LUNCH ENTREES											
✔Capellini Pomodoro	1	380	10	23	2	5	1030	60	n/a	13	3 starch, 2 veg., 2 fat
✔Capellini Primavera	1	350	7	17	3	10	820	58	n/a	14	3 starch, 2 veg., 1 fat
✔Capellini Primavera w/ Chicken	1	510	13	17	4.5	45	1550	59	n/a	39	3 starch, 2 veg., 4 lean meat
✔Chicken Giardino	1	360	9	23	3.5	50	900	47	n/a	23	3 starch, 2 lean meat, 1/2 fat
✔Linguine Alla Marinara	1	330	6	17	0.5	0	710	57	n/a	10	3 starch, 1 carb., 1 fat
✔Shrimp Primavera	1	410	6	18	2.5	125	830	62	n/a	26	3 1/2 starch, 2 veg., 2 lean meat

SIDES

Plain Breadstick	1	140	2	13	0	0	270	26	n/a	5	1 1/2 starch

SOUP

✔ Minestrone	6 oz	100	1	11	0	0	670	18	n/a	5	1 starch

✔ = Healthiest Bets; n/a = not available

Notes

Papa John's Pizza

❖Papa John's provides nutrition information for all of its pizzas and side items in a brochure.

Light 'n Lean Choice

14" Garden Special Pizza, Original Crust
(*2 slices*)

Calories......................596	Sodium (mg)..........1,040
Fat (g) 21	Carbohydrate (g).........72
% calories from fat..32	Fiber (g) 6
Saturated fat (g)........8	Protein (g) 28
Cholesterol (mg).........40	

Exchanges: 4 starch, 2 veg., 2 high-fat meat, 1 fat

Healthy 'n Hearty Choice

14" Pepperoni Pizza, Original Crust
(*3 slices*)

Calories......................930	Sodium (mg)..........2,280
Fat (g) 39	Carbohydrate (g) 105
% calories from fat..38	Fiber (g) 6
Saturated fat (g)......15	Protein (g) 45
Cholesterol (mg).........75	

Exchanges: 6 starch, 3 high-fat meat, 3 fat

Papa John's Pizza

	Amount	Cal.	Fat (g)	% Cal. Fat	Sat. Fat (g)	Chol. (mg)	Sod. (mg)	Carb. (g)	Fiber (g)	Pro. (g)	Servings/Exchanges
ORIGINAL CRUST PIZZAS											
All the Meats	1 slice	410	18	40	7	35	1040	42	3	21	3 starch, 2 high-fat meat
✔Cheese	1 slice	286	9	28	3	18	540	37	2	14	2 1/2 starch, 1 high-fat meat
Garden Special	1 slice	298	11	33	4	20	570	36	3	14	2 starch, 1 veg., 1 high-fat meat
Pepperoni	1 slice	310	13	38	5	25	760	35	2	15	2 starch, 1 high-fat meat, 1/2 fat
Sausage	1 slice	340	13	34	6	25	910	40	2	15	2 1/2 starch, 1 high-fat meat, 1/2 fat

✔ = Healthiest Bets; n/a = not available

(Continued)

ORIGINAL CRUST PIZZAS (Continued)	Amount	Cal.	Fat (g)	% Cal. Fat	Sat. Fat (g)	Chol. (mg)	Sod. (mg)	Carb. (g)	Fiber (g)	Pro. (g)	Servings/Exchanges
The Works	1 slice	369	17	41	6	29	840	37	3	18	2 1/2 starch, 2 medium-fat meat, 1 fat
SIDES											
✔Breadsticks	1 stick	170	3	16	0	0	270	27	1	6	2 starch, 1/2 fat
✔Cheesesticks	1 stick	160	6	34	1.5	10	290	21	1	7	1 1/2 starch, 1 fat
Garlic Sauce	1 Tbsp	75	9	100	1.5	0	115	2	0	0	2 fat
✔Nacho Cheese	1 Tbsp	30	2	60	1.5	8	113	0	0	2	free
✔Pizza Sauce	1 Tbsp	10	1	50	0	0	60	1	1	0	free
THIN CRUST PIZZAS											
All the Meats	1 slice	330	20	55	9	39	919	23	2	15	1 1/2 starch, 2 medium-fat meat, 2 fat
Cheese	1 slice	220	11	45	5	18	480	22	2	9	1 1/2 starch, 1 high-fat meat

Garden Special	1 slice	238	12	45	6	19	540	23	3	9	1 starch, 1 veg., 1 high-fat meat
Pepperoni	1 slice	266	15	51	7	24	580	22	2	11	1 1/2 starch, 1 high-fat meat, 1 fat
Sausage	1 slice	270	15	50	7	29	730	22	2	12	1 1/2 starch, 1 high-fat meat, 1 fat
The Works	1 slice	319	19	54	8	35	760	24	3	14	1 1/2 starch, 1 high-fat meat, 2 fat

✔ = Healthiest Bets; n/a = not available

For all pizzas, 1 slice = 1/8 of a 14" pizza.

Notes

Pizza Hut

❖Pizza Hut provides nutrition information for all its menu items in a brochure.

Light 'n Lean Choice

Medium Ham Pizza, Thin 'N Crispy Crust
(*3 slices*)

Calories...................... 570

Fat (g) 18

  % calories from fat..28

  Saturated fat (g)........9

Cholesterol (mg) 45

Sodium (mg) 1,680

Carbohydrate (g)........ 69

  Fiber (g) 3

Protein (g) 30

Exchanges: 4 1/2 starch, 3 medium-fat meat

Healthy 'n Hearty Choice

Medium Veggie Lover's Pizza, Hand Tossed Crust
(*3 slices*)

Calories.......................720

Fat (g) 21

  % calories from fat..26

  Saturated fat (g)........9

Cholesterol (mg) 60

Sodium (mg) 1,950

Carbohydrate (g).......102

  Fiber (g) 9

Protein (g) 33

Exchanges: 6 starch, 3 veg., 3 fat

Pizza Hut

	Amount	Cal.	Fat (g)	% Cal. Fat	Sat. Fat (g)	Chol. (mg)	Sod. (mg)	Carb. (g)	Fiber (g)	Pro. (g)	Servings/Exchanges
DESSERTS											
✔Apple Dessert Pizza	1 slice	250	5	16	1	0	230	48	2	3	2 starch, 1 carb., 1 fat
✔Cherry Dessert Pizza	1 slice	250	5	16	1	0	220	47	3	3	2 starch, 1 carb., 1 fat
HAND TOSSED CRUST PIZZAS											
✔Beef Topping	1 slice	280	10	32	5	20	860	32	3	15	2 starch, 1 medium-fat meat, 1 fat
✔Cheese	1 slice	280	10	32	5	25	770	32	2	16	2 starch, 1 high-fat meat
✔Chicken Supreme	1 slice	240	6	23	3	25	660	31	3	14	2 starch, 1 lean meat, 1/2 fat
✔Ham	1 slice	230	6	23	3	25	710	30	2	13	2 starch, 1 lean meat, 1/2 fat

(Continued)

✔ = Healthiest Bets; n/a = not available

HAND TOSSED CRUST PIZZAS (Continued)	Amount	Cal.	Fat (g)	% Cal. Fat	Sat. Fat (g)	Chol. (mg)	Sod. (mg)	Carb. (g)	Fiber (g)	Pro. (g)	Servings/Exchanges
Italian Sausage	1 slice	300	12	36	5	30	780	32	3	15	2 starch, 1 high-fat meat
Meat Lover's	1 slice	290	11	34	4.5	35	820	32	3	15	2 starch, 1 high-fat meat
✓Pepperoni	1 slice	260	9	31	4	30	750	31	3	12	2 starch, 1 high-fat meat
Pepperoni Lover's	1 slice	320	13	37	6	35	910	31	4	17	2 starch, 2 medium-fat meat, 1/2 fat
Pork Topping	1 slice	290	11	34	5	25	850	33	3	14	2 starch, 1 high-fat meat
✓Super Supreme	1 slice	290	10	31	4.5	35	830	34	4	15	2 starch, 1 high-fat meat
✓Supreme	1 slice	270	9	30	4.5	25	760	32	3	13	2 starch, 1 high-fat meat
✓Veggie Lover's	1 slice	240	7	26	3	20	650	34	3	11	2 starch, 1 veg., 1 fat
OTHER ENTREES											
Cavatini Pasta	1	480	14	26	6	25	1170	66	9	21	4 1/2 starch, 1 high-fat meat, 1 fat

	Amount	Cal.	Fat (g)	% Fat Cal.	Sat. Fat (g)	Chol. (mg)	Sod. (mg)	Carb. (g)	Fiber (g)	Pro. (g)	Exchanges/Choices
Cavatini Supreme Pasta	1	560	19	31	8	30	1400	73	10	24	5 starch, 1 medium-fat meat, 3 fat
Ham & Cheese Sandwich	1	550	21	34	7	65	2150	57	4	33	4 starch, 3 medium-fat meat, 1 fat
✔Spaghetti w/ Marinara Sauce	1	490	6	11	1	0	730	91	8	18	5 starch, 1 carb., 1 fat
✔Spaghetti w/ Meat Sauce	1	600	13	20	5	25	910	98	9	23	5 1/2 starch, 1 carb., 1 medium-fat meat, 1 1/2 fat
Spaghetti w/ Meatballs	1	850	24	25	10	50	1120	120	10	37	7 starch, 1 carb., 2 medium-fat meat, 3 fat
Supreme Sandwich	1	640	28	39	10	85	2150	62	4	34	4 starch, 3 lean meat, 4 fat
PAN PIZZAS											
Beef Topping	1 slice	310	14	41	5	20	720	31	2	14	2 starch, 1 medium-fat meat, 2 fat

(Continued)

✔ = Healthiest Bets; n/a = not available

PAN PIZZAS (Continued)	Amount	Cal.	Fat (g)	% Cal. Fat	Sat. Fat (g)	Chol. (mg)	Sod. (mg)	Carb. (g)	Fiber (g)	Pro. (g)	Servings/Exchanges
Cheese	1 slice	300	14	42	6	25	610	30	2	15	2 starch, 1 high-fat meat, 1 fat
Chicken Supreme	1 slice	280	11	35	3.5	25	570	32	3	14	2 starch, 1 lean meat, 1 1/2 fat
✔Ham	1 slice	250	9	32	4	10	590	31	2	12	2 starch, 1 lean meat, 1 fat
Italian Sausage	1 slice	350	18	46	6	40	740	31	3	16	2 starch, 1 high-fat meat, 1 1/2 fat
Meat Lover's	1 slice	360	19	48	6	40	870	30	3	17	2 starch, 2 high-fat meat
Pepperoni	1 slice	280	12	39	4.5	20	640	31	3	12	2 starch, 1 high-fat meat
Pepperoni Lover's	1 slice	350	17	44	8	20	800	32	2	17	2 starch, 2 medium-fat meat, 1 fat
Pork Topping	1 slice	300	13	39	5	30	720	31	3	14	2 starch, 1 high-fat meat, 1/2 fat
Super Supreme	1 slice	340	16	42	5	30	790	33	4	15	2 starch, 1 high-fat meat, 1 fat

	Amount	Cal.	Fat (g)	% Cal. Fat	Sat. Fat (g)	Chol. (mg)	Sod. (mg)	Carb. (g)	Fiber (g)	Pro. (g)	Exchanges/Choices
Supreme	1 slice	300	13	39	5	25	670	32	3	13	2 starch, 1 high-fat meat, 1/2 fat
✔Veggie Lover's	1 slice	240	9	34	3.5	10	480	31	3	10	1 1/2 starch, 1 veg., 2 fat
PERSONAL PAN PIZZAS											
Cheese	whole pizza	630	24	34	11	45	1160	76	4	28	5 starch, 2 high-fat meat, 1 fat
Pepperoni	whole pizza	670	29	39	12	60	1250	73	4	29	5 starch, 2 high-fat meat, 2 fat
Supreme	whole pizza	710	31	39	13	60	1380	76	5	32	5 starch, 2 high-fat meat, 2 fat
SIDES											
✔Bread Stick	1	130	4	28	1	0	170	20	1	3	1 starch, 1 fat
✔Bread Stick Dipping Sauce	1 order	30	1	16	0	0	170	5	1	1	free
✔Garlic Bread	1 slice	150	8	48	1.5	0	240	16	1	3	1 starch, 1 1/2 fat
Hot Buffalo Wings	4 wings	210	12	51	3	130	900	4	1	22	3 medium-fat meat
✔Mild Buffalo Wings	5 wings	200	12	54	3.5	150	510	1	1	23	3 medium-fat meat

✔ = Healthiest Bets; n/a = not available

(Continued)

	Amount	Cal.	Fat (g)	% Cal. Fat	Sat. Fat (g)	Chol. (mg)	Sod. (mg)	Carb. (g)	Fiber (g)	Pro. (g)	Servings/Exchanges
STUFFED CRUST PIZZAS											
Beef Topping	1 slice	410	14	31	6	30	1270	49	4	20	3 starch, 2 medium-fat meat, 1 fat
Cheese	1 slice	380	11	26	5	25	1160	49	4	21	3 starch, 2 medium-fat meat
Chicken Supreme	1 slice	390	13	30	6	40	1130	46	4	21	3 starch, 2 lean meat, 1 fat
Ham	1 slice	380	14	33	6	45	1250	43	4	22	3 starch, 2 lean meat, 1 fat
Italian Sausage	1 slice	430	19	40	8	35	1200	46	4	20	3 starch, 2 high-fat meat
Meat Lover's	1 slice	500	23	41	10	60	1510	47	4	25	3 starch, 2 high-fat meat, 1/2 fat
Pepperoni	1 slice	410	17	37	7	40	1250	46	4	20	3 starch, 2 medium-fat meat, 1 fat
Pepperoni Lover's	1 slice	480	22	41	9	60	1440	47	4	24	3 starch, 2 high-fat meat

	Serving										Exchanges
Pork Topping	1 slice	420	16	34	7	30	1290	46	4	22	3 starch, 2 medium-fat meat, 1 fat
Super Supreme	1 slice	470	20	38	8	50	1440	49	5	24	3 starch, 2 high-fat meat
Supreme	1 slice	440	16	33	7	40	1380	51	4	23	3 1/2 starch, 2 medium-fat meat, 1 fat
Veggie Lover's	1 slice	390	14	32	6	25	1140	48	5	18	3 starch, 1 veg., 1 high-fat meat, 1 fat
THE EDGE PIZZA											
✔Chicken Veggie (medium)	1 slice	120	3	23	1	10	310	16	1	6	1 starch, 1 lean meat
✔Chicken Veggie (large)	1 slice	160	4	23	2	10	430	21	2	8	1 1/2 starch, 1 medium-fat meat
✔Meaty (medium)	1 slice	150	7	42	3	15	430	15	1	7	1 starch, 1 medium-fat meat

(Continued)

✔ = Healthiest Bets; n/a = not available

THE EDGE PIZZA (Continued)	Amount	Cal.	Fat (g)	% Cal. Fat	Sat. Fat (g)	Chol. (mg)	Sod. (mg)	Carb. (g)	Fiber (g)	Pro. (g)	Servings/Exchanges
✓Meaty (large)	1 slice	200	10	45	4	25	580	19	1	9	1 starch, 1 medium-fat meat, 1 fat
✓The Works (medium)	1 slice	140	5	32	2	10	360	16	1	6	1 starch, 1 medium-fat meat
✓The Works (large)	1 slice	180	7	35	3	15	470	21	2	8	1 1/2 starch, 1 medium-fat meat
✓Veggie (medium)	1 slice	110	3	20	1	5	250	16	1	4	1 starch, 1/2 fat
✓Veggie (large)	1 slice	140	4	23	1.5	5	340	21	2	6	1 1/2 starch, 1 fat
THE SICILIAN PIZZA											
Beef Topping	1 slice	320	15	42	6	20	930	31	3	13	2 starch, 1 medium-fat meat, 2 fat
Cheese	1 slice	290	13	40	6	10	740	31	2	12	2 starch, 1 medium-fat meat, 1 1/2 fat

										Exchanges/Choices
Chicken Supreme	1 slice	270	10	33	3.5	15	730	32	3	13	2 starch, 1 medium-fat meat, 1 fat
Ham	1 slice	260	10	35	4	15	750	31	2	11	2 starch, 1 medium-fat meat, 1 fat
Italian Sausage	1 slice	330	16	44	6	25	850	32	2	14	2 starch, 1 medium-fat meat, 2 fat
Meat Lover's	1 slice	350	18	46	7	30	990	32	3	15	2 starch, 1 medium-fat meat, 2 1/2 fat
Pepperoni	1 slice	290	13	40	5	20	760	31	2	11	2 starch, 1 medium-fat meat, 1 1/2 fat
Pepperoni Lover's	1 slice	330	17	46	7	30	910	31	2	14	2 starch, 1 medium-fat meat, 2 fat

(Continued)

✔ = Healthiest Bets; n/a = not available

THE SICILIAN PIZZA (Continued)	Amount	Cal.	Fat (g)	% Cal. Fat	Sat. Fat (g)	Chol. (mg)	Sod. (mg)	Carb. (g)	Fiber (g)	Pro. (g)	Servings/Exchanges
Pork Topping	1 slice	320	16	45	6	20	890	31	3	13	2 starch, 1 medium-fat meat, 2 fat
Super Supreme	1 slice	320	16	45	6	25	930	32	3	14	2 starch, 1 medium-fat meat, 2 fat
Supreme	1 slice	310	15	44	6	20	860	32	3	13	2 starch, 1 medium-fat meat, 2 fat
Veggie Lover's	1 slice	270	11	37	3.5	5	670	32	3	10	2 starch, 1 medium-fat meat, 1 fat
THIN 'N CRISPY CRUST PIZZAS											
✔Beef Topping	1 slice	240	11	41	5	20	790	22	2	13	1 1/2 starch, 1 medium-fat meat, 1 fat
✔Cheese	1 slice	210	9	39	4.5	20	530	21	2	12	1 1/2 starch, 1 medium-fat meat, 1 fat

✔Chicken Supreme	1 slice	220	7	29	2.5	25	550	26	2	14	1 1/2 starch, 1 medium-fat meat
✔Ham	1 slice	190	6	28	3	15	560	23	1	10	1 1/2 starch, 1 medium-fat meat
Italian Sausage	1 slice	300	16	48	6	35	740	24	3	15	1 1/2 starch, 1 medium-fat meat, 2 fat
Meat Lover's	1 slice	310	16	46	7	35	900	25	3	16	1 1/2 starch, 2 medium-fat meat, 1 fat
✔Pepperoni	1 slice	220	9	37	4	20	610	22	2	10	1 1/2 starch, 1 high-fat meat
Pepperoni Lover's	1 slice	270	12	40	6	25	780	26	2	15	1 1/2 starch, 2 medium-fat meat
Pork Topping	1 slice	270	13	43	6	25	780	22	2	14	1 1/2 starch, 1 medium-fat meat, 1 1/2 fat

✔ = Healthiest Bets; n/a = not available

(Continued)

THIN 'N CRISPY CRUST PIZZAS (Continued)	Amount	Cal.	Fat (g)	% Cal. Fat	Sat. Fat (g)	Chol. (mg)	Sod. (mg)	Carb. (g)	Fiber (g)	Pro. (g)	Servings/Exchanges
Super Supreme	1 slice	280	13	42	5	30	810	26	4	15	1 1/2 starch, 2 medium-fat meat, 1 1/2 fat
Supreme	1 slice	250	11	40	5	20	710	24	3	13	1 1/2 starch, 1 medium-fat meat, 1 fat
✔ Veggie Lover's	1 slice	170	6	32	2	10	460	23	3	7	1 1/2 starch, 1 fat

✔ = Healthiest Bets; n/a = not available

Notes

Romano's Macaroni Grill

❖Romano's Macaroni Grill provided only its menu.

Light 'n Lean Choice

Insalata della Casa
(*balsamic vinaigrette served on side*)
Pizza Riomaggiore (*split*)

Healthy 'n Hearty Choice

Wine (*1 glass*)
Insalata Verde
Fusilli Vegetali (*split*)
Petti di Pollo Pepe (*split*)

No nutrition information available from restaurant.

Healthier Picks

Lunch Menu

Antipasti
Bruschette Miste (*tomato & basil or mushroom & garlic*)
Mozzarella alla Caprese

Insalate (*order salad dressing on side*)
Insalata Italiana (*hold cheese*)
Zuppa e Insalata (*if broth-based soup*)
Insalata con Pollo
Insalata della Casa
Insalata Gargana

(Continued)

Panini (*Italian sandwiches; hold vegetable chips*)
Galli (*hold pancetta*)
Pollo Cesare (*hold cheese*)

Pizza (*request light cheese; consider splitting and ordering Insalata della Casa*)
Pizza Margherita
Pizza Napoli
Pizza Vegetale
Pizza di Pollo Barbacoda
Pizza Riomaggiore

Pasta
Capellini al Pomodoro
Lasagna alla Bolognese
Spaghettini alla Bolognese
Fusilli Vegetali
Fettuccine con Pollo

Specialita della Casa
Petti di Pollo Pepe (*order with no oil or butter*)

Dinner Menu

Antipasti
Bruschette Miste (*tomato and basil or mushroom and garlic*)
New Zealand Green Lip Mussels (*1/2 dozen on pasta*)
Portabella Mushroom
Mozzarella alla Caprese

Insalate (*order salad dressing on side*)
Insalata Italiana (*hold cheese*)
Insalata della Casa
Spinaci e Aglio
Insalata Gargana
Insalata Verde

Pizza (*request light cheese; consider splitting and ordering Insalata della Casa*)
Pizza Margherita
Pizza Napoli
Pizza Vegetale
Pizza di Pollo Barbacoda
Pizza Riomaggiore

Pasta
Capellini al Pomodoro
Fusilli Vegetali
Fettuccine con Pollo
Linguine alla Pescatora
Lasagna alla Bolognese
Spaghettini alla Bolognese

Pollame (*chicken*)
Petti di Pollo Pepe (*order with no oil or butter*)

Vitello, Manzo (*meats*)
Coscia di Porco (*ham steak*)
Grilled Lamb Chops (*split; order with Fusilli Vegetali*)
Lombatine di Maiale (*grilled center-cut pork chops; split; order with Capellini al Pomodoro*)

Round Table Pizza

❖Round Table Pizza provided nutrition information for its personal-size and large pizzas. Saluté pizzas have 25% less fat than the regular pizzas.

Light 'n Lean Choice

Personal-Size Western BBQ Chicken Supreme Pizza, Thin Crust

Calories.......................590	Sodium (mg)..........1,130
Fat (g) 20	Carbohydrate (g).........60
% calories from fat..31	Fiber (g) 2
Saturated fat (g)......12	Protein (g) 30
Cholesterol (mg) 90	

Exchanges: 4 starch, 3 medium-fat meat, 1 fat

Healthy 'n Hearty Choice

Guinever's Garden Delight, Thin Crust *(4 slices)*

Calories.......................600	Sodium (mg)..........1,000
Fat (g) 24	Carbohydrate (g).........72
% calories from fat..36	Fiber (g) 0
Saturated fat (g)......12	Protein (g) 28
Cholesterol (mg) 60	

Exchanges: 4 starch, 4 medium-fat meat

Round Table Pizza

	Amount	Cal.	Fat (g)	% Cal. Fat	Sat. Fat (g)	Chol. (mg)	Sod. (mg)	Carb. (g)	Fiber (g)	Pro. (g)	Servings/Exchanges
PAN PIZZAS, LARGE											
✔Alfredo Contempo	1/16 pizza	220	7	29	4	25	240	27	0	12	2 starch, 1 medium-fat meat
✔Bacon Super Deli	1/16 pizza	260	14	48	5	25	380	26	0	12	2 starch, 1 medium-fat meat, 2 fat
✔Cheese	1/16 pizza	210	7	30	4.5	20	250	26	0	10	2 starch, 1 medium-fat meat
✔Chicken & Garlic Gourmet	1/16 pizza	230	8	31	4	25	310	27	0	11	2 starch, 1 medium-fat meat, 1/2 fat
✔Classic Pesto	1/16 pizza	230	9	35	4	15	240	27	0	9	2 starch, 1 medium-fat meat, 1 fat

✔ = Healthiest Bets; n/a = not available

(Continued)

PAN PIZZAS, LARGE (Continued)	Amount	Cal.	Fat (g)	% Cal. Fat	Sat. Fat (g)	Chol. (mg)	Sod. (mg)	Carb. (g)	Fiber (g)	Pro. (g)	Servings/Exchanges
✓Garden Pesto	1/16 pizza	230	9	35	4	15	230	28	0	9	2 starch, 1 medium-fat meat, 1 fat
✓Gourmet Veggie	1/16 pizza	220	7	29	3.5	20	230	28	1	9	2 starch, 1 fat
✓Guinever's Garden Delight	1/16 pizza	200	6	27	3.5	15	250	27	0	9	2 starch, 1 fat
✓Italian Garlic Supreme	1/16 pizza	250	11	38	4	25	240	27	0	10	2 starch, 1 medium-fat meat, 1 fat
✓King Arthur's Supreme	1/16 pizza	240	10	38	4	25	320	27	0	10	2 starch, 1 medium-fat meat, 1 fat
Maui Zaui w/ Chili Sauce	1/16 pizza	320	11	31	6	30	500	39	0	15	2 1/2 starch, 1 medium-fat meat, 1 fat
✓Maui Zaui w/ Red Pizza Sauce	1/16 pizza	310	10	29	6	30	490	37	1	15	2 1/2 starch, 1 medium-fat meat, 1 fat

✔Pepperoni	1/16 pizza	220	8	33	3.5	20	240	26	0	9	2 starch, 1 medium-fat meat, 1/2 fat
✔Saluté Cashew Chicken	1/16 pizza	200	5	21	2	15	260	31	0	9	2 starch, 1 lean meat
✔Saluté Chicken & Garlic	1/16 pizza	200	6	27	2.5	20	270	28	0	9	2 starch, 1 lean meat, 1/2 fat
✔Saluté Veggie	1/16 pizza	190	5	24	2.5	10	190	28	1	8	2 starch, 1 medium-fat meat
Steak Supreme w/Creamy Garlic Sauce	1/16 pizza	370	17	41	6	45	460	36	0	17	2 1/2 starch, 1 medium-fat meat, 2 fat
Steak Supreme w/ Red Sauce	1/16 pizza	350	15	39	6	40	490	37	0	17	2 1/2 starch, 1 medium-fat meat, 2 fat
✔Western BBQ Chicken Supreme	1/16 pizza	220	7	27	3.5	30	360	27	0	11	2 starch, 1 lean meat, 1 fat
✔Zesty Santa Fe Chicken	1/16 pizza	240	9	34	4.5	30	360	27	0	11	2 starch, 1 lean meat, 1 fat

(Continued)

✔ = Healthiest Bets; n/a = not available

	Amount	Cal.	Fat (g)	% Cal. Fat	Sat. Fat (g)	Chol. (mg)	Sod. (mg)	Carb. (g)	Fiber (g)	Pro. (g)	Servings/Exchanges
PAN PIZZAS, PERSONAL SIZE											
Bacon Super Deli	whole pizza	920	37	36	17	85	1310	100	2	41	7 starch, 3 medium-fat meat, 4 fat
Buffalo Chicken	whole pizza	880	33	34	14	90	1480	104	2	39	7 starch, 3 lean meat, 5 fat
Cheese	whole pizza	800	26	29	16	70	880	100	2	35	7 starch, 2 medium-fat meat, 3 fat
Chicken & Garlic Gourmet	whole pizza	850	28	30	14	90	1100	106	3	40	7 starch, 3 medium-fat meat, 2 1/2 fat
Classic Pesto	whole pizza	830	29	31	13	55	830	106	3	33	7 starch, 3 lean meat, 4 fat
Garden Pesto	whole pizza	830	29	31	13	55	780	106	4	33	7 starch, 2 medium-fat meat, 4 fat
Gourmet Veggie	whole pizza	810	25	28	13	60	780	108	5	34	7 starch, 2 medium-fat meat, 3 fat

	Serving	Cal									Exchanges
Guinever's Garden Delight	whole pizza	750	21	25	12	50	840	104	3	31	7 starch, 1 medium-fat meat, 3 fat
Italian Garlic Supreme	whole pizza	960	42	39	14	95	900	104	2	39	7 starch, 3 medium-fat meat, 5 fat
King Arthur's Supreme	whole pizza	860	33	35	13	80	1090	103	3	37	7 starch, 2 medium-fat meat, 4 1/2 fat
Pepperoni	whole pizza	810	29	32	12	75	820	100	2	34	7 starch, 2 medium-fat meat, 4 fat
Western BBQ Chicken Supreme	whole pizza	820	22	24	12	90	1200	104	3	37	7 starch, 2 lean meat, 3 fat

THIN CRUST PIZZAS, LARGE

	Serving	Cal									Exchanges
✓ Alfredo Contempo	1/16 pizza	170	7	35	3.5	25	210	17	0	9	1 starch, 1 medium-fat meat

(Continued)

✓ = Healthiest Bets; n/a = not available

THIN CRUST PIZZAS, LARGE (Continued)	Amount	Cal.	Fat (g)	% Cal. Fat	Sat. Fat (g)	Chol. (mg)	Sod. (mg)	Carb. (g)	Fiber (g)	Pro. (g)	Servings/Exchanges
Bacon Super Deli	1/16 pizza	200	13	59	4.5	25	360	16	0	9	1 starch, 1 medium-fat meat, 1 1/2 fat
✓Cheese	1/16 pizza	160	6	34	4	20	240	16	0	7	1 starch, 1 medium-fat meat
✓Chicken & Garlic Gourmet	1/16 pizza	170	7	37	3.5	25	280	17	0	9	1 starch, 1 medium-fat meat
✓Classic Pesto	1/16 pizza	170	8	42	3.5	15	210	18	0	7	1 starch, 1 medium-fat meat, 1/2 fat
✓Garden Pesto	1/16 pizza	170	8	42	3.5	15	200	18	0	7	1 starch, 1 1/2 fat
✓Gourmet Veggie	1/16 pizza	160	7	37	3	15	200	18	0	7	1 starch, 1 medium-fat meat
✓Guinever's Garden Delight	1/16 pizza	150	6	36	3	15	250	18	0	7	1 starch, 1 fat
✓Italian Garlic Supreme	1/16 pizza	200	10	45	4	25	220	17	0	8	1 starch, 1 medium-fat meat, 1 fat
✓King Arthur's Supreme	1/16 pizza	200	10	45	4	25	340	18	0	9	1 starch, 1 medium-fat meat, 1 fat

✔Maui Zaui w/ Chili Sauce	1/16 pizza	180	7	35	3.5	20	330	19	0	9	1 starch, 1 medium-fat meat
✔Maui Zaui w/ Red Pizza Sauce	1/16 pizza	170	7	35	3.5	20	350	18	0	9	1 starch, 1 medium-fat meat
✔Pepperoni	1/16 pizza	170	8	42	3	20	240	17	0	8	1 starch, 1 medium-fat meat
✔Saluté Cashew Chicken	1/16 pizza	150	4	24	2	15	240	21	0	7	1 1/2 starch, 1 lean meat
✔Saluté Chicken & Garlic	1/16 pizza	150	5	30	2.5	20	250	18	0	8	1 starch, 1 lean meat
✔Saluté Veggie	1/16 pizza	140	5	32	2	10	170	19	1	6	1 starch, 1 fat
Steak Supreme w/ Creamy Garlic Sauce	1/16 pizza	210	11	47	4	30	310	17	0	10	1 starch, 1 medium-fat meat, 1 fat
Steak Supreme w/ Red Sauce	1/16 pizza	200	10	45	4	30	340	18	0	10	1 starch, 1 medium-fat meat, 1 fat
✔Western BBQ Chicken Supreme	1/16 pizza	170	6	32	3.5	25	330	17	0	8	1 starch, 1 medium-fat meat

(Continued)

✔ = Healthiest Bets; n/a = not available

THIN CRUST PIZZAS, LARGE (Continued)	Amount	Cal.	Fat (g)	% Cal. Fat	Sat. Fat (g)	Chol. (mg)	Sod. (mg)	Carb. (g)	Fiber (g)	Pro. (g)	Servings/Exchanges
✓Zesty Santa Fe Chicken	1/16 pizza	180	8	40	4	25	310	17	0	9	1 starch, 1 lean meat, 1 fat
THIN CRUST PIZZAS, PERSONAL SIZE											
Bacon Super Deli	whole pizza	690	35	46	16	85	1230	56	1	33	4 starch, 3 medium-fat meat, 4 fat
Buffalo Chicken	whole pizza	660	31	42	14	90	1410	60	2	31	4 starch, 3 medium-fat meat, 3 fat
Cheese	whole pizza	570	24	38	15	70	850	57	2	28	4 starch, 2 medium-fat meat, 3 fat
Chicken & Garlic Gourmet	whole pizza	620	26	38	13	90	1030	62	2	32	4 starch, 3 lean meat, 3 fat
Classic Pesto	whole pizza	610	27	40	13	55	750	62	3	26	4 starch, 2 medium-fat meat, 3 fat

Garden Pesto	whole pizza	610	27	40	12	55	710	63	3	26	4 starch, 2 medium-fat meat, 3 fat
Gourmet Veggie	whole pizza	580	23	36	12	60	710	65	4	26	4 starch, 2 medium-fat meat, 2 1/2 fat
Guinever's Garden Delight	whole pizza	540	20	33	11	50	880	63	3	24	4 starch, 2 medium-fat meat, 2 fat
Italian Garlic Supreme	whole pizza	730	40	49	14	95	830	60	2	31	4 starch, 3 medium-fat meat, 5 fat
King Arthur's Supreme	whole pizza	710	37	47	15	90	1180	61	3	32	4 starch, 3 medium-fat meat, 4 fat
Pepperoni	whole pizza	620	30	44	11	80	830	58	2	28	4 starch, 2 medium-fat meat, 4 fat

(Continued)

✓ = Healthiest Bets; n/a = not available

THIN CRUST PIZZAS, PERSONAL SIZE (Continued)	Amount	Cal.	Fat (g)	% Cal. Fat	Sat. Fat (g)	Chol. (mg)	Sod. (mg)	Carb. (g)	Fiber (g)	Pro. (g)	Servings/Exchanges
Western BBQ Chicken Supreme	whole pizza	590	20	31	12	90	1130	60	2	30	4 starch, 3 medium-fat meat, 1 fat

Notes

Tacos, Burritos, and All Else Mexican

RESTAURANTS

Chi-Chi's

Del Taco

Taco Bell

Taco John's

Taco Time

NUTRITION PROS

- Beans used in Mexican cooking, such as pinto beans and black beans, add soluble fiber. This is the kind of fiber that can make your blood glucose rise more slowly and less high.
- In most of the fast-food Mexican restaurants, ordering is à la carte—an enchilada, a burrito, a Mexican salad. This helps you order less and eat less.
- High-fat items, such as guacamole, cheese, and sour cream, are added onto and not mixed into some dishes. That's a plus because special requests to hold or serve them on the side are mission possible.
- Hot and spicy sauces—red sauce, green sauce, or salsa—add zest without the fat and calories of sour cream, cheese, and guacamole.
- Garlic, cilantro, chilies, and onions add flavor with few calories.

- Mexican cuisine is naturally low in protein. You don't get 8-oz hunks of meat. You find a small amount of protein mixed into dishes.
- Mexican cuisine is naturally high in carbohydrate. Beans, flour or corn tortillas, and rice are the staples of the cuisine.
- Most fast-food Mexican restaurants now fry in 100% vegetable oil. That's better than lard because it contains no cholesterol and less saturated fat. But remember, teaspoon for teaspoon, the calories are the same.
- In the fast-food Mexican restaurants, the "bet-you-can't-eat-just-one" tortilla chips don't greet you at the table.

NUTRITION CONS

- Fried items seem almost unavoidable—tortilla chips, taco shells, tortilla shells (such as salad might be served in), and chimichangas.
- Cheese—shredded, melted, or sauced—is a mainstay ingredient.
- Vegetables are few and far between—a few shreds of lettuce or pieces of tomato.
- Fruit is nowhere to be found.
- High-fiber beans are often served refried. Some restaurants still use lard to make their refried beans.
- The bet-you-can't-eat-just-one tortilla chips are waiting at your table in most sit-down Mexican or Tex-Mex restaurants.

Healthy Tips

★ If the fried tortilla chips greet you when you sit down, hands off. Send them back from whence they came or at least to the opposite side of the table.

★ Use extra salsa and other hot sauces to add flavor with very few calories.

★ Use salsa or another hot sauce as a salad dressing.

★ Don't feel it is a must to order an entree. Choose from appetizers and side dishes to control your portions.

★ Take advantage of ordering à la carte. Mix and match a healthy meal.

★ As a starter, try a cup of black bean soup or chili to fill you up and not out.

★ Make a bowl of black bean soup or chili the main course with a salad on the side.

★ Look for menu items that use soft tortillas rather than crispy fried ones. For example, choose a burrito or an enchilada rather than a taco or a chimichanga.

★ Split an order of an entrée. Fajitas are great to split. They say they're for one, but there's always enough for two.

★ Split a side dish—Mexican rice, refried beans, or black beans—to get more carbohydrates and fiber.

★ Take advantage of lite or nonfat sour cream if it's served.

Get It Your Way

* ★ Hold the guacamole, cheese, and sour cream, or ask for them on the side.
* ★ If a menu item is served with melted cheese, request a light helping.
* ★ Substitute black beans for refried beans (if available).
* ★ Ask for extra tomatoes and lettuce.
* ★ Request extra salsa or other zesty, low-calorie topper.

Chi-Chi's

❖Chi-Chi's provided nutrition information for two
  menu items.

Light 'n Lean Choice

Tortilla Soup (*hold the cheese*)
Mexican Pizza (*order as entree*)

No nutrition information was available for these
items.

Healthy 'n Hearty Choice

Low-Fat Chicken Enchiladas
(*request extra pico de gallo*)
Spanish Rice
Steamed Mexi-Veggies

Calories......................688	Sodium (mg)..............n/a
Fat (g) 19	Carbohydrate (g) ....n/a
% calories from fat..25	Fiber (g) ....n/a
Saturated fat (g) ....n/a	Protein (g) ....n/a
Cholesterol (mg)........n/a	

Exchanges: insufficient nutrition information to
calculate

Healthier Picks

Appetizers
Mexican Pizza (*consider ordering as an entree*)
Grilled Chicken Quesadilla (*hold sour cream and
    guacamole; request double order of salsa; consider
    ordering as an entree*)

(*Continued*)

Vegadilla (*hold sour cream and guacamole; request double order of salsa; consider ordering as an entree*)

Soups and Salads

Taco Salad (*request in bowl instead of fried tortilla shell; try salsa as salad dressing*)

Chajitas Salad (*request in bowl instead of fried tortilla shell; hold sour cream and guacamole; try salsa as salad dressing*)

Tortilla Soup (*hold the cheese*)

Tortilla Soup & Salad (*hold the cheese*)

Dinner Salad (*hold the cheese*)

Sandwiches

Grilled Chicken Sandwich (*substitute Spanish rice for fries*)

Chi-Chi's Burger (*substitute Spanish rice for fries*)

Chajitas Sandwich (*substitute Spanish rice for fries*)

Chi-Chi's Favorites

Twice Grilled BBQ Burritos (*hold the cheese and sweet corn cake*)

El Grande Burritos (*choose beef or chicken; hold the cheese and sweet corn cake*)

Pollo Magnifico (*substitute tortilla for sweet corn cake*)

Enchiladas Conquistador (*order chicken or beef; hold sweet corn cake*)

Low-Fat Chicken Enchiladas*

Low-Fat Grilled Chicken Soft Tacos*

Sizzling Chajitas (*hold guacamole and sour cream; request double order of salsa*)

*See nutrition information in table.

Chi-Chi's

	Amount	Cal.	Fat (g)	% Cal. Fat	Sat. Fat (g)	Chol. (mg)	Sod. (mg)	Carb. (g)	Fiber (g)	Pro. (g)	Servings/Exchanges
Low Fat Chicken Enchiladas	1	688	19	25	n/a	n/a	n/a	n/a	n/a	n/a	insufficient info. to calculate
Low Fat Chicken Soft Taco	1	692	7	9	n/a	n/a	n/a	n/a	n/a	n/a	insufficient info. to calculate

Notes

Del Taco

❖Del Taco provides nutrition information for all its menu items in a brochure.

Light 'n Lean Choice

Tostada Salad
Chicken Soft Taco
Beans 'n Cheese Cup (*split*)

Calories.......................550	Sodium (mg)...........2,065
Fat (g) 23	Carbohydrate (g).........62
% calories from fat..38	Fiber (g) 25
Saturated fat (g)......10	Protein (g) 28
Cholesterol (mg).........48	

Exchanges: 5 starch, 1 veg., 3 medium-fat meat, 1 1/2 fat

Healthy 'n Hearty Choice

Red Burrito
Spicy Jack Quesadilla
Rice Cup

Calories.......................680	Sodium (mg)...........2,180
Fat (g) 22	Carbohydrate (g).........89
% calories from fat..29	Fiber (g) 8
Saturated fat (g)......13	Protein (g) 24
Cholesterol (mg).........47	

Exchanges: 6 starch, 2 medium-fat meat, 1 fat

Del Taco

	Amount	Cal.	Fat (g)	% Cal. Fat	Sat. Fat (g)	Chol. (mg)	Sod. (mg)	Carb. (g)	Fiber (g)	Pro. (g)	Servings/Exchanges
BEVERAGES											
✔Milk, 1% low-fat	1	130	3	18	2	10	150	15	0	10	1 low-fat milk
✔Orange Juice	1	140	0	0	0	0	0	34	1	2	2 fruit
BREAKFAST											
✔Breakfast Burrito	1	260	12	42	6	160	520	26	1	10	2 starch, 1 medium-fat meat, 1 fat
Egg & Bean Burrito	1	610	25	37	13	530	1950	70	14	33	4 1/2 starch, 3 lean meat, 3 fat
Egg & Beef Burrito	1	580	33	51	17	565	1000	42	3	34	3 starch, 4 medium-fat meat, 2 1/2 fat
Egg Burrito	1	450	24	48	13	530	740	39	3	23	2 1/2 starch, 2 lean meat, 5 fat

(Continued)

✔ = Healthiest Bets; n/a = not available

BREAKFAST (*Continued*)	Amount	Cal.	Fat (g)	% Cal. Fat	Sat. Fat (g)	Chol. (mg)	Sod. (mg)	Carb. (g)	Fiber (g)	Pro. (g)	Servings/Exchanges
Steak & Egg Burrito	1	580	34	53	16	560	1270	41	3	33	3 starch, 3 medium-fat meat, 4 fat
BURGERS											
✓Cheeseburger	1	330	13	35	6	35	870	37	3	16	2 1/2 starch, 1 medium-fat meat, 1 1/2 fat
Del Burger	1	380	21	50	5	35	490	35	4	13	2 starch, 1 medium-fat meat, 3 fat
Del Cheeseburger	1	430	25	52	7	45	710	35	4	16	2 starch, 2 medium-fat meat, 3 fat
Double Del Cheeseburger	1	560	35	56	12	85	960	35	4	26	2 starch, 3 medium-fat meat, 4 fat
✓Hamburger	1	280	9	29	3	25	640	37	3	13	2 1/2 starch, 1 medium-fat meat, 1 fat
BURRITOS											
Combo Burrito	1	490	21	39	13	55	1380	53	8	26	3 1/2 starch, 2 medium-fat meat, 2 fat

Del Beef Burrito	1	650	30	42	17	90	1090	42	3	31	3 starch, 3 medium-fat meat, 3 fat
Del Classic Chicken Burrito	1	580	38	59	13	70	1110	42	3	24	3 starch, 2 lean meat, 6 fat
Deluxe Combo Burrito	1	530	25	42	15	60	1390	56	9	27	3 1/2 starch, 2 medium-fat meat, 3 fat
Deluxe Del Beef Burrito	1	590	33	50	19	95	1110	45	4	32	3 starch, 3 medium-fat meat, 3 1/2 fat
Green Burrito	1	280	8	26	5	15	1030	38	6	11	2 1/2 starch, 1 medium-fat meat, 1/2 fat
Macho Beef Burrito	1	1170	62	48	29	190	2190	89	7	60	6 starch, 7 medium-fat meat, 5 fat
Macho Combo Burrito	1	1050	44	38	21	115	2760	113	17	49	7 starch, 3 medium-fat meat, 6 fat
✔ Red Burrito	1	270	8	27	5	15	1020	38	6	11	2 1/2 starch, 1 medium-fat meat, 1/2 fat

✔ = Healthiest Bets; n/a = not available

(Continued)

BURRITOS (Continued)	Amount	Cal.	Fat (g)	% Cal. Fat	Sat. Fat (g)	Chol. (mg)	Sod. (mg)	Carb. (g)	Fiber (g)	Pro. (g)	Servings/Exchanges
Regular Red Burrito	1	390	12	28	9	20	1439	59	11	18	4 starch, 1 medium-fat meat, 1 fat
Regular Green Burrito	1	400	12	27	9	20	1450	59	10	18	4 starch, 1 medium-fat meat, 1 fat
Sonora Chicken Burrito	1	600	40	60	13	80	1230	42	5	24	3 starch, 2 lean meat, 7 fat
Spicy Chicken Burrito	1	480	16	30	10	40	1620	65	8	23	4 starch, 2 medium-fat meat, 1 fat
The Works Burrito	1	480	18	34	11	25	1500	69	9	18	4 1/2 starch, 1 medium-fat meat, 2 1/2 fat
FRENCH FRIES											
Best Value Large Fries	1 order	490	32	59	5	0	380	47	5	5	3 starch, 6 fat
Chili Cheese Fries	1 order	670	46	62	15	45	880	51	5	17	3 1/2 starch, 1 high-fat meat, 7 fat
Deluxe Chili Cheese Fries	1 order	710	49	62	16	50	880	53	6	17	3 1/2 starch, 10 fat
Regular Fries	1 order	350	23	59	4	0	270	34	3	3	2 starch, 4 1/2 fat

	Amount										Exchanges/Choices
Small Fries	1 order	210	14	60	2	0	160	20	2	2	1 starch, 3 fat
NACHOS											
Macho Nachos	1 order	1200	66	50	26	55	2720	130	16	33	8 starch, 1 high-fat meat, 11 fat
Nachos	1 order	380	24	57	8	5	630	40	2	5	2 1/2 starch, 5 fat
QUESADILLAS											
Chicken Quesadilla	1	580	31	48	21	104	1240	41	2	33	2 1/2 starch, 4 medium-fat meat, 2 fat
✓Quesadilla	1	260	12	42	9	30	530	24	1	10	1 1/2 starch, 1 medium-fat meat, 1 fat
Regular Quesadilla	1	500	27	49	20	75	860	39	2	23	2 1/2 starch, 2 medium-fat meat, 3 fat
Spicy Jack Chicken Quesadilla	1	670	30	40	16	105	1300	40	2	32	2 1/2 starch, 4 lean meat, 4 fat

✔ = Healthiest Bets; n/a = not available

(Continued)

QUESADILLAS (Continued)	Amount	Cal.	Fat (g)	% Cal. Fat	Sat. Fat (g)	Chol. (mg)	Sod. (mg)	Carb. (g)	Fiber (g)	Pro. (g)	Servings/Exchanges
✓Spicy Jack Quesadilla	1	250	12	43	7	30	560	23	1	10	1 1/2 starch, 1 medium-fat meat, 1 fat
Spicy Jack Regular Quesadilla	1	490	26	48	17	75	920	38	2	23	2 1/2 starch, 2 medium-fat meat, 3 fat
SALADS											
Deluxe Chicken Salad	1	710	32	41	13	66	2130	75	14	31	4 starch, 3 veg, 2 lean meat, 5 fat
Deluxe Taco Salad	1	760	37	44	17	70	2010	76	14	31	4 starch, 3 veg, 2 medium-fat meat, 5 fat
✓Tostada Salad	1	210	9	39	5	15	640	24	6	9	1 starch, 1 veg., 1 medium-fat meat, 1 fat
SHAKES											
Chocolate (small)	1	620	12	17	9	35	270	89	1	12	1 low-fat milk, 5 carb, 2 fat

Chocolate (large)	1	680	16	21	12	45	350	117	1	16	1 low-fat milk, 6 carb., 2 1/2 fat
Strawberry (small)	1	410	6	13	4	30	220	76	1	11	1 low-fat milk, 4 carb.
Strawberry (large)	1	540	8	13	6	40	280	100	1	14	1 low-fat milk, 5 carb., 1 fat
Vanilla (small)	1	420	7	15	5	35	250	75	0	12	1 low-fat milk, 4 carb.
Vanilla (large)	1	550	10	16	6	50	320	97	0	16	1 low-fat milk, 5 carb., 1 1/2 fat

SIDES

Beans 'n Cheese Cup	1	260	3	10	2	5	1810	44	18	16	3 starch, 1 lean meat
✓Rice Cup	1	160	2	11	1	2	600	28	1	3	2 starch

TACOS

✓Chicken Soft Taco	1	210	12	51	4	30	520	16	1	11	1 starch, 1 medium-fat meat, 1 fat
✓Deluxe Double Beef Soft Taco	1	250	14	50	7	40	440	18	1	12	1 starch, 1 medium-fat meat, 2 fat
✓Deluxe Double Beef Taco	1	240	16	60	8	40	250	13	1	11	1 starch, 1 medium-fat meat, 2 fat
✓Double Beef Soft Taco	1	210	11	47	6	35	430	16	1	12	1 starch, 1 medium-fat meat, 1 fat

✓ = Healthiest Bets; n/a = not available

(Continued)

TACOS (Continued)	Amount	Cal.	Fat (g)	% Cal. Fat	Sat. Fat (g)	Chol. (mg)	Sod. (mg)	Carb. (g)	Fiber (g)	Pro. (g)	Servings/Exchanges
✔Double Beef Taco	1	210	13	56	6	35	240	11	1	11	1 starch, 1 medium-fat meat, 1 1/2 fat
✔Soft Taco	1	160	8	45	4	20	330	16	1	8	1 starch, 1 lean meat, 1 fat
✔Taco	1	160	10	56	4	20	150	11	1	7	1 starch, 1 medium-fat meat, 1 fat

✔ = Healthiest Bets; n/a = not available

Notes

Taco Bell

❖Taco Bell provides nutrition information for all of its menu items in a brochure.

Light 'n Lean Choice

Chicken Fajita Wrap
Pico de Gallo (*2 orders*)
Non-Fat Sour Cream (*1 order*)

Calories......................500	Sodium (mg)..........1,465
Fat (g) 21	Carbohydrate (g).........44
% calories from fat..38	Fiber (g) 3
Saturated fat (g)........6	Protein (g) 21
Cholesterol (mg) 45	

Exchanges: 3 starch, 2 medium-fat meat, 2 fat

Healthy 'n Hearty Choice

Tostada
Soft Taco
Salsa (*1 order*)
Pintos 'n Cheese

Calories......................735	Sodium (mg)..........2,000
Fat (g) 33	Carbohydrate (g).........75
% calories from fat..40	Fiber (g) 25
Saturated fat (g)......14	Protein (g) 33
Cholesterol (mg) 55	

Exchanges: 4 starch, 3 medium-fat meat, 4 fat

(*Continued*)

Taco Bell

	Amount	Cal.	Fat (g)	% Cal. Fat	Sat. Fat (g)	Chol. (mg)	Sod. (mg)	Carb. (g)	Fiber (g)	Pro. (g)	Servings/Exchanges
BEVERAGES											
✓Milk, 2%	8 oz	110	5	65	2.5	15	115	11	0	8	1 low-fat milk
✓Orange Juice	6 oz	80	0	11	0	0	0	18	0	1	1 fruit
BREAKFAST											
Breakfast Cheese Quesadilla	1	380	21	50	9	280	1010	33	1	15	2 starch, 1 high-fat meat, 2 fat
Breakfast Quesadilla with Bacon	1	450	27	55	11	290	1200	33	2	19	2 starch, 2 high-fat meat, 1 fat
Breakfast Quesadilla with Sausage	1	430	25	53	10	285	1090	33	1	17	2 starch, 5 fat
✓Country Breakfast Burrito	1	270	14	47	5	195	690	26	2	8	2 starch, 3 fat

Double Bacon & Egg Burrito	1	480	27	51	9	400	1240	39	2	18	2 1/2 starch, 5 fat
✔Fiesta Breakfast Burrito	1	280	16	51	6	25	580	25	2	9	1 1/2 starch, 3 fat
Grande Breakfast Burrito	1	420	22	47	7	205	1050	43	3	13	3 starch, 4 fat
Hash Brown Nuggets	1	280	18	58	5	0	570	29	1	2	3 starch, 3 1/2 fat

BURRITOS

7-Layer Burrito	1	530	23	40	7	25	1280	66	13	16	4 1/2 starch, 1 high-fat meat, 2 1/2 fat
Bacon Cheeseburger Burrito	1	570	31	48	12	70	1460	46	6	27	3 starch, 3 medium-fat meat, 3 fat
Bean Burrito	1	380	12	28	4	10	1110	55	13	13	3 1/2 starch, 2 fat
BIG BEEF Burrito Supreme	1	520	23	40	10	55	1520	54	11	24	3 1/2 starch, 2 medium-fat meat, 3 fat
BIG CHICKEN Supreme	1	510	24	42	7	95	1900	52	4	23	3 1/2 starch, 2 lean meat, 3 1/2 fat
Burrito Supreme	1	440	19	37	8	35	1230	51	10	17	3 starch, 1 medium-fat meat, 3 fat

(Continued)

✔ = Healthiest Bets; n/a = not available

BURRITOS (Continued)	Amount	Cal.	Fat (g)	% Cal. Fat	Sat. Fat (g)	Chol. (mg)	Sod. (mg)	Carb. (g)	Fiber (g)	Pro. (g)	Servings/Exchanges
Chicken Club Burrito	1	540	32	52	10	80	1250	43	4	20	3 starch, 2 medium-fat meat, 4 fat
✔Chili Cheese Burrito	1	330	13	35	6	35	870	37	5	14	2 1/2 starch, 1 medium-fat meat, 1 1/2 fat
Grilled Chicken	1	410	15	33	4.5	55	1380	50	4	17	3 starch, 1 lean fat meat, 2 fat

CONDIMENTS

	Amount	Cal.	Fat (g)	% Cal. Fat	Sat. Fat (g)	Chol. (mg)	Sod. (mg)	Carb. (g)	Fiber (g)	Pro. (g)	Servings/Exchanges
✔Border Sauce - Fire	1/3 oz	0	0	0	0	0	110	1	0	0	free
✔Border Sauce - Hot	1/3 oz	0	0	0	0	0	85	0	0	0	free
✔Border Sauce - Mild	1/3 oz	0	0	0	0	0	75	0	0	0	free
✔Burger Sauce	1/2 oz/1 Tbsp	60	5	72	1	5	110	2	0	0	1 fat
✔Cheddar Cheese	1/4 oz/1/2 Tbsp	30	2	60	1.5	5	45	0	0	2	free
Club Sauce	1/2 oz/1 Tbsp	80	8	90	1	10	105	1	0	0	1 1/2 fat
✔Green Sauce	1 oz/1 Tbsp	5	0	0	0	0	150	1	0	0	free

✓Guacamole	3/4 oz/1 1/2 Tbsp	35	3	77	0	0	80	1	1	0	1/2 fat
✓Nacho Cheese											
Sauce	2 oz/4 Tbsp	120	10	75	2.5	5	470	5	1	2	2 fat
✓Picante Sauce	1/3 oz	0	0	0	0	0	110	1	0	0	free
✓Pico de Gallo	3/4 oz/1 1/2 Tbsp	5	0	0	0	0	65	1	0	0	free
✓Red Sauce	1 oz	10	0	0	0	0	220	2	0	0	free
✓Sour Cream	3/4 oz/1 1/2 Tbsp	40	4	90	2.5	10	10	1	0	1	1 fat

DESSERTS

Choco Taco Ice Cream	1	310	17	49	10	50	100	37	1	3	2 1/2 carb., 3 fat

FAJITA WRAPS

Chicken Fajita Wrap	1	470	22	42	6	60	1290	51	4	17	3 starch, 1 medium-fat meat, 3 fat
Chicken Fajita Wrap Supreme	1	520	26	45	8	40	1300	53	4	18	3 starch, 2 medium-fat meat, 3 fat
Steak Fajita Wrap	1	470	21	40	6	40	1190	50	3	20	3 starch, 2 medium-fat meat, 2 fat

(Continued)

✓ = Healthiest Bets; n/a = not available

FAJITA WRAPS (Continued)	Amount	Cal.	Fat (g)	% Cal. Fat	Sat. Fat (g)	Chol. (mg)	Sod. (mg)	Carb. (g)	Fiber (g)	Pro. (g)	Servings/Exchanges
Steak Fajita Wrap Supreme	1	510	25	44	8	50	1200	52	3	21	3 1/2 starch, 2 medium-fat meat, 3 fat
✔Veggie Fajita Wrap	1	420	19	41	5	20	980	53	3	10	3 1/2 starch, 2 medium-fat meat, 2 fat
Veggie Fajita Wrap Supreme	1	470	22	45	7	30	990	55	3	11	3 1/2 starch, 4 fat
GORDITAS											
Gordita Fiesta Beef	1	290	13	40	4	25	880	31	3	14	2 starch, 1 medium-fat meat, 1 1/2 fat
Gordita Fiesta Chicken	1	280	12	39	3	45	910	29	3	14	2 starch, 1 lean meat, 2 fat
Gordita Fiesta Steak	1	270	10	33	2.5	25	800	28	2	17	2 starch, 2 medium-fat meat
Gordita Santa Fe Beef	1	370	20	49	4	35	440	33	4	14	2 starch, 1 medium-fat meat, 3 fat
Gordita Santa Fe Chicken	1	360	19	48	2.5	55	470	32	3	15	2 starch, 2 lean meat, 2 1/2 fat

Item	Amt	Cal	Fat (g)	%	Sat Fat (g)	Chol (mg)	Sod (mg)	Carb (g)		Prot (g)	Exchanges
Gordita Santa Fe Steak	1	350	18	46	2.5	35	360	31	2	18	2 starch, 2 medium-fat meat, 1 1/2 fat
Gordita Supreme Beef	1	300	13	39	6	35	390	31	3	14	2 starch, 1 medium-fat meat, 1/2 fat
Gordita Supreme Chicken	1	290	12	37	5	55	420	30	2	15	2 starch, 1 lean meat, 2 fat
Gordita Supreme Steak	1	280	11	35	5	35	310	28	1	18	2 starch, 2 medium-fat meat

OTHER ENTREES

Item	Amt	Cal	Fat (g)	%	Sat Fat (g)	Chol (mg)	Sod (mg)	Carb (g)		Prot (g)	Exchanges
✔ BIG BEEF MexiMelt	1	290	15	48	7	45	850	23	4	16	1 1/2 starch, 3 fat
BIG BEEF Nachos Supreme	1	450	24	50	8	30	810	45	9	14	3 starch, 1 medium-fat meat, 4 fat
✔ Cheese Quesadilla	1	350	18	49	9	50	860	32	2	16	2 starch, 1 medium-fat meat, 2 1/2 fat
Chicken Quesadilla	1	410	21	47	10	90	1170	34	3	23	2 starch, 3 medium-fat meat, 1 fat

(Continued)

✔ = Healthiest Bets; n/a = not available

OTHER ENTREES (Continued)	Amount	Cal.	Fat (g)	% Cal. Fat	Sat. Fat (g)	Chol. (mg)	Sod. (mg)	Carb. (g)	Fiber (g)	Pro. (g)	Servings/Exchanges
Mexican Pizza	1	570	35	57	10	45	1040	42	8	21	3 starch, 2 medium-fat meat, 5 fat
Nachos BellGrande	1	770	39	47	11	35	1310	84	17	21	5 1/2 starch, 1 medium-fat meat, 7 fat
✓Tostada	1	300	15	42	5	15	650	31	12	10	2 starch, 1 medium-fat meat, 2 fat
SALADS											
Taco Salad w/ Salsa	1	850	52	56	15	60	1780	65	16	30	4 starch, 3 medium-fat meat, 7 fat
Taco Salad w/ Salsa w/o Shell	1	420	22	45	11	60	1520	32	15	24	2 starch, 3 medium-fat meat, 1 fat
SIDES											
✓Cinnamon Twists	1 order	140	6	39	0	0	190	19	0	1	1 starch, 1 fat
Mexican Rice	1	190	9	47	3.5	15	760	23	1	5	1 1/2 starch, 2 fat
Nachos	1	320	18	52	4	20	570	34	3	5	2 starch, 3 1/2 fat
✓Pintos 'n Cheese	1	190	9	43	4	15	650	18	10	9	1 starch, 1 medium-fat meat, 1/2 fat

TACOS

										Exchanges
BLT Soft Taco	1	340	23	61	8	40	610	22	2	11	1 1/2 starch, 1 medium-fat meat, 3 1/2 fat
✔ DOUBLE DECKER Taco	1	340	15	40	5	25	750	38	9	14	2 1/2 starch, 1 medium-fat meat, 2 fat
✔ DOUBLE DECKER Taco Supreme	1	390	19	42	8	35	760	40	9	15	2 1/2 starch, 1 medium-fat meat, 3 fat
Grilled Chicken Soft Taco	1	240	12	45	3.5	45	1110	21	3	12	1 1/2 starch, 1 lean meat, 2 fat
Grilled Steak Soft Taco	1	230	10	39	2.5	25	1020	20	2	15	1 starch, 2 medium-fat meat
Grilled Steak Soft Taco Supreme	1	290	14	43	5	35	1040	24	3	16	1 1/2 starch, 2 medium-fat meat, 1 fat
✔ Soft Taco	1	220	10	43	4.5	25	580	21	3	11	1 starch, 1 medium-fat meat, 1 fat

(Continued)

✔ = Healthiest Bets; n/a = not available

TACOS (Continued)	Amount	Cal.	Fat (g)	% Cal. Fat	Sat. Fat (g)	Chol. (mg)	Sod. (mg)	Carb. (g)	Fiber (g)	Pro. (g)	Servings/Exchanges
✓Soft Taco Supreme	1	260	14	48	7	35	590	23	3	12	1 1/2 starch, 1 medium-fat meat, 2 fat
✓Taco	1	180	10	53	4	25	330	12	3	9	1 starch, 1 medium-fat meat, 1 fat
✓Taco Supreme	1	220	14	53	7	35	350	14	3	10	1 starch, 1 medium-fat meat, 2 fat

✓ = Healthiest Bets; n/a = not available

Notes

Taco John's

❖Taco John's provides nutrition information for all its menu items in a brochure.

Light 'n Lean Choice

Chicken Fajita Burrito
Bean Burrito

Calories.......................757	Sodium (mg) 2,413
Fat (g) 23	Carbohydrate (g).......102
% calories from fat..27	Fiber (g) ....n/a
Saturated fat (g)......10	Protein (g) 36
Cholesterol (mg) 67	

Exchanges: 6 1/2 starch, 2 lean meat, 3 fat

Healthy 'n Hearty Choice

Bean Burrito
Soft Shell Tacos
Refried Beans (*split*)

Calories.......................796	Sodium (mg) 1,902
Fat (g) 29	Carbohydrate (g).......107
% calories from fat..33	Fiber (g) ....n/a
Saturated fat (g).....9.9	Protein (g) 38
Cholesterol (mg) 53	

Exchanges: 6 1/2 starch, 2 medium-fat meat, 3 fat

(*Continued*)

Taco John's

	Amount	Cal.	Fat (g)	% Cal. Fat	Sat. Fat (g)	Chol. (mg)	Sod. (mg)	Carb. (g)	Fiber (g)	Pro. (g)	Servings/Exchanges
BURRITOS											
✔Bean Burrito	1	387	11	26	4.5	18	886	57	n/a	15	3 1/2 starch, 2 fat
✔Beef Burrito	1	449	20	40	8.6	52	863	44	n/a	23	3 starch, 1 medium-fat meat, 3 fat
✔Combination Burrito	1	418	16	34	6.5	35	865	50	n/a	19	3 starch, 1 medium-fat meat, 2 fat
Meat & Potato Burrito	1	503	24	43	6.8	25	1341	53	n/a	17	3 1/2 starch, 1 medium-fat meat, 4 fat
✔Super Burrito	1	465	19	37	8.5	41	922	53	n/a	20	3 1/2 starch, 1 medium-fat meat, 3 fat
DESSERTS											
✔Apple Flauta	1	84	1	11	0	0	72	19	n/a	1	1 carb.

✔ Cherry Flauta	1	143	4	25	0.7	0	110	27	n/a	2	1 1/2 carb., 1 fat
✔ Choco Taco	1	320	17	48	11	20	100	38	n/a	3	2 1/2 carb., 3 fat
✔ Churro	1	147	8	49	2	4	160	17	n/a	2	1 carb., 1 1/2 fat
✔ Cream Cheese Flauta	1	181	8	40	3	10	135	27	n/a	2	1 1/2 carb., 1 1/2 fat

FAJITAS

Chicken Fajita Burrito	1	370	12	29	5.2	49	1536	45	n/a	21	3 starch, 2 lean meat, 1 fat
Chicken Fajita Salad (includes bowl, no dressing)	1	557	33	53	9.5	56	1541	44	n/a	22	2 starch, 2 veg, 2 medium-fat meat, 4 1/2 fat
✔ Chicken Fajita Softshell	1	200	7	32	3	33	903	21	n/a	13	1 starch, 1 lean meat, 1 fat

KID'S MEALS

Crispy Taco	1	579	34	53	10	35	789	54	n/a	13	4 starch, 7 fat
Softshell Taco	1	617	33	48	10	35	1037	64	n/a	15	4 starch, 6 1/2 fat

(Continued)

✔ = Healthiest Bets; n/a = not available

	Amount	Cal.	Fat (g)	% Cal. Fat	Sat. Fat (g)	Chol. (mg)	Sod. (mg)	Carb. (g)	Fiber (g)	Pro. (g)	Servings/Exchanges
OTHER ENTREES											
Mexi Rolls with Nacho Cheese	1 order	863	48	50	11	54	1392	72	n/a	30	5 starch, 2 high-fat meat, 5 1/2 fat
Potato Olés Bravo	1 order	579	38	59	7	7	1550	47	n/a	11	3 starch, 7 1/2 fat
Sierra Chicken Fillet Sandwich	1	534	29	49	8	68	1406	40	n/a	30	2 1/2 starch, 3 lean meat, 4 fat
Super Nachos	1 order	919	56	55	13	48	1484	72	n/a	26	5 starch, 2 high-fat meat, 7 fat
Taco Salad (includes bowl, no dressing)	1	584	38	59	11	46	766	43	n/a	20	2 starch, 3 veg., 1 medium-fat meat, 6 1/2 fat
SIDES											
Chili	9.25 oz	350	21	54	9.6	56	865	19	n/a	20	1 starch, 2 lean meat, 3 fat
Nacho Cheese	2 oz/4 Tbsp	300	10	30	0	0	600	0	n/a	5	1 high-fat meat
Nachos	1 order	333	21	57	1.8	0	611	27	n/a	7	2 starch, 4 fat

Potato Olés	1 order	363	23	56	5.4	0	964	38	n/a	3	2 1/2 starch, 4 1/2 fat
Potato Olés (large)	1 order	484	30	56	7	0	1285	50	n/a	4	3 starch, 6 fat
Potato Olés (with Nacho Cheese)	1 order	483	33	61	5.4	0	1564	38	n/a	8	2 1/2 starch, 6 1/2 fat
Refried Beans	9.5 oz	357	9	23	2	17	1032	53	n/a	18	3 1/2 starch, 1 lean meat, 1 fat
✔Sour Cream	1 oz	60	5	75	0	0	15	1	n/a	1	1 fat

TACOS

✔Crispy Tacos	1 order	182	11	54	4.2	26	272	12	n/a	9	1 starch, 1 high-fat meat
✔Softshell Tacos	1 order	230	10	39	4.4	26	520	23	n/a	14	1 1/2 starch, 1 medium-fat meat, 1 fat
✔Taco Bravo	1	346	14	36	5	28	677	39	n/a	15	2 1/2 starch, 1 medium-fat meat, 2 fat
✔Taco Burger	1	280	12	39	5	32	576	28	n/a	15	2 starch, 2 medium-fat meat

✔ = Healthiest Bets; n/a = not available

Taco Time

❖Taco Time provides nutrition information for all of its menu items in a brochure.

Light 'n Lean Choice

Super Shredded Beef Soft Taco
Mexican Rice

Calories.....................527	Sodium (mg)...........1,086
Fat (g) 13	Carbohydrate (g).........68
% calories from fat..22	Fiber (g) 8
Saturated fat (g)........7	Protein (g) 15
Cholesterol (mg).........22	

Exchanges: 4 starch, 1 medium-fat meat, 1 fat

Healthy 'n Hearty Choice

Value Soft Bean Burrito (*single*)
Chicken Soft Taco
Refritos (*refried beans; split*)

Calories.....................864	Sodium (mg)...........1,749
Fat (g) 26	Carbohydrate (g).......118
% calories from fat..27	Fiber (g) 20
Saturated fat (g)......10	Protein (g) 43
Cholesterol (mg).........63	

Exchanges: 8 1/2 starch, 4 lean meat, 2 fat

Taco Time

BURRITOS

	Amount	Cal.	Fat (g)	% Cal. Fat	Sat. Fat (g)	Chol. (mg)	Sod. (mg)	Carb. (g)	Fiber (g)	Pro. (g)	Servings/Exchanges
Casita Burrito, Meat	1	647	31	43	15	89	1233	54	16	40	3 1/2 starch, 4 medium-fat meat, 2 fat
✔Crisp Burrito, Bean	1	427	18	38	5	12	453	53	9	15	3 1/2 starch, 1 lean meat, 3 fat
Crisp Burrito, Chicken	1	422	25	53	8	54	795	32	2	17	2 starch, 2 lean meat, 4 fat
Crisp Burrito, Meat	1	552	30	49	10	58	1000	39	7	34	2 1/2 starch, 4 medium-fat meat, 2 fat
✔Double Soft Bean Burrito	1	506	12	21	6	22	860	77	19	23	5 starch, 1 lean meat, 2 fat
Double Soft Combination Burrito	1	617	23	34	10	63	1343	66	18	39	4 starch, 4 medium-fat meat, 1/2 fat

✔ = Healthiest Bets; n/a = not available

(Continued)

BURRITOS (Continued)	Amount	Cal.	Fat (g)	% Cal. Fat	Sat. Fat (g)	Chol. (mg)	Sod. (mg)	Carb. (g)	Fiber (g)	Pro. (g)	Servings/Exchanges
Double Soft Meat Burrito	1	726	33	41	14	99	1809	55	17	57	3 1/2 starch, 7 lean meat, 2 1/2 fat
✔ Value Soft Bean Burrito	1	380	10	24	4	15	715	58	13	16	4 starch, 1 lean meat, 1 fat
Value Soft Meat Burrito	1	491	21	38	8	56	1197	48	12	31	3 1/2 starch, 3 lean meat, 2 fat
✔ Veggie Burrito	1	491	16	29	6	24	643	70	10	21	4 1/2 starch, 3 fat
CONDIMENTS											
✔ Enchilada Sauce	1 oz/2 Tbsp	12	0	0	0	0	133	3	1	0	free
✔ Guacamole	1 oz/2 Tbsp	29	2	62	0	0	94	2	1	0	free
✔ Hot Sauce	1 oz/2 Tbsp	10	0	0	0	0	120	2	0	0	free
✔ Ranchero Salsa	2 oz/4 Tbsp	21	1	43	0	0	192	3	1	1	free
✔ Sour Cream	1 oz/2 Tbsp	55	5	82	3	19	11	1	0	1	1 fat
✔ Sour Cream Dressing	1.5 oz/3 Tbsp	137	14	92	5	8	207	2	0	1	3 fat

Thousand Island Dressing	1 oz/2 Tbsp	160	16	90	2	10	220	4	0	0	3 fat

DESSERTS

✔Cherry Empanada	1	250	9	32	n/a	0	46	37	n/a	5	2 1/2 carb., 2 fat

OTHER ENTREES

✔Cheese Quesadilla	1	205	11	48	6	30	255	17	1	11	1 starch, 1 high-fat meat
Nachos	1 order	680	38	50	19	78	1250	61	11	26	4 starch, 2 medium-fat meat, 4 fat
Nachos Deluxe	1 order	1048	57	49	23	109	2252	91	17	46	6 starch, 4 medium-fat meat, 7 fat
Taco Cheeseburger	1	633	36	51	10	66	1291	48	7	31	3 starch, 3 medium-fat meat, 4 fat

SALADS

✔Chicken Taco Salad w/o Dressing (regular)	1	370	21	51	7	48	861	27	3	19	2 starch, 2 medium-fat meat, 2 fat

(Continued)

✔ = Healthiest Bets; n/a = not available

SALADS (Continued)	Amount	Cal.	Fat (g)	% Cal. Fat	Sat. Fat (g)	Chol. (mg)	Sod. (mg)	Carb. (g)	Fiber (g)	Pro. (g)	Servings/Exchanges
Taco Salad w/o Dressing (regular)	1	479	28	53	11	63	895	30	7	30	1 starch, 2 veg., 3 medium-fat meat, 2 1/2 fat
Tostada Delight Salad, Meat	1	628	33	47	14	82	1004	48	13	36	3 starch, 4 medium-fat meat, 2 fat
SIDES AND INGREDIENTS											
Cheddar Cheese	0.75 oz	86	7	73	4	22	132	0	0	5	1 high-fat meat
Chips	1 order	266	12	41	3	0	461	35	3	4	2 starch, 2 fat
Crustos	1 order	373	15	36	n/a	0	86	47	n/a	9	3 carb., 3 fat
✓Mexican Rice	4 oz	159	2	11	1	0	530	30	1	3	2 starch
Mexi-Fries (regular)	1 order	266	17	58	n/a	0	799	27	n/a	3	2 starch, 3 fat
Mexi-Fries (large)	1 order	532	34	58	n/a	0	1598	54	n/a	6	3 1/2 starch, 7 fat
✓Refritos	2.5 oz	97	0	0	0	0	101	18	6	6	1 starch

TACOS

	Amount	Cal.	Fat (g)	% Cal. Fat	Sat. Fat (g)	Chol. (mg)	Sod. (mg)	Carb. (g)	Fiber (g)	Prot. (g)	Servings/Exchanges
✔ Chicken Soft Taco	1	387	16	37	6	48	933	41	7	21	3 starch, 2 medium-fat meat, 1 fat
✔ Crisp Taco	1	295	17	52	7	48	609	16	5	22	1 starch, 3 medium-fat meat
Natural Super Taco, Meat	1	627	27	39	13	82	915	60	14	41	4 starch, 4 medium-fat meat, 1 fat
Rolled Soft Flour Taco	1	512	23	40	10	63	1111	46	12	33	3 starch, 3 medium-fat meat, 1 1/2 fat
✔ Super Shredded Beef Soft Taco	1	368	11	27	6	22	556	38	7	12	2 starch, 1 medium-fat meat, 1 fat
✔ Value Soft Taco (single)	1	316	15	43	7	48	599	23	5	24	1 1/2 starch, 3 medium-fat meat

✔ = Healthiest Bets; n/a = not available

Notes

Sit-Down American Fare

RESTAURANTS

Bennigan's

Big Boy Restaurant

Bob Evans Farms

Coco's

Denny's

Perkins Family Restaurant

Ruby Tuesday

Note: Nutrition information provided by most restaurants in this category is far from complete. You might not find a few large chains you expect to see in this chapter because they were unwilling to provide either a menu or nutrition information. The only restaurant willing to tell all is Denny's. Others in the chapter provided some information, mainly for their healthier items. Any nutrition information made available is listed below. In addition, you'll see lists of Healthier Picks for the restaurants that were willing to give us a menu but limited nutrition information.

NUTRITION PROS

- Many sit-down American restaurants have added healthier options to their menus.
- You can pick and choose among the appetizers, salads, soups, and side dishes to put together healthy, portion-controlled meals.

- Healthier preparation methods are available—stir-frying, grilling, and blackening.
- Time and a desire to please is on your side. This makes special requests easier for you and possible for the kitchen.
- Portions are large, but take-home containers are at the ready.
- These restaurants hardly limit their menu to American specialties. They globe trot to bring you Mexican fajitas or salads, Italian pastas or pizzas, and Chinese pot stickers or stir-fry dishes. This helps to widen the variety of healthier choices.
- Raw and cooked vegetables are easier to find here than in fast-food restaurants. Just be careful they aren't drenched in fat or fried.
- Condiments to help you add taste without fat might be found in the kitchen—teriyaki or soy sauce, lemons, limes, a variety of vinegars, ketchup, barbecue sauce, and low-calorie salad dressings. Ask, and maybe you'll receive.

NUTRITION CONS

- Bread, rolls, crackers, or breadsticks and butter might greet you at the table.
- These restaurants love to fry—from fried mozzarella sticks to fried shrimp, chicken fingers, french fries, and onion rings.
- Sandwiches and other entrees may be accompanied by french fries, onion rings, potato chips, or creamy coleslaw.
- Some foods get a healthy start—vegetables, potatoes, or pasta. But then they are drenched in salad

dressing or cheese sauce, or dropped a foot deep in oil and fried.

- Salads can start off healthy but end up with high-fat toppers—avocado, cheese, bacon, or croutons.
- Portions are frequently too big...many are way too BIG.
- Unadulterated fruit is still not plentiful. The apples buried between a double crust are not the healthiest way to count your fruits.
- Cheese is in, on, and around a startling number of menu items—melted cheese on a sandwich, cheese sauce on vegetables or pasta.

Healthy Tips

- ★ Combine a soup, salad, and side dish for a healthy, portion-controlled meal.
- ★ Combine one or two appetizers and a salad for a healthy, portion-controlled meal.
- ★ Share two complementary entrees—pasta topped with a tomato-based sauce or vegetables and a Mexican salad, for example.
- ★ Split everything with your dining partner from appetizer to dessert.
- ★ Order your take-home container when you order your meal. Pack up the portion to take home when your order arrives.

Get It Your Way

★ Ask for your salad dressing on the side—all of the time.

★ Ask that high-fat salad toppers be used lightly or left in the kitchen.

★ Request to substitute high-fat, high-calorie sides with lower-fat, lower-calorie items. Substitute a baked potato for french fries or onion rings, request a sandwich on whole-wheat bread rather than on a croissant, opt for mustard rather than mayonnaise.

★ Request to hold the butter or cheese sauce on vegetables.

★ Leave the fried tortilla shell in which a big salad is served in the kitchen.

★ Request some lemon or lime slices, vinegar, or soy or teriyaki sauce on the side to flavor menu items with few calories.

Bennigan's

❖Bennigan's provided nutrition information for only its "Health Club" menu items.

Light 'n Lean Choice

Dinner Salad
Fat-Free Honey Dijon Salad Dressing
Health Club Vegetable Lasagna

Insufficient nutrition information to calculate.

Healthy 'n Hearty Choice

Oriental Chicken Salad (*split*)
Beef Fajitas, for One (*split*)
Cinnamon Apples (*order for dessert*)

Insufficient nutrition information to calculate.

Healthier Picks

Appetizers
Chicken Quesadillas (*hold guacamole and sour cream; order double salsa; order as an entree*)

Salads
Grilled Chicken Caesar Salad (*request dressing on the side*)
Charleston Chicken Salad (*request dressing on the side and hold cheese*)
Oriental Chicken Salad (*request dressing on the side*)

(*Continued*)

Dinner Salad, traditional (*request dressing on the side*)
(*Choose these salad dressings on the side: Oil &
Vinegar, Fat-Free Ranch, Low-Cal Italian, Fat-Free
Honey Dijon.*)

Entrees

Chicken Teriyaki (*order with two healthy sides*)
Pot of Gold Pot Roast
Grilled Shrimp
Fajitas, all (*hold guacamole and sour cream; order
double salsa*)
Pasta Marinara
Bennigan's Health Club, all*
All American Burger (*substitute a healthy side for
french fries*)
Onion & Mushroom Burger (*hold cheese and mayon-
naise; substitute a healthy side for french fries*)

Sandwiches

Swiss Chicken Sandwich (*hold cheese and mayonnaise; substitute a healthy side for french fries*)
French Dip (*hold cheese; substitute a healthy side for
french fries*)
Turkey O'Toole (*hold cheese; request dressing on the
side; substitute a healthy side for french fries*)
Heapin' Ham 'n' Cheese (*hold cheese; request dressing
on the side; substitute a healthy side for french fries*)
Philly Cheese Steak Sandwich (*hold cheese; request
dressing on the side; substitute a healthy side for
french fries*)

*See nutrition information for these items in table.

Kid's Meals

(*For all: substitute a healthy side for french fries; hold
    the cookie if you don't want your child to have one*)
Billy The Kid Burger
Hot Diggety Dog
Mac 'n' Cheese

Sides

Basket of Four Dinner Rolls
Loaded Baked Potato (*hold the add-ons or order on
    the side*)
Confetti Rice
Roast Vegetables
Southwest Corn
Steamed Broccoli

(*Continued*)

Bennigan's

	Amount	Cal.	Fat (g)	% Cal. Fat	Sat. Fat (g)	Chol. (mg)	Sod. (mg)	Carb. (g)	Fiber (g)	Pro. (g)	Servings/Exchanges
DESSERTS											
Health Club Cookie Sundae	1 order	807	7	8	n/a	n/a	n/a	136	n/a	15	9 cart., 1 fat
ENTREES											
Health Club Chicken Fajitas	1 order	783	15	17	n/a	n/a	n/a	114	n/a	67	7 starch, 3 veg., 6 lean meat
✔Health Club Chicken Platter	1 order	700	9	12	n/a	n/a	n/a	90	n/a	60	6 starch, 6 very lean meat
SANDWICHES											
✔Health Club Chicken Sandwich	1 order	498	8	14	n/a	n/a	n/a	98	n/a	30	6 starch, 3 very lean meat, 1 fat
✔Health Club Club Sandwich	1 order	450	10	20	n/a	n/a	n/a	60	n/a	32	4 starch, 2 lean meat, 1 fat

✔ = Healthiest Bets; n/a = not available

Big Boy Restaurant

❖Big Boy provides nutrition information for the "Health Smart" items on its menu.

Light 'n Lean Choice

From Mini Breakfast:

Fresh Fruit
Hot Cakes 'n Bacon (*short stack of pancakes; substitute ham for bacon*)

Unable to calculate from limited nutrition information provided for these items.

Healthy 'n Hearty Choice

Cabbage Soup (*bowl*)
Breast of Chicken w/ Mozzarella Pita
(*with ranch dressing*)
Rice Pilaf
Fat-Free Frozen Yogurt (*4 fl oz, 1/2 cup*)

Calories......................664		Sodium (mg)..........1,001	
Fat (g) 15		Carbohydrate (g)..........83	
% calories from fat..20		Fiber (g) ....n/a	
Saturated fat (g) ....n/a		Protein (g) 48	
Cholesterol (mg) 91			

Exchanges: 3 starch, 2 carb., 5 very lean meat, 2 1/2 fat

Healthier Picks

Health Smart menu items, all (*see table for nutrition information*)

(*Continued*)

Breakfast (*available any time of day*)

Hot Cakes (*hold butter; request syrup on the side; order with ham or no meat*)

French Toast (*hold butter; request syrup on the side; order with ham or no meat*)

Belgian Waffles (*hold butter; request syrup on the side; order with fresh strawberries*)

Three Egg Omelettes (*order plain, ham, farmer's, vegetarian, or Mexican; hold the cheese and split the omelette*)

Eggs Benedict (*half order; hold the Hollandaise sauce*)

Mini Breakfasts

Bake Shop Mini

Hot Cakes 'n Bacon (*substitute ham for bacon*)

French Toast 'n Bacon (*substitute ham for bacon*)

One Egg, Any Style (*request dry toast with butter on the side*)

The Fresh Start

Cold Cereal (*request fat-free [skim] milk*)

Hot Oatmeal (*request fat-free milk*)

Home-Baked Pastries (*request dry with butter, cream cheese, and/or jam on the side*)

Toasted Homemade Bread

English Muffin

Toasted Bagel

Fresh Fruit

All

Appetizers and Sides

Vegetable of the Day

Rice Pilaf

Baked Potato

Soups and Salads

Chili

Any broth-based soup

Tossed Salad (*request dressing on the side; see nutrition information on healthy salad dressings*)

Chicken Breast Caesar Salad (*request dressing on the side; substitute healthy dressing*)

Burgers and Sandwiches (*all include french fries and coleslaw or tossed salad; substitute french fries with healthy side, and order tossed salad with dressing on the side*)

Big Boy (*hold the cheese and special sauce*)

Brawny Lad (*request bun unbuttered*)

The U.S. Open (*order chicken breast; hold cheese*)

The World Series (*order chicken breast; hold cheese and bacon*)

Slim Jim (*hold the cheese and special sauce*)

Grilled Chicken Breast Sandwich

Turkey Sandwich

The Super Bowl (*order chicken breast, hold cheese*)

Home Cookin' (*all are served with a fresh-baked roll and choice of coleslaw, tossed salad, or Caesar salad; choose the tossed salad with healthy dressing on the side or substitute a healthy side*)

Sirloin Steak

Tender Pork Chops

Grilled Ham Steak

Lemon Pepper Chicken

Boston Cracker Crumb Cod

White Wine & Lemon Cod

Spaghetti Marinara

Hearty Home-Style Side Dishes

Stewed Tomatoes

Sauteed Mushrooms

(*Continued*)

Big Boy Restaurant

	Amount	Cal.	Fat (g)	% Cal. Fat	Sat. Fat (g)	Chol. (mg)	Sod. (mg)	Carb. (g)	Fiber (g)	Pro. (g)	Servings/Exchanges
BREAKFAST											
✓Plain Egg Beaters Omelette	1 order	305	10	30	n/a	0	603	36	n/a	19	2 starch, 2 lean meat, 1 fat
✓Scrambled Egg Beaters	1 order	305	10	30	n/a	0	603	36	n/a	19	2 starch, 2 lean meat, 1 fat
✓Vegetarian Egg Beaters Omelette	1 order	330	10	27	n/a	0	613	40	n/a	21	2 starch, 2 veg., 2 lean meat, 1 fat
DESSERTS											
✓Frozen Yogurt (fat-free)	1 order	118	0	0	n/a	0	60	27	n/a	3	1 1/2 carb.
✓Frozen Yogurt Shake	1 order	158	0	0	n/a	2	120	33	n/a	7	2 carb.
ENTREES											
✓Baked Cod	1 order	744	21	25	n/a	76	655	82	n/a	57	5 1/2 starch, 6 very lean meat, 3 fat

✓Breast of Chicken w/ Mozzarella	1 order	697	20	26	n/a	76	613	80	n/a	50	5 starch, 5 very lean meat, 3 fat
✓Cajun Cod	1 order	736	21	26	n/a	76	745	80	n/a	56	5 starch, 6 very lean meat, 3 fat
✓Chicken & Pasta Primavera	1 order	678	14	19	n/a	65	875	83	n/a	53	5 starch, 2 veg., 5 lean meat, 2 fat
✓Chicken 'n Vegetable Stir Fry	1 order	795	18	20	n/a	65	845	109	n/a	51	6 starch, 3 veg., 4 lean meat, 1 fat
✓Spaghetti Marinara	1 order	589	11	17	n/a	8	784	105	n/a	17	7 starch, 2 fat
✓Vegetable Stir Fry	1 order	616	14	20	n/a	0	774	109	n/a	17	6 starch, 3 veg., 3 fat

PITAS

✓Breast of Chicken w/ Mozzarella (ranch dressing)	1 order	361	11	27	n/a	84	369	23	n/a	41	1 1/2 starch, 5 very lean meat, 1 fat

✔ = Healthiest Bets; n/a = not available

(Continued)

PITAS (Continued)	Amount	Cal.	Fat (g)	% Cal. Fat	Sat. Fat (g)	Chol. (mg)	Sod. (mg)	Carb. (g)	Fiber (g)	Pro. (g)	Servings/Exchanges
✓Turkey Pita (ranch dressing)	1 order	245	6	22	n/a	83	938	23	n/a	25	1 1/2 starch, 3 very lean meat, 1/2 fat

SALAD DRESSINGS

	Amount	Cal.	Fat (g)	% Cal. Fat	Sat. Fat (g)	Chol. (mg)	Sod. (mg)	Carb. (g)	Fiber (g)	Pro. (g)	Servings/Exchanges
✓Fat-Free Oriental Dressing	1 oz/2 Tbsp	20	0	0	n/a	0	189	4	n/a	1	free
✓Italian Dressing (fat free)	1 oz/2 Tbsp	11	0	0	n/a	0	191	3	n/a	0	free
✓Reduced Calorie Ranch	1 oz/2 Tbsp	41	3	66	n/a	8	151	3	n/a	1	1/2 fat

SALADS

	Amount	Cal.	Fat (g)	% Cal. Fat	Sat. Fat (g)	Chol. (mg)	Sod. (mg)	Carb. (g)	Fiber (g)	Pro. (g)	Servings/Exchanges
✓Chicken Breast Salad (w/ roll, margarine)	1 order	523	16	27	n/a	73	654	50	n/a	44	2 starch, 3 veg., 5 lean meat
✓Oriental Chicken Breast Salad (w/ roll, margarine)	1 order	660	20	27	n/a	65	855	73	n/a	48	4 starch, 3 veg., 5 lean meat, 1 fat

✔Tossed Salad	1 order	35	0	0	n/a	0	71	7	n/a	2	1 veg.

SIDES

✔Baked Potato (plain)	1	163	0	0	n/a	0	7	37	n/a	5	2 1/2 starch
✔Dinner Roll	1	210	5	21	n/a	0	340	36	n/a	6	2 starch, 1 fat
✔Promise Margarine	1 order	25	3	108	n/a	0	35	0	n/a	0	1/2 fat
✔Rice Pilaf	1 order	145	3	19	n/a	7	225	26	n/a	3	2 starch, 1/2 fat

SOUPS

✔Cabbage Soup	1 bowl	40	1	23	n/a	0	347	7	n/a	1	1/2 starch

✔ = Healthiest Bets; n/a = not available

Notes

Bob Evans Farms

❖Bob Evans Farms provided nutrition information for several menu items.

Light 'n Lean Choice

Bean Soup (*cup*)
Vegetable Stir Fry
Applesauce

Calories......................503
Fat (g) 8
   % calories from fat..14
   Saturated fat (g) ....n/a
Cholesterol (mg) 20

Sodium (mg) 2,478
Carbohydrate (g).........98
   Fiber (g) ....n/a
Protein (g) 18

Exchanges: 3 starch, 3 veg., 1 fruit, 1 carb., 1 very lean meat, 1 fat

Healthy 'n Hearty Choice

Cajun Catfish (*order one-piece dinner*)
Grilled Vegetables
Long Grain & Wild Rice
Dinner Roll (*1 roll*)

No nutrition information was available from the restaurant for these items.

Healthier Picks

Hotcakes & Such (*all are served with regular syrup and margarine; butter and low-calorie syrup are*

available upon request; ham is the lowest-fat meat
to add to a breakfast order)
French Toast (*option to substitute Egg Beaters for
slight charge*)
Traditional Buttermilk Hotcakes
Blueberry Hotcakes

Omelettes (*split one and ask to substitute dry toast or
English muffin for buttermilk biscuits; you can
substitute Egg Beaters for a slight charge*)
Western (*hold cheese*)
Ham & Cheese (*hold cheese*)
Garden Harvest

Starting Right
Fruit Plate (*substitute dry toast or English muffin for
buttermilk biscuits*)
Lite Sausage Breakfast* (*request cream cheese on the
side*)
Quaker Oatmeal*
Quaker Oatmeal,* with orange juice and a bagel
(*request cream cheese on the side*)

A La Carte
One Egg
Quaker Grits
Toast & Jelly
English Muffin
Bagel (*request cream cheese on the side*)
Breakfast Fruit Cup
Breakfast Ham

(*Continued*)

Salads *(choose yeast-raised dinner rolls* and Oil & Vinegar, Reduced Fat Italian, or Fat-Free Ranch salad dressing)*
Fruit Plate

Sandwiches & Burgers
Pot Roast Sandwich *(hold cheese)*
Grilled Chicken Sandwich
Deluxe Hamburger

Soups & More
Bean Soup *(cup or bowl)**
Beef Vegetable Soup

Entrees *(all are served with buttermilk biscuits or yeast-raised dinner rolls; choose dinner rolls.*)*
Vegetable Harvest Dinner *(choose from healthy sides)*
Spaghetti with Meat Sauce *(hold grilled garlic bread and eat dinner rolls)*
Chicken or Vegetable Stir-Fry*
Homestyle Meat Loaf & Gravy *(order gravy on the side; substitute baked potato for mashed)*
Open-Faced Roast Beef *(substitute baked potato for mashed)*
Turkey & Dressing *(order gravy on the side and use small amount)*
Chicken Monterey *(order smaller one-piece dinner; hold cheese)*
Grilled Chicken* *(order one-piece dinner and healthy side items)*
Apple Barbecued Chicken *(order one-piece dinner; 4 g fat)*
Cajun Catfish *(order one-piece dinner)*

Sides

Fresh Garden Salad
Long Grain & Wild Rice
Grilled Vegetables
Applesauce (*0 g fat*)
Cottage Cheese
Buttered Sweet Corn
Green Beans*
Glazed Baby Carrots
Baked Potato (*0 g fat*)

*See nutrition information for these items in the table that
follows.

(*Continued*)

Bob Evans Farms

	Amount	Cal.	Fat (g)	% Cal. Fat	Sat. Fat (g)	Chol. (mg)	Sod. (mg)	Carb. (g)	Fiber (g)	Pro. (g)	Servings/Exchanges
BREAKFAST											
✔French Toast	1 slice	161	3	17	n/a	59	362	27	n/a	6	2 starch, 1/2 fat
Lite Sausage Link	1	104	6	52	n/a	20	297	0	n/a	12	2 lean meat
✔Oatmeal	1 order	252	4	14	n/a	0	854	44	n/a	11	3 starch, 1 fat
ENTREES											
Chicken Stir Fry	1 order	531	11	19	n/a	123	1819	61	n/a	50	3 1/2 starch, 2 veg., 5 very lean meat, 1 fat
✔Grilled Chicken Breast	1 order	285	6	19	n/a	147	128	0	n/a	53	9 very lean meat
Vegetable Stir Fry	1 order	319	7	20	n/a	14	1723	61	n/a	10	3 starch, 3 veg., 1 fat

SIDES

Dinner Rolls, plain	2	320	8	23	n/a	0	1260	72	n/a	10	5 starch, 1 1/2 fat
Green Beans	1 order	55	1	16	n/a	6	675	9	n/a	5	2 veg.

SOUPS

✔Bean Soup	1 cup	104	1	9	n/a	6	655	17	n/a	8	1 starch, 1 very lean meat
✔Bean Soup	1 bowl	146	1	6	n/a	8	921	23	n/a	12	1 1/2 starch, 1 very lean meat

✔ = Healthiest Bets; n/a = not available

Notes

Coco's

❖Coco's provided nutrition information for several menu items.

Light 'n Lean Choice

Gardenburger Dinner
(*Gardenburger with pasta salad*)

Calories	800	Sodium (mg) 1,520
Fat (g)	36	Carbohydrate (g) 103
% calories from fat	41	Fiber (g) 17
Saturated fat (g)	6	Protein (g) 25
Cholesterol (mg)	9	

Exchanges: 6 starch, 2 veg., 7 fat

Healthy 'n Hearty Choice

Fresh Catch Dinner
(*red snapper; rice pilaf; green garden salad, with
Catalina salad dressing; dinner bread;
Promise margarine*)

Calories	800	Sodium (mg) 1,780
Fat (g)	30	Carbohydrate (g) 102
% calories from fat	34	Fiber (g) 8
Saturated fat (g)	6	Protein (g) 36
Cholesterol (mg)	110	

Exchanges: 7 starch, 3 very lean meat, 5 fat

Coco's

	Amount	Cal.	Fat (g)	% Cal. Fat	Sat. Fat (g)	Chol. (mg)	Sod. (mg)	Carb. (g)	Fiber (g)	Pro. (g)	Servings/Exchanges
BEVERAGES											
✓Milk, 2%	8 oz	130	5	35	n/a	25	130	13	n/a	10	1 low-fat milk
✓Milk, nonfat	8 oz	90	0	0	n/a	5	120	12	n/a	9	1 fat-free milk
BREAKFAST											
✓Fresh Oatmeal Breakfast	1 order	470	3	6	0.5	0	560	107	6	9	7 starch, 1/2 fat
✓Low Cholesterol Breakfast	1 order	500	6	11	1	5	720	103	11	18	7 starch, 1 fat
✓Oatmeal, w/ salt	6 oz	150	3	18	n/a	0	420	27	n/a	5	2 starch, 1/2 fat
Omelette Primaver	1 order	770	50	58	16	620	1230	50	9	33	3 starch, 1 veg., 3 medium-fat meat, 7 fat

✓ = Healthiest Bets; n/a = not available

(Continued)

BREAKFAST (Continued)	Amount	Cal.	Fat (g)	% Cal. Fat	Sat. Fat (g)	Chol. (mg)	Sod. (mg)	Carb. (g)	Fiber (g)	Pro. (g)	Servings/Exchanges
✔S&W 70% Calorie Reduced Pancake Syrup	2 oz/4 Tbsp	60	0	0	n/a	0	105	15	n/a	0	1 carb.
✔Sunny Fresh Select Eggs, Scrambled	2 eggs	80	3	34	n/a	100	190	2	n/a	13	2 very lean meat
CONDIMENTS											
✔Italian Dressing (low fat, reduced calorie)	3 oz/6 Tbsp	160	9	51	n/a	0	916	16	n/a	1	1 carb., 2 fat
✔Promise Spread	1/2 Tbsp	25	3	108	n/a	0	35	0	n/a	0	1/2 fat
DESSERTS											
Apple Pie (reduced fat, made with NutraSweet)	1/5 pie	550	26	43	n/a	n/a	620	72	n/a	n/a	5 carb., 5 fat
Apple Pie (regular)	1/5 pie	780	43	50	n/a	n/a	710	92	n/a	n/a	6 carb., 8 fat

Cherry Pie (reduced fat, made with NutraSweet)	1/5 pie	650	30	42	n/a	n/a	660	89	n/a	n/a	6 carb., 6 fat
Cherry Pie (regular)	1/5 pie	810	44	49	n/a	n/a	700	98	n/a	n/a	6 1/2 carb., 9 fat
✓Muffin (low fat)	1	250	2	7	n/a	n/a	460	n/a	n/a	n/a	insufficient info. to calculate

DINNERS

Fresh Catch Dinner	1 order	800	30	34	6	110	1780	102	8	36	7 starch, 3 very lean meat, 5 fat
Gardenburger	1 order	800	36	41	6	9	1520	103	17	25	6 starch, 2 veg., 7 fat
Stir Fry Chicken Dinner	1 order	1270	36	26	8	175	5450	117	15	65	7 starch, 3 veg., 5 lean meat, 4 fat
Teriyaki Chicken Dinner	1 order	820	12	13	3	145	3800	111	13	71	7 starch, 7 very lean meat, 1 fat

✔ = Healthiest Bets; n/a = not available

(Continued)

DINNERS (Continued)	Amount	Cal.	Fat (g)	% Cal. Fat	Sat. Fat (g)	Chol. (mg)	Sod. (mg)	Carb. (g)	Fiber (g)	Pro. (g)	Servings/Exchanges
Teriyaki Chicken Sandwich	1 order	1080	39	33	15	175	4020	113	7	69	7 1/2 starch, 7 lean meat, 3 1/2 fat

SIDES

	Amount	Cal.	Fat (g)	% Cal. Fat	Sat. Fat (g)	Chol. (mg)	Sod. (mg)	Carb. (g)	Fiber (g)	Pro. (g)	Servings/Exchanges
✔Cottage Cheese (low fat)	1/2 cup	90	3	30	n/a	15	390	4	n/a	14	2 very lean meat

✔ = Healthiest Bets; n/a = not available

Notes

Denny's

❖Denny's provided nutrition information for all of its menu items.

Light 'n Lean Choice

Waffle
Syrup (*2 Tbsp*)
Banana/Strawberry Medley

Calories......................508	Sodium (mg)..............223
Fat (g) 21	Carbohydrate (g).........74
% calories from fat..37	Fiber (g) 2
Saturated fat (g)........4	Protein (g) 8
Cholesterol (mg) 146	

Exchanges: 1 1/2 starch, 2 fruit, 1 1/2 carb., 4 fat

Healthy 'n Hearty Choice

Grilled Chicken Sandwich
Carrots in Honey Glaze
Side Garden Salad with Fat Free Honey Mustard
Dressing (*2 Tbsp*)
Applesauce

Calories......................800	Sodium (mg)..........2,310
Fat (g) 26	Carbohydrate (g).......104
% calories from fat..29	Fiber (g) 10
Saturated fat (g)........6	Protein (g) 38
Cholesterol (mg) 93	

Exchanges: 3 1/2 starch, 3 veg., 1 fruit, 1 carb., 3 lean meat, 2 fat

(*Continued*)

Denny's

APPETIZERS

	Amount	Cal.	Fat (g)	% Cal. Fat	Sat. Fat (g)	Chol. (mg)	Sod. (mg)	Carb. (g)	Fiber (g)	Pro. (g)	Servings/Exchanges
Buffalo Chicken Strips	1 order	734	42	51	4	96	1673	43	0	48	3 starch, 6 lean meat, 5 fat
Buffalo Wings (12)	1 order	856	54	57	17	500	5552	1	1	92	12 lean meat, 3 1/2 fat
Chicken Quesadilla	1 order	827	55	60	23	181	1982	43	2	50	3 starch, 6 medium-fat meat, 5 fat
Chicken Strips (5), fried	1 order	720	33	41	4	95	1666	56	0	47	4 starch, 7 lean meat, 2 fat
Mozzarella Sticks (8), with sauce	1 order	756	43	51	24	48	5423	56	7	37	4 starch, 4 medium-fat meat, 4 1/2 fat
Onion Ring Basket (7)	1 order	824	50	55	12	14	2173	83	1	11	5 1/2 starch, 10 fat
Sampler	1 order	1405	80	51	24	75	5305	124	4	47	8 starch, 3 high-fat meat, 10 fat

BEVERAGES

	Serving Size	Cal.	Fat (g)	% Fat	Sat. Fat (g)	Chol. (mg)	Sod. (mg)	Carb. (g)	Fiber (g)	Pro. (g)	Servings/Exchanges
✔ Apple Juice	10 oz	126	0	0	0	0	24	33	0	0	2 fruit
Chocolate Milk	10 oz	235	9	34	6	22	189	30	0	9	1 whole milk, 1 carb.
Chocolate Shake/Malt	10 oz	579	27	42	17	108	278	77	0	12	1 whole milk, 4 carb., 2 fat
French Vanilla Coffee	8 oz	76	1	12	1	2	4	16	0	0	1 carb.
✔ Grapefruit Juice	10 oz	115	0	0	0	0	0	29	0	1	2 fruit
Hazelnut Coffee	8 oz	66	1	14	1	2	4	14	0	0	1 carb.
Hot Chocolate	8 oz	90	2	20	0	0	155	18	0	4	1 carb.
Irish Cream Coffee	8 oz	73	1	12	1	2	4	16	0	0	1 carb.
Lemonade	16 oz	150	0	0	0	0	38	35	0	0	2 carb.
✔ Milk, 2% (regular size)	10 oz	151	6	36	4	22	152	15	0	10	1 low-fat milk
✔ Orange Juice	10 oz	126	0	0	0	0	31	31	0	2	2 fruit
✔ Raspberry Iced Tea	16 oz	78	0	0	0	0	0	21	0	0	1 1/2 carb.

✔ = Healthiest Bets; n/a = not available

(Continued)

BEVERAGES (Continued)	Amount	Cal.	Fat (g)	% Cal. Fat	Sat. Fat (g)	Chol. (mg)	Sod. (mg)	Carb. (g)	Fiber (g)	Pro. (g)	Servings/Exchanges
✓Tomato Juice	10 oz	56	0	0	0	0	921	11	2	2	2 veg.
Vanilla Shake/Malt	11 oz	581	27	42	17	108	236	77	0	11	1 whole milk, 4 carb., 2 fat
BREAKFAST											
All American Slam	15 oz	1028	87	76	21	724	1924	24	2	48	1 1/2 starch, 6 medium-fat meat, 11 fat
Bacon (4 slices)	1 order	162	18	100	5	36	640	1	0	12	2 high-fat meat
✓Bagel, dry, whole	1	235	1	4	0	0	495	46	0	9	3 starch
Big Texas Chicken Fajita Skillet	1	1184	88	67	33	679	2406	43	5	59	2 1/2 starch, 1 veg., 7 high-fat meat, 3 1/2 fat
Biscuit & Sausage Gravy	1	570	38	60	10	24	1475	45	0	11	3 starch, 7 1/2 fat
Blueberry Muffin	1	309	14	41	0	0	190	42	0	4	3 starch, 3 fat
Canadian Bacon	1 order	110	5	41	2	43	1039	1	0	17	2 lean meat

Canadian Scramble Skillet	1	842	62	66	25	642	2183	34	3	50	2 starch, 6 high-fat meat
✔ Cereal, dry	1	100	0	0	0	0	276	23	1	2	1 1/2 starch
Chicken Fried Steak & Eggs	1	723	56	70	18	452	1505	31	8	28	2 starch, 3 medium-fat meat, 8 fat
✔ Egg Beaters	1 order	71	5	67	1	1	138	1	0	5	1 medium-fat meat
Eggs Benedict	1	860	56	59	23	525	1943	55	3	35	3 1/2 starch, 3 medium-fat meat, 8 fat
✔ English Muffin, dry, whole	1	125	1	7	0	0	198	24	1	5	1 1/2 starch
Farmer's Omelette	1	912	69	68	19	633	1816	38	3	34	2 starch, 1 veg., 4 medium-fat meat, 10 fat
French Slam	1	1029	71	62	20	777	1428	58	2	44	4 starch, 5 medium-fat meat, 9 fat

(Continued)

✔ = Healthiest Bets; n/a = not available

BREAKFAST (Continued)	Amount	Cal.	Fat (g)	% Cal. Fat	Sat. Fat (g)	Chol. (mg)	Sod. (mg)	Carb. (g)	Fiber (g)	Pro. (g)	Servings/Exchanges
French Toast, plain (2 slices)	1 order	510	25	44	6	317	413	51	2	19	3 1/2 starch, 1 medium-fat meat, 4 fat
✔ Grits	1	80	0	0	0	0	520	18	0	2	1 starch
✔ Ham	1	94	3	29	1	23	761	2	0	15	2 very lean meat
Ham'n'Cheddar Omelette	1	743	55	67	10	657	1518	24	2	36	1 1/2 starch, 5 medium-fat meat, 6 fat
Hashed Browns	1 order	218	14	58	2	0	424	20	2	2	1 starch, 3 fat
Hashed Browns, Covered	1 order	318	23	65	7	30	604	21	2	9	1 1/2 starch, 4 1/2 fat
Hashed Browns, Covered & Smothered	1 order	359	26	65	7	30	790	26	2	9	2 starch, 5 fat
Hotcakes, plain (3)	1 order	491	7	13	1	0	1818	95	3	12	6 carb., 1 fat
✔ Junior Waffle Supreme	1	190	11	52	2	73	102	20	0	3	1 starch 2 fat

Meat Lover's Sampler	1	806	62	69	17	481	2211	24	2	42	1 1/2 starch, 5 medium-fat meat, 7 fat
Meat Lover's Skillet	1	1344	108	72	37	673	3063	34	3	59	2 starch, 8 high-fat meat, 4 fat
Moons Over My Hammy	1	807	48	54	8	430	2247	46	2	44	3 starch, 5 medium-fat meat, 4 1/2 fat
✓ Oatmeal	1	100	2	18	0	0	175	18	3	5	1 starch
✓ One Egg	1	134	12	81	3	205	61	1	0	6	1 medium-fat meat, 1 fat
Original Grand Slam	1	795	50	57	14	460	2237	65	2	34	4 starch, 3 medium-fat meat, 5 fat
Pork Chop & Eggs	1	555	36	58	9	469	968	21	2	33	1 1/2 starch, 4 medium-fat meat, 3 fat
Porterhouse Steak & Eggs	1	1223	95	70	32	570	1369	21	< 2	70	1 1/2 starch, 9 medium-fat meat, 8 fat

(Continued)

✓ = Healthiest Bets; n/a = not available

BREAKFAST (Continued)	Amount	Cal.	Fat (g)	% Cal. Fat	Sat. Fat (g)	Chol. (mg)	Sod. (mg)	Carb. (g)	Fiber (g)	Pro. (g)	Servings/Exchanges
✔ Reduced Calorie Syrup	1.5 oz	23	0	0	0	0	96	6	0	0	1/2 carb.
Sausage (4 links)	1 order	354	32	81	2	64	944	0	0	16	2 high-fat meat, 2 fat
Sausage Patties	1 order	506	47	84	15	76	760	2	0	18	3 high-fat meat, 3 fat
Sausage Supreme Skillet	1	1170	96	74	31	620	2371	36	4	40	2 starch, 1 veg., 5 high-fat meat, 8 fat
Scram Slam	1	974	80	74	23	694	1750	30	4	42	4 starch, 5 medium-fat meat, 11 fat
Senior Belgian Waffle Slam	1	399	33	74	8	302	612	12	0	16	1 starch, 2 medium-fat meat, 4 fat
Senior Omelette	1	623	47	68	10	439	1194	27	3	23	2 starch, 2 medium-fat meat, 7 fat

											Exchanges
Senior Starter	1	336	24	64	5	205	541	36	2	11	2 1/2 starch, 1 medium-fat meat, 3 fat
Senior Triple Play	1	537	25	42	6	409	1445	64	2	20	4 starch, 1 medium-fat meat, 4 fat
Sirloin Steak & Eggs	1	808	64	71	18	476	952	21	2	37	1 1/2 starch, 5 medium-fat meat, 8 fat
Slim Slam w/out syrup	1	495	12	22	3	34	1746	98	1	34	6 1/2 starch, 2 medium-fat meat
Slim Slam with syrup	1	638	12	17	3	34	1772	98	1	34	6 1/2 starch, 3 lean meat, 1/2 fat
Southern Slam	1	1065	84	71	23	484	2449	47	0	37	3 starch, 4 medium-fat meat, 13 fat

(*Continued*)

✔ = Healthiest Bets; n/a = not available

BREAKFAST (Continued)	Amount	Cal.	Fat (g)	% Cal. Fat	Sat. Fat (g)	Chol. (mg)	Sod. (mg)	Carb. (g)	Fiber (g)	Pro. (g)	Servings/Exchanges
Super/Play It Again Slam	1	1192	75	57	21	690	3555	98	3	51	6 1/2 starch, 5 medium-fat meat, 8 fat
✔Syrup	1.5 oz/3 Tbsp	143	0	0	0	0	26	36	0	0	2 1/2 carb.
T-bone Steak & Eggs	1	1045	82	71	26	530	1191	21	2	56	1 1/2 starch, 7 medium-fat meat, 9 fat
✔Toast, dry	1 slice	92	1	10	0	0	166	17	1	3	1 starch
Ultimate Omelette	1	780	62	72	14	639	1360	29	4	31	1 1/2 starch, 1 veg, 4 medium-fat meat, 8 fat
Veggie-Cheese Omelette	1	714	53	67	10	644	955	29	4	28	1 1/2 starch, 1 veg., 3 medium-fat meat, 8 fat
✔Waffle, plain	1	304	21	62	3	146	200	23	0	7	1 1/2 starch, 4 fat

CONDIMENTS

✔ BBQ Sauce	1.5 oz	47	1	19	0	0	595	11	0	0	1 starch
✔ Brown Gravy	1 oz/2 Tbsp	13	0	0	0	0	184	2	0	0	free
✔ Chicken Gravy	1 oz/2 Tbsp	14	1	35	1	2	139	2	0	0	free
✔ Country Gravy	1 oz/2 Tbsp	17	1	53	0	0	93	2	0	0	free
✔ Cream Cheese	1 oz/2 Tbsp	100	10	90	6	31	90	1	0	2	2 fat
Horseradish Sauce	1.5 oz/3 Tbsp	170	20	106	3	43	227	3	0	1	4 fat
✔ Sour Cream	1.5 oz/3 Tbsp	91	9	89	6	19	23	2	0	1	2 fat
Whipped Margarine	0.5 oz/1 Tbsp	87	10	103	2	0	117	0	0	0	2 fat

DESSERTS

Apple Pie	1 slice	430	20	42	5	5	390	59	1	3	4 carb., 4 fat
Apple Pie with Equal	1 slice	370	20	49	5	5	360	43	2	3	3 carb., 4 fat

(Continued)

✔ = Healthiest Bets; n/a = not available

DESSERTS (Continued)	Amount	Cal.	Fat (g)	% Cal. Fat	Sat. Fat (g)	Chol. (mg)	Sod. (mg)	Carb. (g)	Fiber (g)	Pro. (g)	Servings/Exchanges
Banana Split Sundae	1	894	43	43	19	78	177	121	6	15	7 carb., 8 1/2 fat
✔Blueberry Topping	3 oz	105	0	0	0	0	15	26	0	0	2 carb.
Cheesecake Pie	1 slice	470	27	52	13	90	280	48	0	8	3 carb., 5 fat
Cherry Pie	1 slice	540	21	35	5	5	430	83	2	5	5 1/2 carb., 4 fat
✔Cherry Topping	3 oz/6 Tbsp	86	0	0	0	0	5	21	0	0	1 1/2 carb.
Chocolate Cake	1 slice	370	17	41	4	29	374	53	2	4	3 1/2 carb., 3 fat
Chocolate Peanut Butter Pie	1 slice	653	39	54	19	27	319	64	3	12	4 carb., 8 fat
Chocolate Topping	2 oz/4 Tbsp	317	25	71	0	0	83	27	0	2	1 1/2 carb., 5 fat
Double Scoop/Sundae	1	375	27	65	12	74	86	29	0	6	2 carb., 5 fat
Dutch Apple Pie	1 slice	440	19	39	5	0	290	65	1	3	4 carb., 4 fat
French Silk Pie	1 slice	650	43	60	26	165	220	60	2	6	4 carb., 8 1/2 fat
✔Fudge Topping	2 oz/4 Tbsp	201	10	45	7	3	96	30	1	1	2 carb., 2 fat

German Chocolate Pie	1 slice	580	33	51	18	15	460	66	2	7	4 1/2 carb, 6 1/2 fat
Hot Fudge Cake Sundae	1	587	38	50	11	62	486	83	3	9	5 1/2 carb, 7 1/2 fat
Ice Cream Float	12 oz	280	10	32	6	0	109	47	0	3	3 carb, 2 fat
Key Lime Pie	1 slice	600	27	41	15	35	300	79	0	10	5 carb, 5 fat
Lemon Meringue Pie	1 slice	460	17	33	4	95	310	71	1	5	5 carb, 3 fat
Single Scoop/Sundae	1	188	14	67	6	37	43	14	0	3	1 carb, 3 fat
✔Strawberry Topping	3 oz/6 Tbsp	115	1	8	0	0	12	26	1	1	2 carb.
✔Whipped Cream	2 oz/4 Tbsp	23	2	78	0	7	3	2	0	0	free

DINNERS, PLATTERS, ETC.

Battered Cod Dinner	1	732	47	58	7	105	1335	48	3	30	3 starch, 3 lean meat, 8 fat
✔Charleston Chicken Dinner	1	327	18	50	4	65	993	16	1	25	1 starch, 3 lean meat, 2 fat
✔Chicken Fried Steak	1	265	17	58	8	27	668	14	1	15	1 starch, 2 medium-fat meat, 1 fat

(Continued)

✔ = Healthiest Bets; n/a = not available

DINNERS, PLATTERS, ETC. (Continued)	Amount	Cal.	Fat (g)	% Cal. Fat	Sat. Fat (g)	Chol. (mg)	Sod. (mg)	Carb. (g)	Fiber (g)	Pro. (g)	Servings/Exchanges
Chicken Strips (5)	1 order	635	25	35	1	95	1510	55	0	47	3 1/2 starch, 5 lean meat, 2 fat
Chicken Strips (plain)	1 order	568	26	41	4	70	1239	45	0	9	3 starch, 1 lean meat, 4 1/2 fat
Five Star Philly	1	657	29	40	8	97	652	55	4	41	3 1/2 starch, 4 medium-fat meat, 2 fat
✓Grilled Chicken Breast Dinner	1	130	4	28	1	67	566	0	0	24	3 very lean meat
✓Grilled Chicken Dinner (fit fare)	1	130	4	28	1	67	560	0	0	24	3 very lean meat
Grilled Choped Steak	1	400	26	59	11	91	447	12	2	30	1 carb., 4 medium-fat meat, 1 fat
✓Grilled Alaskan Salmon Dinner	1	210	4	17	1	101	103	1	0	43	4 very lean meat
Pork Chop Dinner	1	386	24	56	8	121	844	0	0	39	6 lean meat, 1 fat
Porterhouse Steak	1	708	54	69	24	161	713	0	0	56	8 medium-fat meat, 3 fat
Pot Roast Dinner	1	260	11	38	4	140	1085	5	0	39	6 lean meat

	Amount	Calories	Fat (g)	% Cal. Fat	Sat. Fat (g)	Chol. (mg)	Sodium (mg)	Carb. (g)	Fiber (g)	Protein (g)	Exchanges/Choices
Roast Turkey & Stuffing	1	701	27	35	1	100	2346	63	0	47	4 starch, 6 lean meat, 2 fat
Senior Battered Cod (fried)	1	465	34	66	5	68	743	25	1	15	1 1/2 starch, 2 lean meat, 5 1/2 fat
✔Senior Chicken Fried Steak	1	341	18	48	8	27	943	29	2	16	2 carb., 2 lean meat, 2 fat
✔Senior Grilled Chicken Breast	1	219	6	25	1	67	880	16	0	26	1 carb., 3 lean meat
✔Senior Liver, with bacon & onions	1	322	19	53	5	270	643	20	2	22	1 veg., 1 carb., 3 medium-fat meat, 1 fat
✔Senior Pork Chop	1	193	12	56	4	60	422	0	0	19	3 lean meat, 1 fat
✔Senior Pot Roast	1	149	6	36	2	71	818	6	0	20	3 lean meat
Senior Turkey & Stuffing	1	596	25	38	1	51	1750	61	0	29	4 starch, 2 lean meat, 4 fat
Shrimp Dinner (fried)	1	558	32	52	6	135	1114	49	3	19	3 starch, 2 lean meat, 5 fat
Sirloin Steak Dinner	1	271	21	70	9	62	273	0	0	22	3 medium-fat meat, 1 fat

✔ = Healthiest Bets; n/a = not available

(Continued)

DINNERS, PLATTERS, ETC. (Continued)	Amount	Cal.	Fat (g)	% Cal. Fat	Sat. Fat (g)	Chol. (mg)	Sod. (mg)	Carb. (g)	Fiber (g)	Pro. (g)	Servings/Exchanges
Steak and Shrimp Dinner	1	645	42	59	14	150	1143	31	2	36	2 starch, 4 medium-fat meat, 4 fat
T-Bone Steak Dinner	1	530	40	68	18	121	534	0	0	42	6 medium-fat meat, 2 fat
FRUIT											
✔Banana	1	110	0	0	0	0	0	29	4	1	2 fruit
✔Banana/Strawberry Medley	4 oz	108	1	8	0	0	6	27	2	1	2 fruit
✔Cantaloupe	3 oz	32	0	0	0	0	16	8	1	1	1/2 fruit
✔Fresh Fruit Mix	3 oz	36	0	0	0	0	16	9	1	1	1/2 fruit
✔Grapefruit	1/2	60	0	0	0	0	0	16	6	1	1 fruit
✔Grapes	3 oz	55	1	16	0	0	0	15	1	1	1 fruit
✔Honeydew	3 oz	31	0	0	0	0	22	8	1	1	1/2 fruit

KID'S MEALS

	Amount	Cal	Fat (g)	% Fat Cal	Sat Fat (g)	Chol (mg)	Sod (mg)	Carb (g)	Fiber (g)	Pro (g)	Servings/Exchanges
BURGERlicious	1	296	17	52	6	28	368	24	1	13	1 1/2 starch, 2 medium-fat meat, 1 fat
BURGERlicious w/ cheese	1	341	20	53	6	40	580	24	1	15	1 1/2 starch, 2 medium-fat meat, 2 fat
DENNYSAUR Chicken Nuggets	1	260	9	31	0	35	1088	27	0	18	2 starch, 2 medium-fat meat, 1/2 fat
FRENCHtastic Slam	1	452	33	66	9	311	664	22		19	1 1/2 starch, 2 high-fat meat, 2 1/2 fat
Junior GRAND SLAM	1	397	25	57	7	230	1118	33	1	17	2 starch, 2 high-fat meat, 1 fat
PIGS in a Blanket	1	479	21	39	7	32	1684	63	2	16	4 starch, 1 high-fat meat, 2 fat
PIZZA PARTY	1	400	15	34	3	10	1090	47	7	18	3 starch, 1 high-fat meat, 1 fat
SHRIMPsational Basket	1	291	16	49	3	68	774	27	2	10	2 starch, 1 lean meat, 2 1/2 fat

(Continued)

✔ = Healthiest Bets; n/a = not available

KID'S MEALSS (Continued)	Amount	Cal.	Fat (g)	% Cal. Fat	Sat. Fat (g)	Chol. (mg)	Sod. (mg)	Carb. (g)	Fiber (g)	Pro. (g)	Servings/Exchanges
SMILEY-FACE Hot Cakes w/out meat	1	344	9	24	3	13	1014	62	2	7	4 starch, 2 fat
SMILEY-FACE Hot Cakes with meat	1	463	22	43	7	38	1410	63	2	14	4 starch, 1 high-fat meat, 2 fat
THE BIG Cheese	1	334	20	54	2	24	828	28	2	9	2 starch, 2 high-fat meat
WACKY WAFFLES	1	215	12	50	3	78	102	23	0	4	1 1/2 starch, 2 fat
SALAD DRESSINGS											
Blue Cheese	1 oz/2 Tbsp	124	12	87	4	18	405	4	0	4	1 high-fat meat
Caesar	1 oz/2 Tbsp	142	15	95	2	2	340	1	0	1	3 fat
✔Creamy Italian	1 oz/2 Tbsp	106	10	85	2	0	306	4	0	0	2 fat
✔Fat Free Honey Mustard	1 oz/2 Tbsp	38	0	0	0	0	121	9	0	0	1/2 carb.
✔French	1 oz/2 Tbsp	106	10	85	2	7	274	3	0	0	2 fat

✓Oriental Peanut	1 oz/2 Tbsp	106	8	36	1	0	399	6	0	1	1/2 carb., 1 1/2 fat
✓Ranch	1 oz/2 Tbsp	101	11	98	2	8	215	1	0	1	2 fat
✓Reduced Calorie French	1 oz/2 Tbsp	76	5	59	1	0	265	8	0	0	1/2 carb., 1 fat
✓Reduced Calorie Italian	1 oz/2 Tbsp	23	1	39	0	0	515	3	0	0	free
✓Thousand Island	1 oz/2 Tbsp	104	10	87	2	21	208	2	0	0	2 fat

SALADS

Buffalo Chicken Salad	1	615	37	54	8	88	1258	36	3	39	2 1/2 starch, 5 lean meat, 4 fat
Fried Chicken Salad	1	506	31	55	8	94	1174	30	3	38	1 starch, 2 veg, 4 lean meat, 4 fat
✓Garden Chicken Delite	1	277	5	16	1	67	785	30	6	30	1 starch, 2 veg, 3 lean meat
Grilled Chicken Caesar	1	655	47	65	9	86	1728	23	4	37	1 starch, 2 veg, 4 lean meat, 7 fat

(Continued)

✓ = Healthiest Bets; n/a = not available

SALADS (Continued)	Amount	Cal.	Fat (g)	% Cal. Fat	Sat. Fat (g)	Chol. (mg)	Sod. (mg)	Carb. (g)	Fiber (g)	Pro. (g)	Servings/Exchanges
Oriental Chicken Salad	1	568	26	41	5	67	1656	49	7	33	2 veg., 2 1/2 starch, 4 lean meat 3 fat
Side Caesar	1	338	25	67	5	7	725	20	3	8	1/2 starch, 2 veg., 5 fat
✓ Side Garden Salad	1	113	4	32	1	0	147	16	3	3	3 veg., 1 fat

SANDWICHES AND BURGERS

	Amount	Cal.	Fat (g)	% Cal. Fat	Sat. Fat (g)	Chol. (mg)	Sod. (mg)	Carb. (g)	Fiber (g)	Pro. (g)	Servings/Exchanges
Bacon Cheddar Burger	1	935	63	61	25	164	1732	43	3	53	3 starch, 6 lean meat, 9 fat
Bacon, Letuce & Tomato	1	634	46	65	8	54	1116	37	2	18	2 starch, 1 veg., 2 high-fat meat 5 fat
Big Texas BBQ Burger	1	929	58	56	24	163	2271	53	3	53	3 1/2 starch, 6 medium-fat meat 5 1/2 fat
Charleston Chicken	1	632	32	46	7	81	1967	53	4	35	3 1/2 starch, 4 lean meat, 3 fat

											Exchanges
Chicken Melt	1	520	29	50	5	39	1096	43	2	26	3 starch, 2 medium-fat meat, 4 fat
Classic Burger	1	673	40	53	15	106	1142	42	3	37	3 starch, 4 medium-fat meat, 4 fat
Classic Burger w/ Cheese	1	836	53	57	19	137	1595	43	3	47	3 starch, 5 medium-fat meat, 5 1/2 fat
Club	1	718	38	48	7	75	1666	62	3	32	4 starch, 3 medium-fat meat, 4 1/2 fat
Delidinger	1	852	45	48	6	80	3142	62	3	56	4 starch, 6 medium-fat meat, 3 fat
Deluxe Grilled Cheese	1	482	26	49	2	1	1135	44	2	18	3 starch, 2 high-fat meat, 1 fat
Fisherman's Choice	1	905	56	56	8	69	1704	74	4	29	5 starch, 2 lean meat, 10 fat

(Continued)

✓ = Healthiest Bets; n/a = not available

SANDWICHES AND BURGERS (Continued)	Amount	Cal.	Fat (g)	% Cal. Fat	Sat. Fat (g)	Chol. (mg)	Sod. (mg)	Carb. (g)	Fiber (g)	Pro. (g)	Servings/Exchanges
Garden Burger	1	665	33	44	8	36	1051	75	8	18	5 starch, 1 lean meat, 6 fat
✓Garden Burger (patty only)	1	172	4	17	2	20	424	25	5	8	1 1/2 starch, 1 lean meat
Grilled Chicken	1	509	19	34	5	83	1809	52	3	34	4 starch, 3 lean meat, 2 fat
Grilled Chicken, Fit Fare	1	434	9	19	3	82	1705	56	4	35	3 1/2 starch, 4 lean meat
Ham & Swiss on Rye	1	533	31	52	4	36	1638	40	5	23	2 1/2 starch, 2 medium-fat meat, 4 fat
Patty Melt	1	695	44	57	13	114	1007	39	2	38	2 1/2 starch, 4 medium-fat meat, 5 fat
Senior Grilled Cheese Deluxe	1	482	26	49	2	1	1135	44	2	18	3 starch, 1 high-fat meat, 3 fat
Senior Ham & Swiss	1	497	30	54	4	36	1537	34	4	22	2 starch, 2 medium-fat meat, 4 fat
Senior Turkey Sandwich	1	476	26	49	3	57	1107	39	5	23	2 1/2 starch, 2 lean meat, 4 fat

The Super Bird	1	620	32	46	5	60	1880	48	2	35	3 starch, 4 lean meat, 4 fat
Turkey Breast, on multigrain	1	476	26	49	3	57	1107	39	3	23	2 1/2 starch, 2 lean meat, 4 fat

SIDES

✔ Applesauce	3 oz	60	0	0	0	0	13	15	1	0	1 fruit
✔ Baked Potato, plain	1	186	0	0	0	0	14	43	4	4	3 starch
Biscuit, plain	1	375	22	53	5	0	750	40	0	5	2 1/2 starch, 4 fat
✔ Broccoli in butter sauce	4 oz	50	2	36	2	5	280	7	3	3	2 veg.
✔ Carrots in honey glaze	4 oz	80	3	34	1	0	220	12	3	1	1 veg., 1/2 carb, 1/2 fat
✔ Corn in butter sauce	4 oz	120	4	30	2	5	260	19	3	3	1 starch, 1 fat
✔ Cornbread Stuffing, plain	2 oz	182	9	45	0	0	405	20	0	4	1 starch, 2 fat
✔ Cottage Cheese	3 oz/6 Tbsp	72	3	38	2	10	281	2	0	9	1 lean meat
✔ Dinner Roll	1	132	2	14	0	0	265	26	1	4	2 starch
French Fries (with sandwich)	1 order	323	14	39	3	0	133	44	0	5	3 starch, 3 fat

✔ = Healthiest Bets; n/a = not available

(Continued)

SIDES (Continued)	Amount	Cal.	Fat (g)	% Cal. Fat	Sat. Fat (g)	Chol. (mg)	Sod. (mg)	Carb. (g)	Fiber (g)	Pro. (g)	Servings/Exchanges
French Fries, unsalted	1 order	323	14	39	3	0	130	44	0	5	3 starch, 3 fat
✔Green Beans with bacon	4 oz	60	4	60	2	5	390	6	3	1	1 veg. 1 fat
✔Green Peas in butter sauce	4 oz	100	2	18	2	5	360	14	4	5	1 starch
✔Grilled Mushrooms	2 oz	14	0	0	0	0	0	2	1	2	free
Herb Toast	1 order	200	11	50	2	0	372	21	1	4	1 1/2 starch, 2 fat
✔Mashed Potatoes, plain	6 oz	105	1	9	0	0	378	21	2	3	1 1/2 starch
Onion Rings	1 order	264	16	55	4	4	695	27	0	3	2 starch, 3 fat
✔Rice Pilaf	3 oz	112	2	16	0	0	328	21	0	2	1 1/2 starch
Seasoned Fries	1 order	261	12	41	3	0	556	35	0	5	2 starch, 2 fat
✔Sliced Tomatoes	3 slices	13	0	0	0	0	6	3	1	1	free
SOUPS											
Cheese	8 oz	293	23	71	13	19	895	13	4	6	1 carb. 4 1/2 fat

✔Chicken Noodle	8 oz	60	2	30	0	10	640	8	0	2	1/2 starch
Clam Chowder	8 oz	214	11	46	9	5	903	22	1	5	1 1/2 carb., 2 fat
Cream of Broccoli	8 oz	193	12	56	9	0	818	15	2	4	1 carb., 2 fat
Cream of Potato	8 oz	222	12	49	9	0	761	23	2	4	1 1/2 starch, 2 fat
✔Split Pea	8 oz	146	6	37	2	5	819	18	2	8	1 carb., 1 fat
✔Vegetable Beef	8 oz	79	1	11	1	5	820	11	2	6	1 starch

✔ = Healthiest Bets; n/a = not available

Notes

Perkins Family Restaurant

❖Perkins provided a small amount of nutrition information for a few menu items.

Light 'n Lean Choice

Short Stack, 3 buttermilk pancakes (*split*)
Fresh Fruit

No nutrition information available from restaurant for these items.

Healthy 'n Hearty Choice

Grilled Lemon Chicken Bread Bowl Salad
Fruit Pie (*split*)

No nutrition information available from restaurant for these items.

Healthier Picks

Traditional Favorites
Classic Egg Favorites (*order one egg, lean smoked ham, and toast*)

Premium Omelettes (*split and order with toast*)
Everything Omelette (*hold cheese*)
Ham & Cheese (*hold cheese*)

Pancakes Plus (*low-calorie syrup and margarine/butter blend available upon request*)
Short Stack

Belgian Waffle (*hold powdered sugar*)
French Toast (*hold powdered sugar*)

Burgers and Super Sandwiches (*all are served with choice of french fries or salad; choose salad*)
Hamburger
Chicken Supreme (*hold cheese and bacon*)

Bread Bowl Salads (*low-calorie dressing available upon request*)
Grilled Lemon Chicken
Chef
Grilled Teriyaki Chicken
Chicken Caesar
Taco Salad (*hold crispy tortilla shell; hold sour cream and guacamole; use green chili sauce as salad dressing*)
Perkin's Dinner Salad

Soup of the Day (*choose broth-based*)

Grille & Oven Baked Classics
Cajun Chicken Grille
Lemon Pepper Chicken
Lemon Pepper Grilled Roughy

Pasta Selections
Linguine Marinara

(*Continued*)

Perkins Family Restaurant

	Amount	Cal.	Fat (g)	% Cal. Fat	Sat. Fat (g)	Chol. (mg)	Sod. (mg)	Carb. (g)	Fiber (g)	Pro. (g)	Servings/Exchanges
BREAKFAST											
Egg-stra Low Fat Burrito Breakfast, w/ fresh fruit	1 order	n/a	15	n/a	n/a	0	1850	n/a	n/a	n/a	insufficient info. to calculate
Egg-stra Low Fat Burrito Breakfast w/ low fat muffin	1 order	n/a	18	n/a	n/a	0	1850	n/a	n/a	n/a	insufficient info. to calculate
Oatmeal, w/ 4 oz. 2% milk	1 1/2 pkg.	n/a	n/a	n/a	n/a	4	n/a	n/a	n/a	n/a	insufficient info. to calculate
DESSERTS											
Brownie	1	280	1	3	n/a	n/a	n/a	n/a	n/a	n/a	insufficient info. to calculate

LOW FAT MUFFINS

Banana	1	330	3	8	n/a	n/a	n/a	n/a	insufficient info. to calculate
Blueberry	1	270	3	10	n/a	n/a	n/a	n/a	insufficient info. to calculate
Honey Bran	1	270	3	10	n/a	n/a	n/a	n/a	insufficient info. to calculate
Plain	1	300	3	9	n/a	n/a	n/a	n/a	insufficient info. to calculate

Notes

Ruby Tuesday

❖Ruby Tuesday provided some nutrition
  information for several of its menu items.

Light 'n Lean Choice

Spicy Chicken Fajita Salad
(*hold fried tortilla bowl and cheese*)

No nutrition information available from restaurant
for this item.

Healthy 'n Hearty Choice

Shrimp & Veggie Pasta

Calories	762	Sodium (mg)	1,680
Fat (g)	9	Carbohydrate (g)	128
% calories from fat	11	Fiber (g)	n/a
Saturated fat (g)	n/a	Protein (g)	6
Cholesterol (mg)	n/a		

Exchanges: insufficient information to calculate

Healthier Picks

Starters & Snacks
Chicken Quesadilla
Ruby's Soup of the Day (*if broth-based*)

Entree Salads (*request dressing on the side*)
Salad Bar Extravaganza (*choose mainly fresh vegetables and apply salad dressing gingerly*)*

BBQ Chicken Salad (*hold crisp tortilla strips and cheese*)

Ruby's Caesar Salad, chicken or shrimp (*hold Parmesan cheese*)

Spicy Chicken Fajita Salad (*hold fried tortilla bowl and cheese*)

Combos
Fit 'n Trim Low-Fat Stuffed Potato*

Potato* & Soup (*broth-based*)

Potato* & Salad Bar

Sizzling Fajitas (*hold sour cream, cheese, and guacamole; order double salsa*)
Classic Steak Fajitas

Shrimp Fajitas

Grilled Chicken Fajitas

Triple Play Fajitas

Combination Classic Steak & Grilled Chicken Fajitas

Great Burgers (*substitute salad bar or baked potato for fries*)
BBQ Cheeseburger (*hold cheese*)

Alpine Burger (*hold cheese*)

All-American Burger

Sicilian Burger (*hold cheese*)

Un-Burgers
Gold Coast Turkey Burger (*hold bacon and cheese*)

Turkey Pub Burger (*hold cheese and Thousand Island dressing*)

Veggie Burger (*hold cheese and sour cream dill dressing*)

Sensational Sandwiches
Grilled Cajun Chicken Sandwich (*hold remoulade sauce*)

(*Continued*)

BBQ Chicken 'n Cheese Sandwich (*hold cheese*)
Super Duper Chicken Sandwich (hold cheese and
    bacon)
Herb-Grilled Chicken Sandwich*

Ruby's Originals
Cowboy Grill, chicken or steak (*hold tumbleweed
    onion straws*)
Chicken or Shrimp Stir-Fry*
Grilled Chicken Breast, Teriyaki* or Cajun-Grilled
    (*order with steamed vegetables and rice pilaf*)
Broiled Norwegian Salmon (*lemon pepper or Cajun
    spices; served with rice pilaf and vegetable*)

Pasta
Shrimp & Veggie Pasta*

Signature Substitutions
Steamed Vegetables
Baked Potato
Rice

Fabulous Desserts
Our Fabulous Fat-Free Sundaes (*chocolate or
    strawberry*)*

*Denotes Fit 'n Trim items that are lower in fat. See nutrition
information for these items in the table. Ruby Tuesday also offers
a variety of nonfat salad dressings, Promise light margarine,
Hellmann's light mayonnaise, and fat-free ice cream.

Ruby Tuesday

	Amount	Cal.	Fat (g)	% Cal. Fat	Sat. Fat (g)	Chol. (mg)	Sod. (mg)	Carb. (g)	Fiber (g)	Pro. (g)	Servings/Exchanges
DESSERTS											
Fat Free Fudge Sundae	1	675	0	0	n/a	n/a	37	132	n/a	n/a	insufficient info. to calculate
Fat Free Strawberry Sundae	1	646	0	0	n/a	n/a	25	118	n/a	n/a	insufficient info. to calculate
ENTREES											
Chicken Stir-Fry	1	834	1	1	n/a	n/a	1980	161	n/a	6	insufficient info. to calculate
Chicken Stuffwich	1	874	7	7	n/a	n/a	1460	189	n/a	n/a	Insufficient data to calculate
Herb Grilled Chicken Sandwich	1	538	7	12	n/a	n/a	1320	85	n/a	6	insufficient info. to calculate
Shrimp & Veggie Pasta	1	762	9	11	n/a	n/a	1680	128	n/a	6	insufficient info. to calculate
Shrimp Stir-Fry	1	770	1	1	n/a	n/a	1900	160	n/a	4	insufficient info. to calculate

(*Continued*)

ENTRIES (Continued)	Amount	Cal.	Fat (g)	% Cal. Fat	Sat. Fat (g)	Chol. (mg)	Sod. (mg)	Carb. (g)	Fiber (g)	Pro. (g)	Servings/Exchanges
Teriyaki Chicken	1	516	3	5	n/a	n/a	1650	80	n/a	24	insufficient info. to calculate
Tilapia (3 1/2 oz. fillet only)	1	98	2	9	0	0	520	n/a	n/a	19	3 very lean meat
SIDES											
Lowfat Baked Potato	1	587	4	2	n/a	n/a	710	375	n/a	n/a	insufficient info. to calculate

Notes

Steak Houses

RESTAURANTS

Golden Corral

Outback Steakhouse

Quincy's Family Steakhouse

Note: Very little nutrition information is made available by most steak houses. You probably will not spot a few large chains you expect to find in this chapter because they were unwilling to provide either a menu or nutrition information. The only restaurant to tell all is Quincy's Family Steakhouse. The restaurants in the chapter provided only the nutrition information listed below.

NUTRITION PROS

- The upside of the "food bar" in many steak houses is the low-fat, low-calorie raw vegetables: lettuce, spinach, carrots, broccoli, cucumbers, tomatoes, mushrooms, and more.
- Lean cuts of beef, broiled or grilled chicken breast, and seafood prepared low-fat are available at most steak houses.
- Lean cuts of beef on many steak house menus are filet mignon, sirloin tips, sirloin, or chopped sirloin.
- Healthy low-fat starches are available, but make sure they're not doused in fat before they reach your lips.
- Smaller portions of protein are available. Look for portions that are 5–8 oz. These weights are for raw portions. You will get about 4–6 oz cooked.

■ Fresh or canned fruit is often available if there is a "food bar."

NUTRITION CONS

■ The downside of the "food bar" in many steak houses is the high-fat, high-calorie minefields at the salad trough: pasta salad, fruit ambrosia, potato salad, fried Chinese noodles, tuna or seafood salad, creamy coleslaw, nuts, seeds, and olives.

■ High-fat and high-calorie creamy and mayonnaise-based salad dressings are plentiful, and it's easy to ladle on too much. Keep in mind that the ladle in most salad dressings holds two tablespoons.

■ Higher-fat cuts of beef on many steak house menus are rib eye, prime rib, porterhouse, T-bone, and Delmonico.

■ Chicken and seafood is often fried. You need to read descriptions carefully and ask questions before you order to avoid the fried items.

■ Large portions of protein are the norm—10 to 16 oz (raw weight) is not a rarity. Unfortunately, that amount of protein can serve at least three people.

Healthy Tips

* Use a dab or two of high-fat, high-calorie salad dressing and dilute it with vinegar or lemon wedges.
* Take a stroll around the "food bar" to size-up your choices before you start to fill your plate.
* Ask your dining partner to go to the food bar for you so that you can avoid temptation. Just specify what you want on your salad.
* Order a take-home container when you order your meal. Pack up what you want to save when your order arrives. Then you won't be tempted to cut into tomorrow's lunch or dinner. Remember: Out of sight is out of mind.
* Try menu items such as beef or chicken kabobs or sirloin tips, which may be a smaller quantity of protein.
* Use the split technique: One person of a dining duo orders a lean 6–8 oz steak, chicken, or fish item, with a baked potato and a trip to the food bar. The other orders just the baked potato and a trip to the food bar. Once the order arrives, split the protein down the middle.
* Order beef as you like it done, but trim it well before you dig in.

Get It Your Way

* Ask if the chef puts butter on the meats when cooking them. If the answer is yes, ask that yours be cooked without it.
* When you order a baked potato, make sure you have the high-fat add-ons—butter, sour cream, bacon bits—on the side or left in the kitchen.
* Replace a buttery slice of bread or cheese bread with an unadulterated piece of bread or dinner roll.
* If you order a salad, order salad dressing on the side.
* If you split a piece of meat, ask them to split it in the kitchen.
* Ask for a doggie bag to be delivered with your meal.

Golden Corral

❖Golden Corral provided only its menu.

Light 'n Lean Choice

Sirloin Tips (*5 oz*)
Baked Potato (*with 2 Tbsp sour cream*)
Salad Bar (*broccoli, mushrooms, raisins,
tomatoes, and cucumbers*)
Fat-Free Dressing (*2 Tbsp*)

No nutrition information provided by restaurant.

Healthy 'n Hearty Choice

Petite Sirloin
Rice Pilaf
Yeast Roll (*1, with 1 tsp butter*)
Salad Bar (*spinach, shredded carrots, diced egg,
green pepper rings, and cauliflower*)
Fat-Free Dressing (*2 Tbsp*)

No nutrition information provided by restaurant.

Healthier Picks

Entrees
Petite Sirloin
Sirloin Tips (*5 oz*)
Grilled Chicken Breast
1/4 Rotisserie Chicken (*white meat*)
Spaghetti with Meat Sauce

(*Continued*)

Hot Buffet Items

Yeast Rolls
5-Grain Bread
Soup (*broth-based*)
Rice Pilaf
Baked Potato (*healthier add-ons: chives, spring onions, onions, salsa*)
Mashed Potatoes
Broccoli & Cauliflower (*hold cheese sauce*)
Green Beans
Corn

Cold Buffet Items

All vegetables
Pickles
Cottage Cheese
Fat-Free Dressings
Diced Egg
Fresh Fruit
Raisins
Pineapple Tidbits
Diced Ham or Turkey
Saltines

Sweet Spot

Vanilla Soft Serve
Yogurt
Sugar-Free Fruit Crisp
Sugar-Free Chocolate Pudding or Jell-O

Outback Steakhouse

❖Outback Steakhouse provided nutrition
 information for only its "Tangy Tomato" No-Oil
 salad dressing.

Light 'n Lean Choice

Grilled Shrimp On The Barbie
(appetizer, order as main course)
Jacket Potato, with butter *(1 tsp)*
Fresh Veggies
House Salad with Tangy Tomato No-Oil Dressing
(2 Tbsp)

Only no-oil salad dressing nutrition information was
provided by restaurant.

Healthy 'n Hearty Choice

The Outback Special
(12-oz center-cut sirloin; split)
Jacket Potato, with sour cream *(2 Tbsp)*
Fresh Veggies
House Salad with regular salad dressing *(2 Tbsp)*

No nutrition information for these items was provided by restaurant.

Healthier Picks

Lunches
The Outbacker *(hold cheese; substitute baked potato
  for Aussie chips)*

(Continued)

No Rules Burger (*add grilled onions, sautéed mushrooms, lettuce and tomato, BBQ sauce, and/or pickles and onions; substitute baked potato for Aussie chips*)

Barbie Chook 'N Bacon (*hold bacon and/or cheese; substitute baked potato for Aussie chips*)

Sweet Chook O' Mine (*hold bacon and/or cheese; substitute baked potato for Aussie chips*)

For Children
Boomerang Cheese Burger
Mac A Roo 'N Cheese

Appetizers
Grilled Shrimp On The Barbie (*good for entree too*)

Entrees
Jackeroo Chops (*take one chop home*)
Lobster Tails (*take one tail home; order with house salad, baked potato, and fresh veggies*)
Victoria's Filet (*9-oz tenderloin; order with house salad, baked potato, and fresh veggies*)
Chicken On The Barbie (*order house salad*)
Botany Bay Fish O' The Day (*order house salad*)

Salads
Chook-N-Caesar Salad (*request dressing on the side*)
Brisbane Caesar Salad (*request dressing on the side*)
Soup 'N Salad, if soup is broth-based (*request dressing on the side*)

Sides
Sautéed 'Shrooms
Jacket Potato
Grilled Onions
Fresh Veggies
House Salad

Outback Steakhouse

	Amount	Cal.	Fat (g)	% Cal. Fat	Sat. Fat (g)	Chol. (mg)	Sod. (mg)	Carb. (g)	Fiber (g)	Pro. (g)	Servings/Exchanges
✓Tangy Tomato No-Oil Salad Dressing	1 oz/2 Tbsp	45	0	0	0	0	140	10	0	0	1/2 carb.

✓ = Healthiest Bets; n/a = not available

Notes

Quincy's Family Steakhouse

❖Quincy's Family Steakhouse provided nutrition information for all of its menu items.

Light 'n Lean Choice

Junior Sirloin Steak (*5.5 oz*)
Corn, Broccoli Spears
Yeast Roll, with butter (*1 tsp*)

Calories	529	Sodium (mg)	855
Fat (g)	20	Carbohydrate (g)	58
% calories from fat	34	Fiber (g)	n/a
Saturated fat (g)	5	Protein (g)	32
Cholesterol (mg)	79		

Exchanges: 3 1/2 starch, 1 veg., 4 lean meat, 1/2 fat

Healthy 'n Hearty Choice

Vegetable Beef Soup
Sirloin Tips w/Pepper & Onions
Baked Potato, with butter (*1 tsp*)
Salad Bar (*tomatoes, mushrooms, red cabbage,*
alfalfa sprouts, and onions)
Light Thousand Island Dressing (*2 Tbsp*)
Fruit from salad bar (*cantaloupe,*
pineapple chunks, and honeydew)

Calories	713	Sodium (mg)	1,568
Fat (g)	19	Carbohydrate (g)	101
% calories from fat	24	Fiber (g)	n/a
Saturated fat (g)	4	Protein (g)	45
Cholesterol (mg)	93		

Exchanges: 2 starch, 3 veg., 2 fruit, 1 1/2 carb., 4 lean meat, 1 fat

Quincy's Family Steakhouse

	Amount	Cal.	Fat (g)	% Cal. Fat	Sat. Fat (g)	Chol. (mg)	Sod. (mg)	Carb. (g)	Fiber (g)	Pro. (g)	Servings/Exchanges
BEEF ENTREES											
Chopped Steak	1	499	42	76	20	89	348	0	n/a	31	4 medium-fat meat, 4 fat
Country Steak w/ Gravy	1	530	25	42	7	54	1161	44	n/a	32	3 starch, 3 medium-fat meat, 2 fat
Cowboy Steak	1	580	33	51	15	176	1308	9	n/a	61	1/2 carb., 9 lean meat, 1 fat
✓Filet w/ Bacon	1	340	17	45	7	124	311	2	n/a	48	7 lean meat
✓Junior Sirloin Steak	1	194	10	46	5	69	199	0	n/a	25	3 lean meat
✓Large Sirloin Steak	1	368	20	49	9	119	390	2	n/a	46	7 lean meat
NY Strip Steak	1	450	26	52	13	148	156	1	n/a	53	8 lean meat

✓ = Healthiest Bets; n/a = not available

(Continued)

BEEF ENTRÉES (Continued)	Amount	Cal.	Fat (g)	% Cal. Fat	Sat. Fat (g)	Chol. (mg)	Sod. (mg)	Carb. (g)	Fiber (g)	Pro. (g)	Servings/Exchanges
Porterhouse Steak	1	683	46	61	23	154	346	0	n/a	67	10 medium-fat meat
✔Regular Sirloin Steak	1	285	16	51	7	71	317	0	n/a	34	5 lean meat
Ribeye Steak	1	452	29	58	13	116	156	0	n/a	48	7 medium-fat meat
✔Sirloin Tips w/ Mushroom Gravy	1	196	7	32	3	64	578	5	n/a	28	4 lean meat
✔Sirloin Tips w/ Pepper & Onions	1	203	8	35	3	63	793	4	n/a	27	1 veg, 4 lean meat
Smothered Strip Steak	1	622	41	59	16	148	239	12	n/a	55	2 veg, 7 medium-fat meat, 1 fat
T-Bone Steak	1	521	35	60	18	118	265	0	n/a	51	7 medium-fat meat
BREAKFAST											
✔Bacon	1 order	35	3	77	1	5	100	0	n/a	2	1/2 fat
Corned Beef Hash	1 order	210	15	64	8	45	795	11	n/a	10	1 starch, 1 medium-fat meat, 2 fat

Country Ham	1 order	90	6	60	2	35	1100	1	n/a	9	1 medium-fat meat
✔Escalloped Apples	3.5 oz	120	2	15	0	0	20	26	n/a	0	1 1/2 carb.
✔Oatmeal	1 oz	175	2	10	0	0	285	18	n/a	4	1 starch
✔Pancakes	1 order	95	3	28	1	30	250	12	n/a	3	1 starch, 1/2 fat
Sausage Gravy	4 oz	70	6	77	2	10	150	3	n/a	2	1 fat
Sausage Links	1 order	225	22	88	8	20	390	0	n/a	7	1 high-fat meat, 2 fat
Sausage Patties	1 order	230	23	90	9	45	350	0	n/a	7	1 high-fat meat, 2 1/2 fat
✔Scrambled Eggs	1 order	95	7	66	2	215	270	1	n/a	7	1 medium-fat
Steak Fingers	1 order	360	25	63	11	50	690	18	n/a	16	1 starch, 2 medium-fat meat, 3 fat
✔Syrup	1 oz/2 Tbsp	75	0	0	0	0	15	20	n/a	0	1 carb.

DESSERTS

✔Apple Cobbler	1	255	8	28	2	5	285	49	n/a	1	3 carb., 1 fat

(Continued)

✔ = Healthiest Bets; n/a = not available

DESSERTS (Continued)	Amount	Cal.	Fat (g)	% Cal. Fat	Sat. Fat (g)	Chol. (mg)	Sod. (mg)	Carb. (g)	Fiber (g)	Pro. (g)	Servings/Exchanges
Banana Pudding	1	240	12	45	9	10	240	30	n/a	3	2 carb., 2 fat
✔Brownie Pudding Cake	1 slice	310	5	15	1	0	395	66	n/a	4	4 carb., 1 fat
✔Caramel Topping	1 oz/2 Tbsp	105	1	9	1	0	120	24	n/a	0	1 1/2 carb.
Cherry Cobbler	1	410	8	18	2	5	185	55	n/a	1	4 1/2 carb., 1 1/2 fat
✔Chocolate Chip Cookie	1	60	8	120	1	5	35	8	n/a	1	1/2 carb., 1 1/2 fat
✔Frozen Yogurt	4 oz	135	2	13	1	5	85	25	n/a	5	2 carb.
✔Fudge Topping	1 oz/2 Tbsp	105	4	34	1	0	75	15	n/a	1	1 carb., 1 fat
✔Peach Cobbler	1	305	8	24	2	5	190	50	n/a	1	3 carb., 1 1/2 fat
✔Sugar Cookie	1	60	3	45	1	5	30	8	n/a	1	1/2 carb., 1/2 fat
OTHER ENTREES											
✔Grilled Chicken (regular)	1	120	2	15	0	55	540	1	n/a	25	4 very lean meat
✔Grilled Salmon	1	228	4	16	1	109	112	1	n/a	46	7 very lean meat

✔Homestyle Chicken Fillet	1	217	9	37	2	25	682	21	n/a	13	1 1/2 starch, 1 lean meat, 1 fat
Roasted BBQ Chicken	1	941	65	62	17	340	1548	21	n/a	70	1 carb., 10 lean meat, 7 fat
Roasted Herb Chicken	1	875	65	67	17	340	1238	4	n/a	70	10 lean meat, 7 fat
Southern Breaded Shrimp	1	546	31	51	6	135	821	47	n/a	19	3 starch, 1 lean meat, 5 fat
Steak & Shrimp	1	677	39	52	12	170	816	33	n/a	48	2 starch, 4 medium-fat meat, 4 fat

SALAD DRESSINGS

Bleu Cheese	1 oz/2 Tbsp	155	16	93	3	10	165	2	n/a	2	3 fat
French	1 oz/2 Tbsp	125	12	86	1	0	500	4	n/a	0	2 fat
✔Honey Mustard	1 oz/2 Tbsp	100	6	54	1	0	220	10	n/a	2	1/2 carb., 1 fat
Italian	1 oz/2 Tbsp	135	14	93	2	0	230	3	n/a	0	3 fat
✔Light Creamy Italian	1 oz/2 Tbsp	65	4	55	0	0	485	8	n/a	2	1/2 carb., 1 fat
✔Light French	1 oz/2 Tbsp	85	4	42	0	0	285	13	n/a	2	1 carb., 1 fat

(Continued)

✔ = Healthiest Bets; n/a = not available

SALAD DRESSINGS (Continued)	Amount	Cal.	Fat (g)	% Cal. Fat	Sat. Fat (g)	Chol. (mg)	Sod. (mg)	Carb. (g)	Fiber (g)	Pro. (g)	Servings/Exchanges
✔Light Italian	1 oz/2 Tbsp	20	2	90	0	0	485	2	n/a	2	free
✔Light Thousand Island	1 oz/2 Tbsp	65	4	55	0	20	340	8	n/a	2	1/2 carb, 1 fat
Parmesan Peppercorn	1 oz/2 Tbsp	150	14	84	0	0	280	4	n/a	1	3 fat
Ranch	1 oz/2 Tbsp	110	11	90	2	10	195	1	n/a	1	2 fat
SANDWICHES											
1/3 pound Hamburger	1	565	33	53	16	66	603	32	n/a	32	2 starch, 4 medium-fat meat, 2 1/2 fat
Bacon Cheese Burger	1	663	41	56	17	87	997	33	n/a	37	2 starch, 4 medium-fat meat, 4 fat
Grilled Chicken Sandwich	1	324	4	11	1	55	1183	39	n/a	33	2 1/2 starch, 4 very lean meat
Philly Cheese Steak	1	588	30	46	11	87	1684	38	n/a	37	2 1/2 starch, 4 medium-fat meat, 2 fat

										Exchanges
✔ Smothered Steak Sandwich	1	429	15	31	6	69	846	36	n/a	34	2 1/2 starch, 4 lean meat, 1/2 fat
Spicy BBQ Chicken Sandwich	1	368	5	12	1	55	1608	45	n/a	34	3 starch, 4 very lean meat
SIDES											
✔ Baked Potato (plain)	1	115	0	0	0	0	0	30	n/a	5	2 starch
✔ Banana Nut Bread	1 slice	165	7	38	1	5	195	22	n/a	2	1 1/2 carb, 1 fat
✔ BBQ Beans	4 oz	114	1	8	0	1	604	21	n/a	4	1 1/2 starch
Biscuit	1	270	15	50	4	11	610	29	n/a	5	2 starch, 3 fat
✔ Broccoli Spears	4 oz	34	0	0	0	0	50	5	n/a	3	1 veg.
✔ Broccoli Spears (w/1 oz. cheese sauce)	5 oz	58	5	78	2	11	212	1	n/a	2	1 veg., 1 fat
✔ Cinnamon Apples	4 oz	172	5	26	1	0	149	34	n/a	0	2 carb., 1 fat
✔ Corn	4 oz	96	1	9	0	0	271	24	n/a	3	1 1/2 starch

✔ = Healthiest Bets; n/a = not available

(Continued)

SIDES (Continued)	Amount	Cal.	Fat (g)	% Cal. Fat	Sat. Fat (g)	Chol. (mg)	Sod. (mg)	Carb. (g)	Fiber (g)	Pro. (g)	Servings/Exchanges
✔ Cornbread	1 piece	140	5	32	1	0	340	19	n/a	3	1 starch, 1 fat
✔ Green Beans	4 oz	61	4	59	1	0	796	6	n/a	1	1 veg., 1 fat
✔ Mashed Potatoes	4 oz	54	6	100	1	0	195	11	n/a	1	1 starch, 1 fat
✔ Rice Pilaf	4 oz	119	2	15	0	0	1283	23	n/a	2	1 1/2 starch
Steak Fries	1 order	358	19	48	6	0	245	45	n/a	5	3 starch, 4 fat
✔ Yeast Roll	1	160	4	23	1	0	285	29	n/a	1	2 starch, 1 fat
SOUPS											
Chili with Beans	6 oz	235	11	42	2	15	920	21	n/a	13	1 1/2 starch, 1 lean meat, 1 1/2 fat
✔ Clam Chowder	6 oz	180	9	45	1	0	835	21	n/a	3	1 1/2 carb., 2 fat
✔ Cream of Broccoli	6 oz	170	10	53	1	0	770	18	n/a	2	1 carb., 2 fat
✔ Vegetable Beef	6 oz	90	2	20	1	0	325	14	n/a	5	1 carb.

✔ = Healthiest Bets; n/a = not available

Sweets, Desserts, and Frozen Treats

RESTAURANTS

Baskin Robbins

Bresler's Ice Cream

Carvel Ice Cream Bakery

Freshëns Premium Yogurt

I Can't Believe It's Yogurt

TCBY

The Scoop: Nutrition information is for 4-fluid-ounce servings. Yes, that's small, but it is the industry standard for providing nutrition information. In many cases the nutrition information is only for vanilla or several flavors. Nutrition information for other flavors can vary slightly. Flavors that have nuts, fudge, or chocolate pieces will most likely have more calories. Several companies base their nutrition information on an average of all flavors.

Just Desserts: The dessert choices are based on between 150 and 350 calories each, rather than the criteria given on page 42.

NUTRITION PROS

- Small portions are an option.
- Some restaurants offer a kiddie size. That's sometimes enough to satisfy your sweet tooth.

(Continued)

- Healthier toppings are easy to spot: fresh fruit, granola, nuts, or raisins.
- Low-fat, fat-free, and/or sugar-free frozen treats abound.
- Desserts are easy to split. Just ask for two forks or spoons.
- You are watching the server's every move. Make sure they make every move you want.

NUTRITION CONS

- Indulgence is easy.
- Unhealthy toppers are plentiful: candy bar pieces, cookies, hot fudge, or butterscotch.
- Sometimes the low-fat, fat-free, and/or sugar-free desserts are not that much lower in calories than the regular varieties.
- Often the low-fat or fat-free products are higher in carbohydrates. The fat gets swapped for carbohydrates.
- Fruit smoothies or shakes are often light on the "real fruit" and heavy on the sugar.

Healthy Tips

- ★ Don't think kiddie size is just for kids. It's a great small size for calorie counters too.
- ★ Order one dessert and two spoons. You'll quickly realize that just a few bites quiets your sweet tooth.

Get It Your Way

★ Low-fat or fat-free; frozen yogurt, light ice cream, or sorbet; and kiddie and small— options are aplenty for calorie or fat watchers.

Baskin Robbins

❖Baskin Robbins provided nutrition information for all its menu items.

Light 'n Lean Choice

Neon Sour Apple Ice

Calories......................110	Sodium (mg)...............10
Fat (g) 0	Carbohydrate (g).........27
% calories from fat ...0	Fiber (g) 0
Saturated fat (g)........0	Protein (g) 0
Cholesterol (mg) 0	

Exchanges: 1 1/2 carb.

Healthy 'n Hearty Choice

Chocolate Regular Deluxe Ice Cream

Calories......................150	Sodium (mg)...............60
Fat (g) 9	Carbohydrate (g).........18
% calories from fat..54	Fiber (g) 0
Saturated fat (g)........6	Protein (g) 2
Cholesterol (mg) 30	

Exchanges: 1 carb., 2 fat

Baskin Robbins

BEVERAGES

	Amount	Cal.	Fat (g)	% Cal. Fat	Sat. Fat (g)	Chol. (mg)	Sod. (mg)	Carb. (g)	Fiber (g)	Pro. (g)	Servings/Exchanges
✔Cappuccino Blast w/ Whipped Cream (regular)	16 oz	320	14	39	8	60	120	44	0	6	2 carb., 1 fat-free milk, 3 fat
✔Cappuccino Nonfat Blast (large)	24 oz	270	0	0	0	0	195	60	0	9	3 carb., 1 fat-free milk
Chocolate Blast w/ Whipped Cream (regular)	16 oz	500	14	25	9	50	240	92	0	8	5 carb., 1 fat-free milk, 3 fat
Chocolate Nonfat Blast (regular)	16 oz	340	0	0	0	0	210	80	0	8	4 1/2 carb., 1 fat-free milk

✔ = Healthiest Bets; n/a = not available

(*Continued*)

BEVERAGES (Continued)	Amount	Cal.	Fat (g)	% Cal. Fat	Sat. Fat (g)	Chol. (mg)	Sod. (mg)	Carb. (g)	Fiber (g)	Pro. (g)	Serving/Exchanges
Lowfat Cappuccino Blast (w/ lowfat milk)	16 oz	240	2	8	1.5	10	125	51	0	6	2 1/2 carb., 1 fat-free milk
Lowfat Cappuccino Blast (w/ lowfat milk)	24 oz	360	3	8	2	15	190	77	1	9	4 carb., 1 fat-free milk
Lowfat Cappuccino Blast (w/ nonfat milk)	16 oz	230	1	4	0	5	125	51	0	6	2 1/2 carb., 1 fat-free milk
Lowfat Cappuccino Blast (w/ nonfat milk)	24 oz	340	1	3	0.5	5	190	77	1	10	4 carb., 1 fat-free milk
Mocha Cappuccino Blast w/ Whipped Cream (regular)	16 oz	360	12	30	8	50	140	56	0	6	3 carb., 1 fat-free milk, 2 fat
✓Mocha Cappuccino Nonfat Blast (regular)	16 oz	240	0	0	0	0	150	52	0	6	2 1/2 carb., 1 fat-free milk

FROZEN YOGURT SMOOTHIES

Aloha Berry Banana, hardscoop (regular)	16 oz	320	3	8	1	5	110	71	3	6	4 carb, 1 fat-free milk
Aloha Berry Banana, hardscoop (scoopersize)	24 oz	440	3	6	1.5	10	200	95	4	11	5 carb, 1 1/2 fat-free milk, 1/2 fat
Aloha Berry Banana, soft serve (regular)	16 oz	310	2	6	0.5	5	135	70	4	7	4 carb., 1 fat-free milk
Aloha Berry Banana, soft serve (scoopersize)	24 oz	400	2	5	1	5	190	91	4	10	5 carb, 1 fat-free milk
Bora Berry Bora, hardscoop (regular)	16 oz	380	0	0	0	0	150	88	4	8	5 carb, 1 fat-free milk
Bora Berry Bora, hardscoop (scoopersize)	24 oz	570	0	0	0	0	225	129	6	12	7 carb, 1 1/2 fat-free milk

✔ = Healthiest Bets; n/a = not available

(Continued)

FROZEN YOGURT SMOOTHIES (Continued)	Amount	Cal.	Fat (g)	% Cal. Fat	Sat. Fat (g)	Chol. (mg)	Sod. (mg)	Carb. (g)	Fiber (g)	Pro. (g)	Servings/Exchanges
Bora Berry Bora, soft serve (regular)	16 oz	340	0	0	0	10	150	76	4	8	4 carb., 1 fat-free milk
Bora Berry Bora, soft serve (scoopersize)	24 oz	480	0	0	0	15	210	111	6	9	6 1/2 carb., 1 fat-free milk
Calypso Berry, hardscoop (regular)	16 oz	320	0	0	0	0	150	70	4	6	4 carb, 1 fat-free milk
Calypso Berry, hardscoop (scoopersize)	24 oz	600	0	0	0	0	255	135	6	12	8 carb, 1 1/2 fat-free milk
Calypso Berry, soft serve (regular)	16 oz	320	0	0	0	0	150	70	4	6	4 carb, 1 fat-free milk
Calypso Berry, soft serve (scoopersize)	24 oz	480	0	0	0	0	210	105	3	9	6 carb., 1 fat-free milk

	Amount	Cal	Fat (g)	% Cal. Fat	Sat. Fat (g)	Chol. (mg)	Sod. (mg)	Carb. (g)	Fiber (g)	Pro. (g)	Servings/Exchanges
Copa Banana, hardscoop (regular)	16 oz	340	0	0	0	0	140	76	2	8	4 carb., 1 fat-free milk
Copa Banana, hardscoop (scoopersize)	24 oz	510	0	0	0	0	210	114	3	12	6 1/2 carb., 1 1/2 fat-free milk
✓ Copa Banana, soft serve (regular)	16 oz	280	0	0	0	10	130	60	2	8	3 carb., 1 fat-free milk
Copa Banana, soft serve (scoopersize)	24 oz	390	0	0	0	0	180	90	3	9	5 carb., 1 fat-free milk
Peach, hardscoop (regular)	16 oz	280	1	3	0	5	160	60	3	10	3 carb., 1 fat-free milk
Peach, hardscoop (scoopersize)	24 oz	390	1	2	0.5	5	250	84	4	14	4 1/2 carb., 1 1/2 fat-free milk
Peach, soft serve (regular)	16 oz	220	1	4	0.5	5	160	46	4	9	2 carb., 1 fat-free milk

✓ = Healthiest Bets; n/a = not available

(Continued)

FROZEN YOGURT SMOOTHIES (Continued)	Amount	Cal.	Fat (g)	% Cal. Fat	Sat. Fat (g)	Chol. (mg)	Sod. (mg)	Carb. (g)	Fiber (g)	Pro. (g)	Servings/Exchanges
Peach, soft serve (scoopersize)	24 oz	290	2	6	1	5	230	60	4	12	3 carb., 1 fat-free milk
Strawberry, hardscoop (regular)	16 oz	370	1	2	0	5	160	81	3	8	4 1/2 carb., 1 fat-free milk
Strawberry, hardscoop (scoopersize)	24 oz	530	1	2	0	5	240	117	4	12	6 1/2 carb., 1 1/2 fat-free milk
Strawberry, soft serve (regular)	16 oz	320	1	3	0.5	5	160	70	4	7	4 carb., 1 fat-free milk
Strawberry, soft serve (scoopersize)	24 oz	450	1	2	1	5	230	96	4	10	5 1/2 carb., 1 fat-free milk
Sunset Orange, hardscoop (scoopersize)	24 oz	510	0	0	0	0	210	114	6	12	6 1/2 carb., 1 1/2 fat-free milk
Sunset Orange, hardscoop (regular)	16 oz	340	0	0	0	0	150	76	4	8	4 carb., 1 fat-free milk

Sunset Orange, soft serve (scoopersize)	24 oz	420	0	0	0	15	195	93	6	12	5 1/2 carb., 1 1/2 fat-free milk
✔ Sunset Orange, soft serve (regular)	16 oz	300	0	0	0	10	140	64	4	8	5 1/2 carb., 1 fat-free milk
Tropical Tango, hardscoop (scoopersize)	24 oz	560	1	0	0.5	5	240	124	3	12	7 1/2 carb., 1 1/2 fat-free milk
Tropical Tango, hardscoop (regular)	16 oz	400	1	2	0	5	160	89	3	8	5 carb., 1 fat-free milk
Tropical Tango, soft serve (scoopersize)	24 oz	480	2	0	1	5	230	104	4	10	6 carb., 1 fat-free milk
Tropical Tango, soft serve (regular)	16 oz	350	1	0	0.5	5	160	77	3	7	4 carb., 1 fat-free milk

(Continued)

✔ = Healthiest Bets; n/a = not available

	Amount	Cal.	Fat (g)	% Cal. Fat	Sat. Fat (g)	Chol. (mg)	Sod. (mg)	Carb. (g)	Fiber (g)	Pro. (g)	Servings/Exchanges
FROZEN YOGURTS											
✔Maui Brownie Madness	1/2 cup	140	3	19	1	5	80	26	1	4	1 1/2 carb., 1/2 fat
✔Perils of Praline	1/2 cup	140	3	19	1.5	5	105	25	0	4	1 1/2 carb., 1/2 fat
FROZONE KIDS FLAVORS											
✔Dirt 'N Worms	1/2 cup	160	8	45	4.5	25	80	22	0	2	1 1/2 carb., 1 fat
✔Eerrie I Scream	1/2 cup	150	8	48	5	25	45	18	0	2	1 carb., 1 1/2 fat
✔Ocean Commotion	1/2 cup	150	7	42	4.5	25	40	20	0	1	1 carb., 1 fat
✔Pink Bubblegum	1/2 cup	150	8	48	5	30	40	19	0	2	1 carb., 1 1/2 fat
✔Star, Stripes, Explod	1/2 cup	150	8	48	4.5	25	40	19	0	2	1 carb., 1 1/2 fat
ICES											
✔Daquiri	1/2 cup	110	0	0	0	0	10	28	0	0	2 carb.
✔Neon Sour Apple	1/2 cup	110	0	0	0	0	10	27	0	0	1 1/2 carb.

	Serving Size	Calories	Fat (g)	Cal. Fat	Sat. Fat (g)	Chol. (mg)	Sodium (mg)	Carb. (g)	Fiber (g)	Protein (g)	Exchanges
✔The Mask	1/2 cup	120	0	0	0		10	29	0	0	2 carb.
✔Watermelon	1/2 cup	110	0	0	0		10	28	0	0	2 carb.
LOW-FAT ICE CREAMS											
✔Carmel Apple ALaMod	1/2 cup	100	2	18	1	5	75	20	0	3	1 carb.
✔Espresso 'N Cream	1/2 cup	100	3	27	1	5	60	18	1	3	1 carb., 1/2 fat
NO ADDED SUGAR ICE CREAMS											
✔Call Me Nuts	1/2 cup	110	2	16	1	5	55	21	1	3	1 1/2 carb.
✔Cherry Cordial	1/2 cup	100	2	18	1.5	5	55	18	0	3	1 carb.
✔Mad About Chocolate	1/2 cup	100	2	18	1	5	40	19	0	3	1 carb.
✔Pineapple Coconut	1/2 cup	90	2	20	1	5	60	16	0	3	1 carb.
✔Thin Mint	1/2 cup	100	3	27	1.5	5	65	16	0	3	1 carb., 1/2 fat
NON-FAT ICE CREAMS											
✔Berry Innocent Cheese	1/2 cup	110	0	0	0	0	100	24	0	3	1 1/2 carb.

✔ = Healthiest Bets; n/a = not available

(Continued)

NON-FAT ICE CREAMS (Continued)	Amount	Cal.	Fat (g)	% Cal. Fat	Sat. Fat (g)	Chol. (mg)	Sod. (mg)	Carb. (g)	Fiber (g)	Pro. (g)	Servings/Exchanges
✔Check-It-Out-Cherry	1/2 cup	100	0	0	0	0	90	22	0	3	1 1/2 carb.
✔Jamoca Swirl	1/2 cup	110	0	0	5	5	105	23	0	3	1 1/2 carb.
REGULAR DELUXE ICE CREAMS											
✔Banana Strawberry	1/2 cup	130	7	48	4.5	25	40	17	0	2	1 carb., 1 fat
✔Baseball Nut	1/2 cup	160	9	51	5	30	55	18	0	2	1 carb., 2 fat
✔Black Walnut	1/2 cup	160	11	62	5	30	45	13	1	3	1 carb., 2 fat
✔Cherries Jubilee	1/2 cup	140	7	45	4.5	30	40	16	0	2	1 carb., 1 fat
✔Chocolate	1/2 cup	150	9	54	6	30	60	18	0	2	1 carb., 2 fat
Chocolate Almond	1/2 cup	180	11	55	5	30	55	17	1	3	1 carb., 2 fat
✔Chocolate Chip	1/2 cup	150	10	60	6	35	45	15	0	2	1 carb., 2 fat
✔Chocolate Chip Cookie Dough	1/2 cup	170	9	48	6	35	70	20	0	2	1 carb., 2 fat

✔Chocolate Fudge	1/2 cup	160	9	51	6	30	80	21	0	2	1 carb., 2 fat
✔Chocolate Mousse Royale	1/2 cup	170	10	53	5	25	60	20	1	2	1 carb., 2 fat
Chocolate Raspberry Truffle	1/2 cup	180	9	45	6	30	60	23	0	3	1 1/2 carb., 2 fat
✔Chunky Heath Bar	1/2 cup	170	10	53	6	30	70	19	0	2	1 carb., 2 fat
Cookies N Cream	1/2 cup	170	11	58	7	30	80	16	0	2	1 carb., 2 fat
✔Egg Nog	1/2 cup	150	8	48	5	40	45	16	0	2	1 carb., 1 1/2 fat
✔Everybody's Favorite Candy Bar	1/2 cup	170	9	48	5	30	90	20	0	2	1 carb., 2 fat
✔French Vanilla	1/2 cup	160	10	56	6	70	45	14	0	2	1 carb., 2 fat
Fudge Brownie	1/2 cup	170	11	58	6	25	75	19	1	3	1 carb., 2 fat
✔German Chocolate Cake	1/2 cup	180	10	50	6	25	75	20	0	3	1 carb., 2 fat
✔Gold Medal Ribbon	1/2 cup	150	8	48	5	30	95	20	0	2	1 carb., 1 1/2 fat
✔Jamoca	1/2 cup	140	9	58	5	35	45	14	0	2	1 carb., 1 1/2 fat

✔ = Healthiest Bets; n/a = not available

(*Continued*)

REGULAR DELUXE ICE CREAMS (Continued)	Amount	Cal.	Fat (g)	% Cal. Fat	Sat. Fat (g)	Chol. (mg)	Sod. (mg)	Carb. (g)	Fiber (g)	Pro. (g)	Servings/Exchanges
✔Jamoca Almond Fudge	1/2 cup	160	9	51	4.5	25	40	17	0	3	1 carb_ 2 fat
✔Lemon Custard	1/2 cup	150	8	48	5	45	55	16	0	2	1 carb_ 1 1/2 fat
✔Mint Chocolate Chip	1/2 cup	150	10	60	6	35	45	15	0	3	1 carb_ 2 fat
Old Fashion Butter Pecan	1/2 cup	160	11	62	6	35	50	13	0	2	1 carb_ 2 fat
✔Oregon Blackberry	1/2 cup	140	8	51	5	30	50	16	0	2	1 carb_ 1 1/2 fat
Peanut Butter N Chocolate	1/2 cup	180	12	60	6	30	95	16	1	3	1 carb_ 2 fat
Pistachio Almond	1/2 cup	170	12	64	5	30	45	13	1	3	1 carb_ 2 fat
✔Pralines N Cream	1/2 cup	160	9	51	5	30	85	19	0	2	1 carb_ 2 fat
✔Pumpkin Pie	1/2 cup	130	7	48	4.5	30	50	16	0	2	1 carb_ 1 fat
✔Quarterback Crunch	1/2 cup	160	10	56	7	30	75	18	0	2	1 carb_ 2 fat
✔Reeses Peanutbutter	1/2 cup	180	11	55	6	30	70	17	0	3	1 carb_ 2 fat
✔Rocky Road	1/2 cup	170	10	53	5	30	60	19	0	3	1 carb_ 2 fat

✔Rum Raisin	1/2 cup	140	7	45	4.5	30	40	18	0	2	1 carb., 1 fat
✔Strawberry Cheesecake	1/2 cup	150	9	54	5	35	65	17	0	2	1 carb., 2 fat
Tripple Chocolate Passion	1/2 cup	180	11	55	7	35	70	21	0	3	1 carb., 2 fat
✔Vanilla	1/2 cup	140	8	51	5	40	40	14	0	3	1 carb., 1 1/2 fat
✔Very Berry Strawberry	1/2 cup	130	7	48	4	25	40	16	0	1	1 carb., 1 fat
✔Winter White Chocolate	1/2 cup	150	9	54	6	25	50	18	0	2	1 carb., 2 fat
✔World Class Chocolate	1/2 cup	160	9	51	5	30	55	18	0	2	1 carb., 2 fat

SHEET CAKES

Cookies N Cream/Chocolate Crunch/White Sponge	118 g	340	19	50	10	40	260	39	1	5	2 1/2 carb., 4 fat
Vanilla/Brownie	134 g	370	19	46	8	65	260	45	1	6	3 carb., 4 fat

SHERBETS

✔Blue Raspberry	1/2 cup	120	2	15	1	5	30	25	0	1	1 1/2 carb.

✔ = Healthiest Bets; n/a = not available

(Continued)

SHERBETS (Continued)	Amount	Cal.	Fat (g)	% Cal. Fat	Sat. Fat (g)	Chol. (mg)	Sod. (mg)	Carb. (g)	Fiber (g)	Pro. (g)	Servings/Exchanges
✔Orange	1/2 cup	120	2	15	1	5	25	26	0	1	1 1/2 carb.
✔Rainbow	1/2 cup	120	2	15	1	5	25	26	0	1	1 1/2 carb.
✔Tangerine Pineapple	1/2 cup	120	1	8	0.5	5	25	22	0	1	1 1/2 carb.
SORBETS											
Mixed Berry Lemonade	1/2 cup	110	0	0	0	0	10	28	0	0	2 carb.
Pink Raspberry Lemon	1/2 cup	120	0	0	0	0	10	29	0	0	2 carb.

✔ = Healthiest Bets; n/a = not available

Notes

Bresler's Ice Cream

❖Bresler's Ice Cream provides nutrition information for some of its menu items in a brochure.

Light 'n Lean Choice

Chocolate Nonfat Soft-Serve Ice Cream
(4 fl oz, 1/2 cup)

Calories......................120	Sodium (mg)...............85
Fat (g) 0	Carbohydrate (g).........26
% calories from fat ...0	Fiber (g) 1
Saturated fat (g)........0	Protein (g) 5
Cholesterol (mg) 0	

Exchanges: 1 1/2 carb.

Healthy 'n Hearty Choice

Chunky Chocolate Brownie Low-Fat Ice Cream
(4 fl oz, 1/2 cup)

Calories......................130	Sodium (mg)...............70
Fat (g) 3	Carbohydrate (g).........27
% calories from fat..21	Fiber (g) 1
Saturated fat (g)........1	Protein (g) 3
Cholesterol (mg).........<5	

Exchanges: 1 1/2 carb.

(Continued)

Bresler's Ice Cream

	Amount	Cal.	Fat (g)	% Cal. Fat	Sat. Fat (g)	Chol. (mg)	Sod. (mg)	Carb. (g)	Fiber (g)	Pro. (g)	Servings/Exchanges
LOW-FAT ICE CREAM											
Cherry and Chocolate	1/2 cup	130	3	21	2	0	65	26	0	3	1 1/2 carb., 1/2 fat
Chunky Chocolate Brownie	1/2 cup	130	3	21	1	<5	70	27	1	3	1 1/2 carb., 1/2 fat
✔Mango Kiwi Swirl	1/2 cup	110	1	8	0	<5	50	24	0	3	1 1/2 carb.
✔Mocha Irish Cream	1/2 cup	130	3	21	2	0	70	25	1	3	1 1/2 carb., 1/2 fat
NONFAT SOFT-SERVE ICE CREAM											
Chocolate	1/2 cup	120	0	0	0	0	85	26	1	5	1 1/2 carb.
Vanilla	1/2 cup	120	0	0	0	<5	85	26	0	5	1 1/2 carb.

✔ = Healthiest Bets; n/a = not available

Carvel Ice Cream Bakery

❖Carvel Ice Cream Bakery provided nutrition
information for some of its menu items.

Light 'n Lean Choice

Chocolate No-Fat Ice Cream
(4 fl oz, 1/2 cup)

Calories......................120	Sodium (mg)................40
Fat (g) 0	Carbohydrate (g).........28
% calories from fat ...0	Fiber (g) 0
Saturated fat (g)........0	Protein (g) 2
Cholesterol (mg) 0	

Exchanges: 1 1/2 carb.

Healthy 'n Hearty Choice

Chocolate Ice Cream
(4 fl oz, 1/2 cup)

Calories......................190	Sodium (mg).............100
Fat (g) 10	Carbohydrate (g).........22
% calories from fat..47	Fiber (g) 0
Saturated fat (g)........6	Protein (g) 4
Cholesterol (mg) 25	

Exchanges: 1 1/2 carb., 2 fat

(Continued)

Carvel Ice Cream Bakery

	Amount	Cal.	Fat (g)	% Cal. Fat	Sat. Fat (g)	Chol. (mg)	Sod. (mg)	Carb. (g)	Fiber (g)	Pro. (g)	Servings/Exchanges
✔Chocolate Ice Cream	4 oz	190	10	47	6	25	100	22	0	4	1 1/2 carb., 2 fat
✔Chocolate No-Fat Ice Cream	4 oz	120	0	0	0	0	40	28	0	2	1 1/2 carb.
✔Sherbet	4 oz	140	1	6	0.5	5	45	31	0	2	2 carb.
✔Vanilla Ice Cream	4 oz	200	10	45	6	40	110	21	0	5	1 1/2 carb., 2 fat
✔Vanilla No-Fat Ice Cream	4 oz	120	0	0	0	0	55	25	0	4	1 1/2 carb.

✔ = Healthiest Bets; n/a = not available

Notes

Freshëns Premium Yogurt

❖Freshëns Premium Yogurt provided nutrition
information for some of its menu items.

Light 'n Lean Choice

Sugar Free Frozen Yogurt, any flavor
(4 fl oz, 1/2 cup)

Calories........................74	Sodium (mg)...............72
Fat (g) 0	Carbohydrate (g).........16
% calories from fat ...0	Fiber (g).................n/a
Saturated fat (g)........0	Protein (g) 4
Cholesterol (mg) 0	

Exchanges: 1 carb.

Healthy 'n Hearty Choice

Nonfat Frozen Yogurt, any flavor
(4 fl oz, 1/2 cup)

Calories........................108	Sodium (mg)...............72
Fat (g) 0	Carbohydrate (g).........24
% calories from fat ...0	Fiber (g).................n/a
Saturated fat (g)........0	Protein (g) 4
Cholesterol (mg) 0	

Exchanges: 1 1/2 carb.

(Continued)

Freshëns Premium Yogurt

	Amount	Cal.	Fat (g)	% Cal. Fat	Sat. Fat (g)	Chol. (mg)	Sod. (mg)	Carb. (g)	Fiber (g)	Pro. (g)	Servings/Exchanges
✓ Lowfat Frozen Yogurt	4 oz	114	0	0	0	0	80	24	n/a	4	1 1/2 carb.
✓ Nonfat Frozen Yogurt	4 oz	108	0	0	0	0	72	24	n/a	4	1 1/2 carb.
Sugar Free Frozen Yogurt	4 oz	74	0	0	0	0	72	16	n/a	4	1 carb.

✓ = Healthiest Bets; n/a = not available
Numbers of calories shown are averages.

Notes

I Can't Believe It's Yogurt

❖I Can't Believe It's Yogurt provides nutrition
information for some of its menu items in a
brochure.

Light 'n Lean Choice

Sorbet, kid's size
(4 fl oz, 1/2 cup)

Calories........................90	Sodium (mg).................0
Fat (g) 0	Carbohydrate (g).........22
% calories from fat ...0	Fiber (g) 0
Saturated fat (g)........0	Protein (g) 0
Cholesterol (mg) 0	

Exchanges: 1 carb.

Healthy 'n Hearty Choice

Original Frozen Yogurt
(4 fl oz, 1/2 cup)

Calories........................120	Sodium (mg) 90
Fat (g) 3	Carbohydrate (g).........21
% calories from fat..23	Fiber (g) 0
Saturated fat (g)........2	Protein (g) 3
Cholesterol (mg) 20	

Exchanges: 1 1/2 carb.

(Continued)

I Can't Believe It's Yogurt

	Amount	Cal.	Fat (g)	% Cal. Fat	Sat. Fat (g)	Chol. (mg)	Sod. (mg)	Carb. (g)	Fiber (g)	Pro. (g)	Servings/Exchanges
✓Nonfat Frozen Yogurt	4 oz	90	0	0	0	0	70	20	0	3	1 carb.
✓Nonfat Frozen Yogurt with NutraSweet	4 oz	90	0	0	0	0	75	18	0	3	1 carb.
✓Original Frozen Yogurt	4 oz	120	3	23	2	20	90	21	0	3	1 1/2 carb., 1/2 fat
✓Sorbet	4 oz	90	0	0	0	0	0	22	0	0	1 carb.
✓Yoglacé	4 oz	45	0	0	0	5	30	12	0	2	1 1/2 carb.

✓ = Healthiest Bets; n/a = not available

Notes

TCBY

❖TCBY provides nutrition information for some of
its items in a brochure.

Light 'n Lean Choice

Nonfat Frozen Yogurt, soft-serve
(4 fl oz, 1/2 cup)

Calories......................110
Fat (g) 0
    % calories from fat ...0
    Saturated fat (g)........0
Cholesterol (mg).........<5

Sodium (mg) 60
Carbohydrate (g)..........23
    Fiber (g) 0
Protein (g) 4

Exchanges: 1 1/2 carb.

Healthy 'n Hearty Choice

Nonfat Ice Cream, hand-dipped
(4 fl oz, 1/2 cup)

Calories......................120
Fat (g) 0
    % calories from fat ...0
    Saturated fat (g)........0
Cholesterol (mg)...........0

Sodium (mg) 55
Carbohydrate (g)..........26
    Fiber (g) 1
Protein (g) 3

Exchanges: 1 1/2 carb.

(Continued)

TCBY

	Amount	Cal.	Fat (g)	% Cal. Fat	Sat. Fat (g)	Chol. (mg)	Sod. (mg)	Carb. (g)	Fiber (g)	Pro. (g)	Servings/Exchanges
HAND-DIPPED											
✔96% Fat Free Frozen Yogurt	1/2 cup	140	3	19	1.5	5	70	26	0	3	1 1/2 carb., 1/2 fat
✔No Sugar Added Lowfat Ice Cream	1/2 cup	110	3	22	1.5	10	60	19	0	3	1 carb.
✔Nonfat Frozen Yogurt	1/2 cup	120	0	0	0	0	60	25	1	4	1/2 carb.
✔Nonfat Ice Cream	1/2 cup	120	0	0	0	0	55	26	1	3	1 1/2 carb.
SOFT-SERVE											
✔96% Fat Free Frozen Yogurt	1/2 cup	140	3	19	2	15	60	23	0	4	1 1/2 carb., 1 fat
✔No Sugar Added Nonfat Yogurt	1/2 cup	80	0	0	0	0	35	20	0	4	1 carb.

✔Nonfat & Nondairy Sorbet	1/2 cup	100	0	0	0	0	30	24	0	0	1 1/2 carb., 1 fat
✔Nonfat Frozen Yogurt	1/2 cup	110	0	0		<5	60	23	0	4	1 1/2 carb., 1/2 fat

✔ = Healthiest Bets; n/a = not available

Notes
_____
_____
_____
_____
_____
_____
_____
_____
_____
_____
_____